Pediatric Office Emergency Medicine (POEM) Training Module

Pediatric Office Emergency Medicine (POEM) Training Module

Editors

Suresh Gupta MD
Professor and Senior Consultant
Co-Chairman & Co-Director
Pediatric Emergency, Critical Care, Allergy & Pulmonology
Institute of Child Health, Sir Ganga Ram Hospital
New Delhi, India

Ruchira Gupta MD
Senior Consultant
Department of Pediatrics
Kailash Hospital and Heart Center
Noida, Uttar Pradesh, India
National Joint Secretary Liaison 2024–2025

Forewords

Vasant M Khalatkar
Neelam Mohan
GV Basavaraja
Yogesh N Parikh
Atanu Bhadra

JAYPEE

JAYPEE BROTHERS MEDICAL PUBLISHERS
The Health Sciences Publisher
New Delhi | London

Jaypee Brothers Medical Publishers (P) Ltd

Headquarters
Jaypee Brothers Medical Publishers (P) Ltd
EMCA House, 23/23-B
Ansari Road, Daryaganj
New Delhi 110 002, India
Landline: +91-11-23272143, +91-11-23272703
+91-11-23282021, +91-11-23245672
Email: jaypee@jaypeebrothers.com

Corporate Office
Jaypee Brothers Medical Publishers (P) Ltd
4838/24, Ansari Road, Daryaganj
New Delhi 110 002, India
Phone: +91-11-43574357
Fax: +91-11-43574314
Email: jaypee@jaypeebrothers.com

Overseas Office
JP Medical Ltd.
83, Victoria Street, London
SW1H 0HW (UK)
Phone: +44 20 3170 8910
Fax: +44 (0)20 3008 6180
Email: info@jpmedpub.com

Website: www.jaypeebrothers.com
Website: www.jaypeedigital.com

Pediatric Office Emergency Medicine (POEM) Training Module

First Edition: **2025**

ISBN: 978-93-6616-618-6

Printed at: Samrat Offset Pvt. Ltd.

PEDIATRIC OFFICE EMERGENCY MEDICINE (POEM)
TRAINING MODULE

National Advisors

Dr Vasant M Khalatkar
Dr Neelam Mohan
Dr GV Basavaraja

National Convenor

Dr Ruchira Gupta

National Scientific Director

Dr (Prof) Suresh Gupta

National Chief Coordinators

Dr Yogesh N Parikh
Dr Atanu Bhadra
Dr Vineet Tyagi

National Team of Experts

Dr Ajit Saxena
Dr Arvind Garg
Dr Cyprian D'Souza
Dr Dibyendu Raychaudhuri
Dr Mahesh Mohite
Dr Maninder Dariwal
Dr Manisha Sawant
Dr Mihit Sarkar
Dr Minhaj
Dr Mullai Balaji
Dr Swathi Rao
Dr Vinod Ratageri
Dr Vivek Goswami

FOREWORD

As the President of the Indian Academy of Pediatrics (IAP), I am proud to introduce the *Pediatric Office Emergency Medicine (POEM) Training Module*, a crucial resource tailored for pediatricians in office practice and those serving in peripheral areas of India. This comprehensive module addresses the unique challenges faced by healthcare providers in managing pediatric emergencies, providing essential algorithms for resuscitation and medical emergency pathways. From neonatal resuscitation to the management of acute conditions such as croup, asthma, and anaphylaxis, this training module equips practitioners with the knowledge and skills necessary to respond effectively in critical situations.

Additionally, the module outlines practical procedures that pediatricians may need to perform in their offices, including eye and ENT interventions, gastrointestinal and genitourinary procedures, and minor surgical techniques. By emphasizing both emergency preparedness and hands-on management strategies, this resource empowers pediatricians to deliver timely care, ultimately enhancing patient outcomes across diverse settings. I encourage all practitioners to engage with this material actively, as it stands as a testament to our commitment to excellence in child health and our dedication to serving the needs of our youngest patients.

Vasant M Khalatkar
President, 2025
Indian Academy of Pediatrics

FOREWORD

As the President Elect of the Indian Academy of Pediatrics (IAP), I am delighted to endorse the *Pediatric Office Emergency Medicine (POEM) Training Module*, a significant contribution to pediatric healthcare education. This module is specifically designed for pediatricians practicing in office settings and those in peripheral areas of India, addressing the critical need for structured guidance in managing pediatric emergencies. The comprehensive content, which includes resuscitation pathways, medical emergency protocols, and practical procedures, will empower practitioners with the skills and knowledge necessary to respond effectively to a wide range of urgent situations.

The structured approach of this module not only enhances the clinical competence of pediatricians but also fosters a culture of preparedness and confidence in emergency care. By integrating evidence-based algorithms and procedural guidelines, we aim to equip healthcare professionals with the tools they need to ensure optimal outcomes for their young patients. I encourage all pediatricians to engage with this invaluable resource, as it reflects our commitment to advancing child health and improving emergency care across India. Together, let us strive to provide the highest standard of care for our children in times of need.

Neelam Mohan
President Elect, 2025
Indian Academy of Pediatrics

FOREWORD

The essence of primary pediatric practice lies not just in managing routine illnesses, but also in skillfully handling minor emergencies that require immediate intervention. These situations, though not life-threatening, can cause significant distress to both children and parents, and their proper management in the office setting can prevent unnecessary hospital visits and complications.

This *Pediatric Office Emergency Medicine (POEM) Training Module* is a comprehensive guide to managing common office emergencies and performing essential procedures in a primary care setting. From removing foreign bodies from the eyes, ears, and nose to managing minor trauma and from handling genital emergencies to treating simple lacerations, this manual covers the complete spectrum of procedures that every practicing pediatrician should be confident in performing.

The procedures detailed in this book are specifically chosen for their relevance to daily practice. Whether it is managing an epistaxis, reducing a paraphimosis, treating a paronychia, or splinting a fracture, each procedure is presented with clear, practical guidelines that can be implemented in any office setting. Special attention has been given to common scenarios like pulled elbow, foreign body removal, and minor surgical procedures that form a significant part of outpatient pediatric emergencies.

What makes this first edition particularly valuable is its focus on procedures that can be safely performed in an office setting with basic equipment. The module includes sections on various routes of drug administration and essential emergency procedures like activated charcoal administration and management of stings, making it an indispensable resource for primary care pediatricians.

I strongly encourage all pediatricians to master these procedures as they represent the cornerstone of competent office-based emergency care. This knowledge not only enhances the quality-of-care we provide but also builds confidence in managing common pediatric emergencies effectively.

GV Basavaraja
Past President, 2024
Indian Academy of Pediatrics

FOREWORD

In the bustling world of pediatric practice, mastering office procedures is an art that transforms everyday challenges into manageable solutions. From a stuck bead in a toddler's nose to a distressing paraphimosis, these seemingly minor emergencies demand swift, skilled intervention.

The *Pediatric Office Emergency Medicine (POEM) Training Module* serves as a beacon for practitioners navigating these daily challenges. This practical guide empowers pediatricians with step-by-step expertise in managing common office emergencies, from deftly removing foreign bodies to skillfully handling minor trauma, from precise drug administration to managing acute genital emergencies.

This manual stands out for its laser focus on procedures that can be performed confidently in any office setting, requiring only basic equipment. For our colleagues practicing in peripheral areas, this knowledge proves invaluable, often eliminating the need for distant referrals and providing immediate relief to distressed young patients.

By mastering these essential procedures, we not only enhance our clinical capabilities but also provide timely, accessible care right where it is needed most—in our offices.

Yogesh N Parikh
National Secretary General
Indian Academy of Pediatrics (2024–2025)

Atanu Bhadra
National Treasurer
Indian Academy of Pediatrics (2024–2025)

PREFACE

In the dynamic field of pediatric medicine, the ability to respond effectively to emergencies is crucial. We are proud to present the *Pediatric Office Emergency Medicine (POEM) Training Module*—a comprehensive resource tailored for pediatricians practicing in office settings and those serving in peripheral areas of India.

This module is the result of collaborative efforts from a dedicated team within the Indian Academy of Pediatrics (IAP). It includes essential algorithms for pediatric resuscitation, medical emergency pathways, and practical procedures for common pediatric emergencies. Each section provides clear, evidence-based guidelines that empower healthcare providers to manage urgent situations with confidence.

Recognizing that many pediatricians work in environments with limited access to advanced medical facilities, this training module aims to equip practitioners with the necessary tools to deliver high-quality care in their communities. From neonatal resuscitation to managing acute asthma and foreign body ingestion, this resource addresses a wide range of scenarios encountered in daily practice.

We hope this module serves not only as a practical guide but also fosters a culture of preparedness and continuous learning among pediatric healthcare providers. We extend our deepest gratitude to all contributors who made this project possible, and we encourage readers to engage actively with the content to enhance pediatric emergency care across India.

Suresh Gupta
Ruchira Gupta

ACKNOWLEDGMENTS

We would like to express our sincere gratitude to the leadership of the Indian Academy of Pediatrics (IAP) for their instrumental support in developing the *Pediatric Office Emergency Medicine (POEM) Training Module*. Special recognition goes to Dr Vasant M Khalatkar, President (2025); Dr Neelam Mohan, President Elect (2025); Dr GV Basavaraja, Past President (2024); Dr Yogesh N Parikh, National Secretary General (2024–2025); and Dr Atanu Bhadra, National Treasurer (2024–2025). Their collective vision and strategic guidance have been crucial in bringing this critical educational initiative to life, demonstrating a profound commitment to advancing pediatric emergency care across India.

The core development of the module was made possible by an exceptional team of dedicated medical professionals who brought their extensive expertise to the project. Drs Ajit Saxena, Arvind Garg, Vinod Ratageri, Mahesh Mohite, Maninder Dariwal, Vineet Tyagi, Vivek Goswami, Dibyendu Raychaudhuri, Manisha Sawant, Mihit Sarkar, Minhaj, Cyprian D'Souza, Swathi Rao, and Mullai Balaji worked collaboratively to create a comprehensive and practical training resource. Their collective efforts ensure that the module will provide pediatricians working in diverse settings with critical knowledge and skills to manage emergency medical situations effectively.

We extend our heartfelt thanks to Mr Naman Singh (Development Editor) from M/s Jaypee Brothers Medical Publishers (P) Ltd, New Delhi, India, whose meticulous editing and drafting were instrumental in shaping the final manual, and to Indopharma for their generous financial and logistical support. These contributions exemplify the collaborative spirit and shared commitment to improving pediatric health care, ultimately aiming to enhance patient outcomes and provide the highest standard of emergency medical care for children across India.

CONTENTS

SECTION 1: PEDIATRIC RESUSCITATION PATHWAYS

1. Neonatal Resuscitation Algorithm 3
2. Pediatric Basic Life Support Algorithm for Healthcare Providers: Single Rescuer 4
3. Pediatric Basic Life Support Algorithm for Healthcare Providers: Two or More Rescuers 5
4. Pediatric Cardiac Arrest Algorithm 6
5. Pediatric Bradycardia with a Pulse Algorithm 7
6. Pediatric Tachycardia with a Pulse Algorithm 8

SECTION 2: MEDICAL EMERGENCY PATHWAYS

1. Emergency Preparedness in Pediatric Office Practice 11
2. Management of Croup in Children 15
3. Acute Asthma in Office Practice 19
4. Bronchiolitis and its Management 24
5. Nontraumatic Chest Pain in Children and Adolescents: Approach and Initial Management 28
6. Evaluation and Management of Syncope in Pediatric Patients 32
7. Brief Resolved Unexplained Events in Pediatric Emergency Management 36
8. Anaphylaxis and its Management Based on Current World Allergy Organization Guidelines 40
9. Emergency Management of the Pediatric Patient with Convulsive Status Epilepticus 45
10. Management of Mild Head Injury in Children 50
11. Emergency Department Approach to Nontraumatic Headache in Children 54
12. Excessive Crying in Infants and its Management 58
13. Management of a Febrile Infants below 3 Months of Age 63
14. Rabies Postexposure Prophylaxis Protocol in India 67
15. Management of Foreign Body Ingestion in Children 71
16. Common Household Poisoning 75

SECTION 3: PEDIATRIC OFFICE EMERGENCY PROCEDURES

PART 1: EYE AND ENT

1. Management of Nasal Foreign Body in Children 87
2. Procedure for Management of Epistaxis in Children 91
3. Procedure for Management of Nasal Injury in Children 95
4. Procedure for Management of Foreign Body in Ear in Children 98
5. Procedure for Management of Cerumen Impaction in Children 101
6. Procedure for Management of Ocular Foreign Body in Children 104
7. Procedure for Eye Drop Administration in Children 108

PART 2: GIT AND GENITOURINARY

8. Procedure for Management of Paraphimosis in Children 111
9. Procedure for Zipper Injury in Children 114
10. Procedure for Detorsion of Testes in Children 117
11. Manual Reduction of Obstructed Inguinal Hernia 121
12. Procedure for Rectal Prolapse Reduction in Children 124
13. Management of Constipated Stool Impaction in Children 127
14. Procedure for Umbilical Granuloma in Children 131

PART 3: MINOR SURGICAL EMERGENCIES

15. Procedure for Ring Removal in Children 134
16. Procedure for Subungual Hematoma in Children 137
17. Procedure for Management of Paronychia in Children 141
18. Management of Ingrowing Toenail in Children 144
19. Procedure for Management of Fingernail and Toenail Avulsion in Children 148
20. Procedure for Fishhook Removal in Children 151
21. Procedure for Management of Hair Tourniquets in Children 155
22. Superficial Splinter Removal in Children 158
23. Management of Warts and Calluses in Children 162
24. Management of Simple Lacerations in Children 165
25. Management of Simple Tongue and Lip Lacerations in Children 171
26. Procedure for Management of Pencil Point Puncture in Children 175

PART 4: TRAUMA AND ORTHOPEDIC

27. First Aid Splint for Children with Fracture 178
28. Procedure for Management of Pulled Elbow in Children 182
29. Procedure for Management of Clavicle Fracture in Children 186

30. Procedure for Management of Ankle Sprain in Children ... 190
31. Procedure for Management of Avulsed Tooth in Children ... 194

PART 5: POISONING AND MORE

32. Administration of Activated Charcoal in Children ... 198
33. Gastric Lavage for Poisoning in Children ... 201
34. Management of Hymenoptera and Bee Stings in Children ... 204
35. Procedure for Rabies Immune Globulin Administration in Children ... 207
36. Intranasal Administration of Midazolam and Fentanyl in Children ... 211
37. Buccal Drug Administration in Children ... 214
38. Making Intramuscular Injections Pain Free in Children ... 217
39. Rectal Drug Administration in Children ... 220

Index ... 225

SECTION 1

Pediatric Resuscitation Pathways

1. Neonatal Resuscitation Algorithm
2. Pediatric Basic Life Support Algorithm for Healthcare Providers: Single Rescuer
3. Pediatric Basic Life Support Algorithm for Healthcare Providers: Two or More Rescuers
4. Pediatric Cardiac Arrest Algorithm
5. Pediatric Bradycardia with a Pulse Algorithm
6. Pediatric Tachycardia with a Pulse Algorithm

CHAPTER 1

Neonatal Resuscitation Algorithm

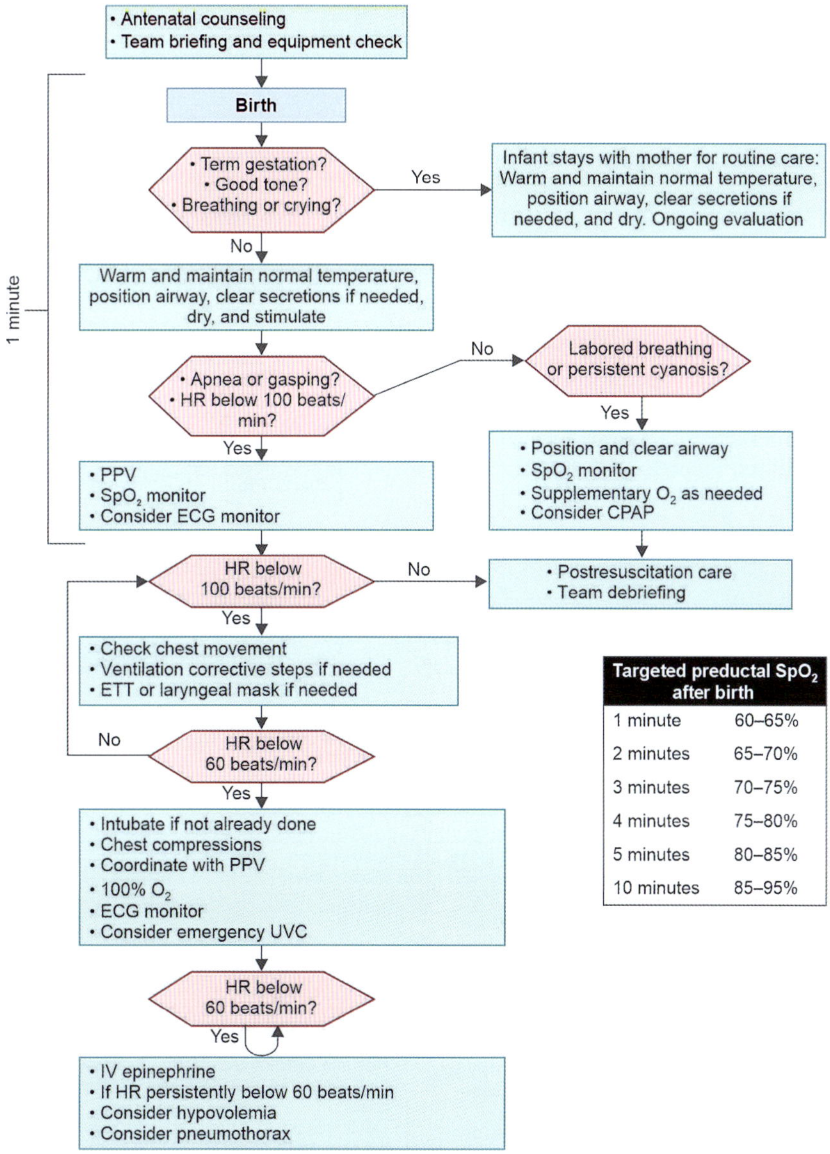

Targeted preductal SpO_2 after birth	
1 minute	60–65%
2 minutes	65–70%
3 minutes	70–75%
4 minutes	75–80%
5 minutes	80–85%
10 minutes	85–95%

(CPAP: continuous positive airway pressure; ECG: electrocardiogram; ETT: endotracheal tube; HR: heart rate; PPV: pulse pressure variation; SpO_2: oxygen saturation; UVC: umbilical venous catheter)

Source: © 2020 American Heart Association.

CHAPTER 2

Pediatric Basic Life Support Algorithm for Healthcare Providers: Single Rescuer

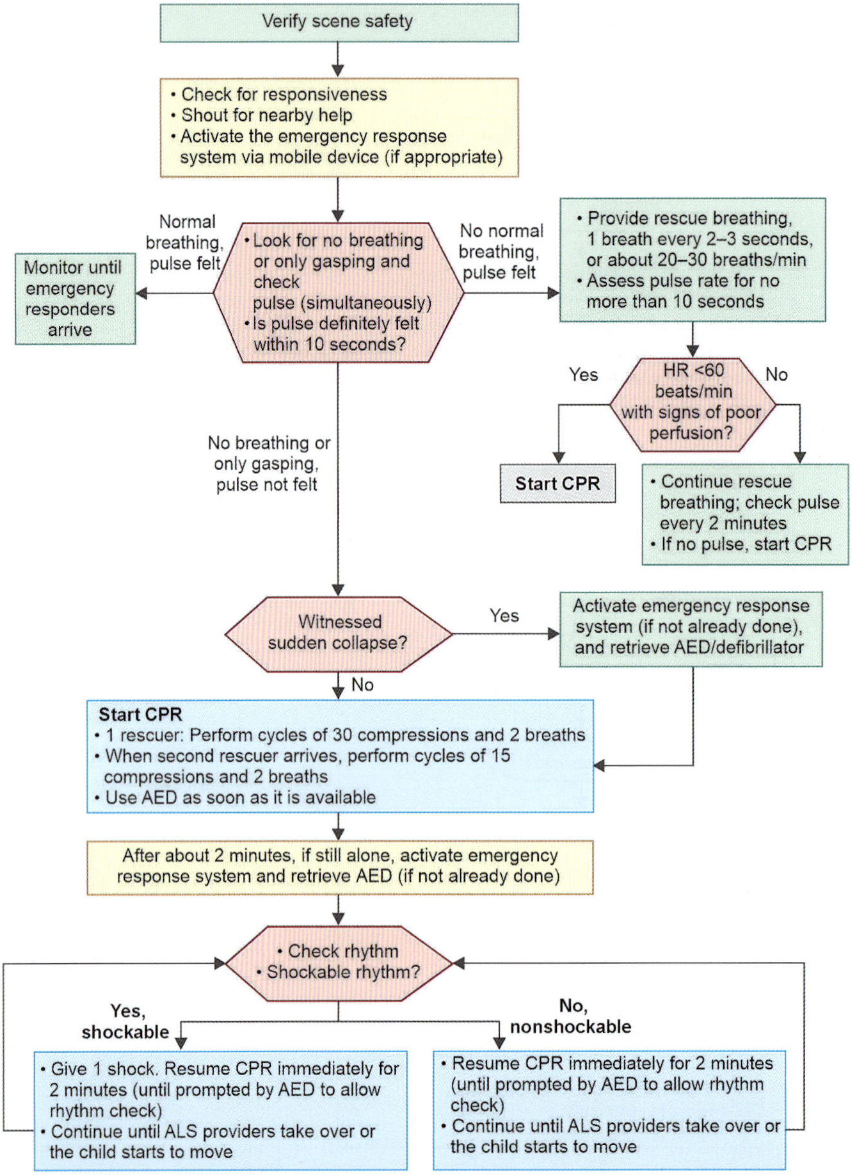

(AED: automated external defibrillator; ALS: advanced life support; CPR: cardiopulmonary resuscitation)

Source: © 2020 American Heart Association.

CHAPTER 3

Pediatric Basic Life Support Algorithm for Healthcare Providers: Two or More Rescuers

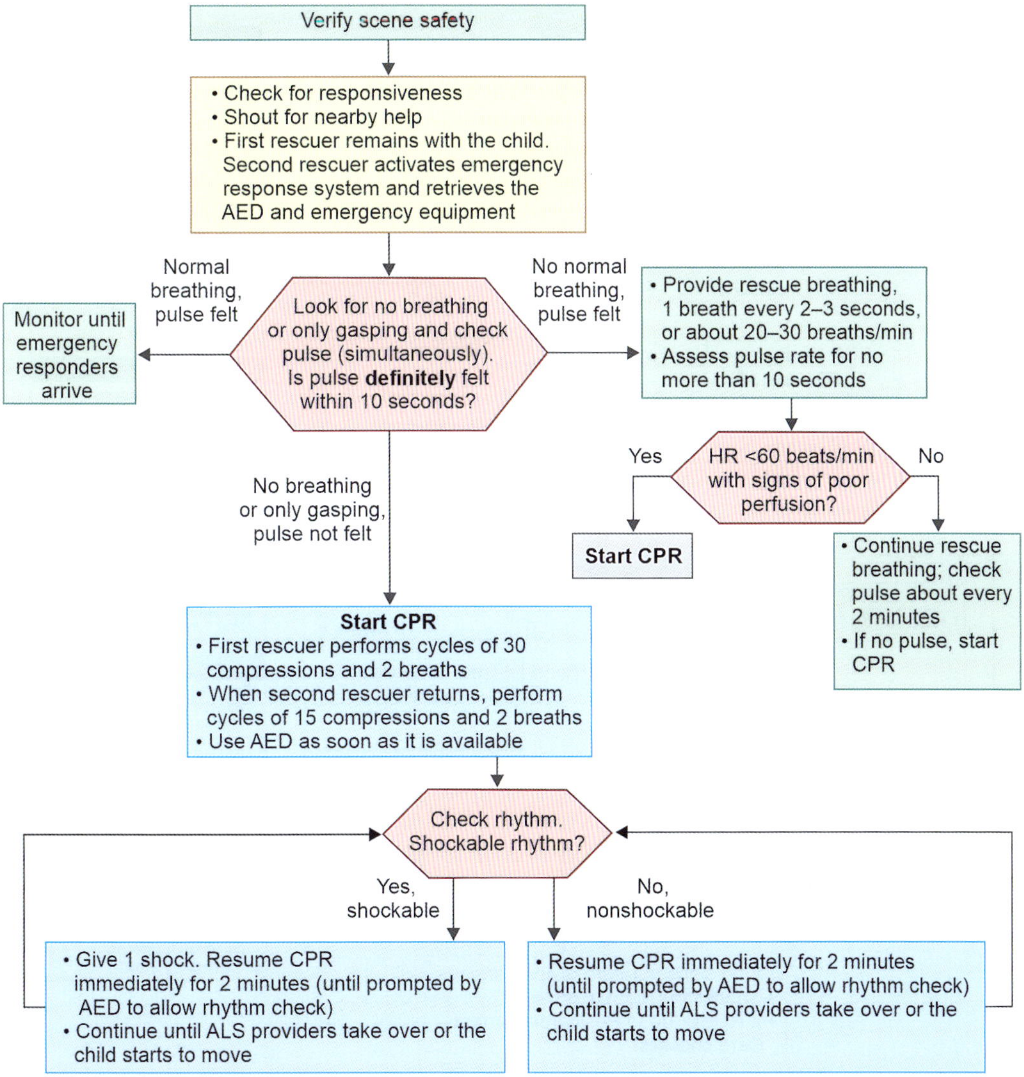

(AED: automated external defibrillator; ALS: advanced life support; CPR: cardiopulmonary resuscitation; HR: heart rate)

Source: © 2020 American Heart Association.

CHAPTER 4

Pediatric Cardiac Arrest Algorithm

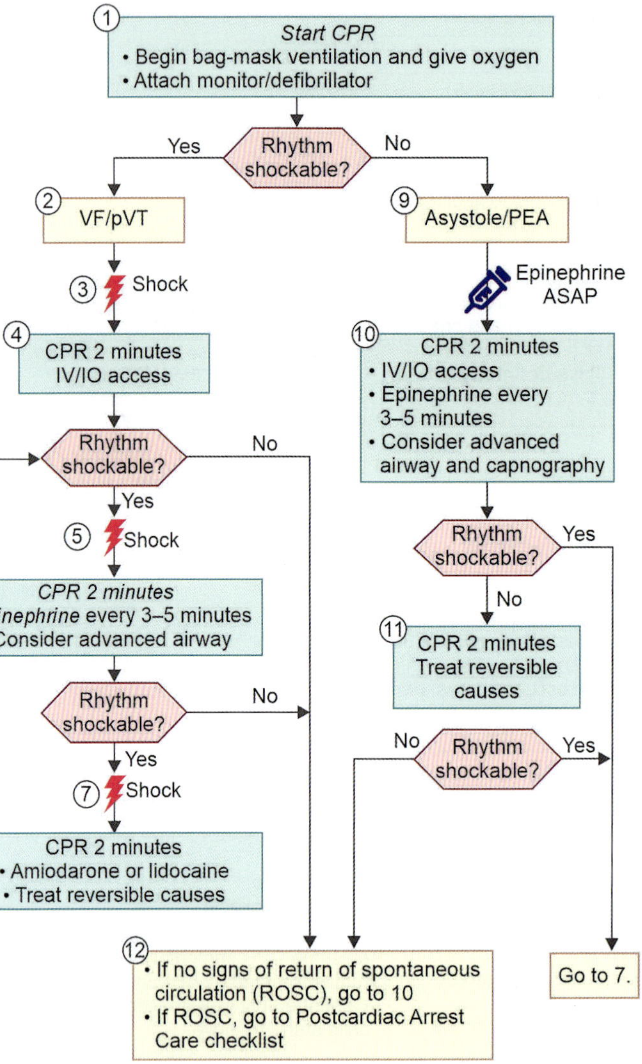

CPR quality

- Push hard (≥⅓ of anteroposterior diameter of chest) and fast (100–120/min) and allow complete chest recoil
- Minimize interruptions in compressions
- Change compressor every 2 minutes, or sooner if fatigued
- If no advanced airway, 15:2 compression–ventilation ratio
- If advanced airway, provide continuous compressions and give a breath every 2–3 seconds

Shock energy for defibrillation

- First shock 2 J/kg
- Second shock 4 J/kg
- Subsequent shocks ≥4 J/kg, maximum 10 J/kg or adult dose

Drug therapy

- **Epinephrine IV/IO dose:**
  - 0.01 mg/kg (0.1 mL/kg of the 0.1 mg/mL concentration).
  - Max dose 1 mg.
  - Repeat every 3–5 minutes. If no IV/IO access, may give endotracheal dose: 0.1 mg/kg (0.1 mL/kg of the 1 mg/mL concentration).
- **Amiodarone IV/IO dose:** 5 mg/kg bolus during cardiac arrest. May repeat up to 3 total doses for refractory VF/pulseless VT
  or
  Lidocaine IV/IO dose:
  Initial: 1 mg/kg loading dose

Advanced airway

- Endotracheal intubation or supraglottic advanced airway
- Waveform capnography or capnometry to confirm and monitor ET tube placement

Reversible causes

- Hypovolemia
- Hypoxia
- Hydrogen ion (acidosis)
- Hypoglycemia
- Hypo-/hyperkalemia
- Hypothermia
- Tension pneumothorax
- Tamponade, cardiac
- Toxins
- Thrombosis, pulmonary
- Thrombosis, coronary

(ASAP: as soon as possible; CPR: cardiopulmonary resuscitation; ET: endotracheal; IV/IO: intravenous/Intraosseous; PEA: pulseless electrical activity; pVT: portal vein thrombosis; VF: ventricular fibrillation; VT: ventricular tachycardia)

Source: © 2020 American Heart Association

CHAPTER 5

Pediatric Bradycardia with a Pulse Algorithm

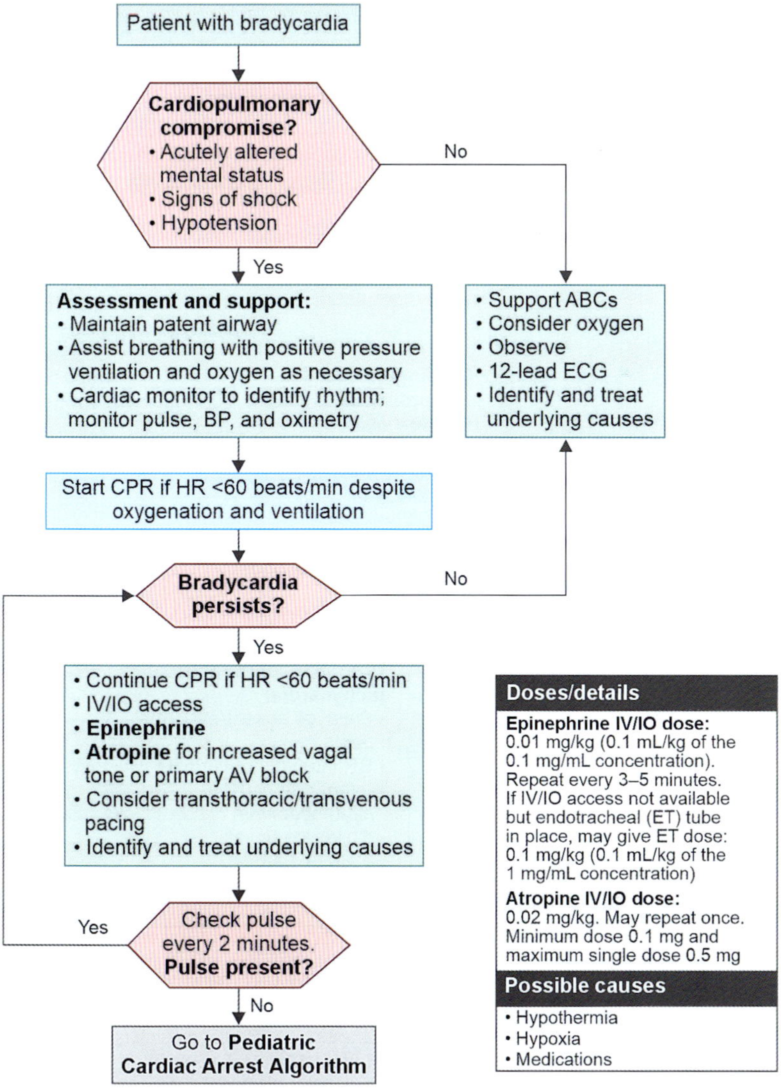

(ABC: airway, breathing, and circulation; AV: atrioventricular; BP: blood pressure; CPR: cardiopulmonary resuscitation; ECG: electrocardiogram; HR: heart rate; IV/IO: intravenous/intraosseous)

Source: © 2020 American Heart Association.

CHAPTER **6**

Pediatric Tachycardia with a Pulse Algorithm

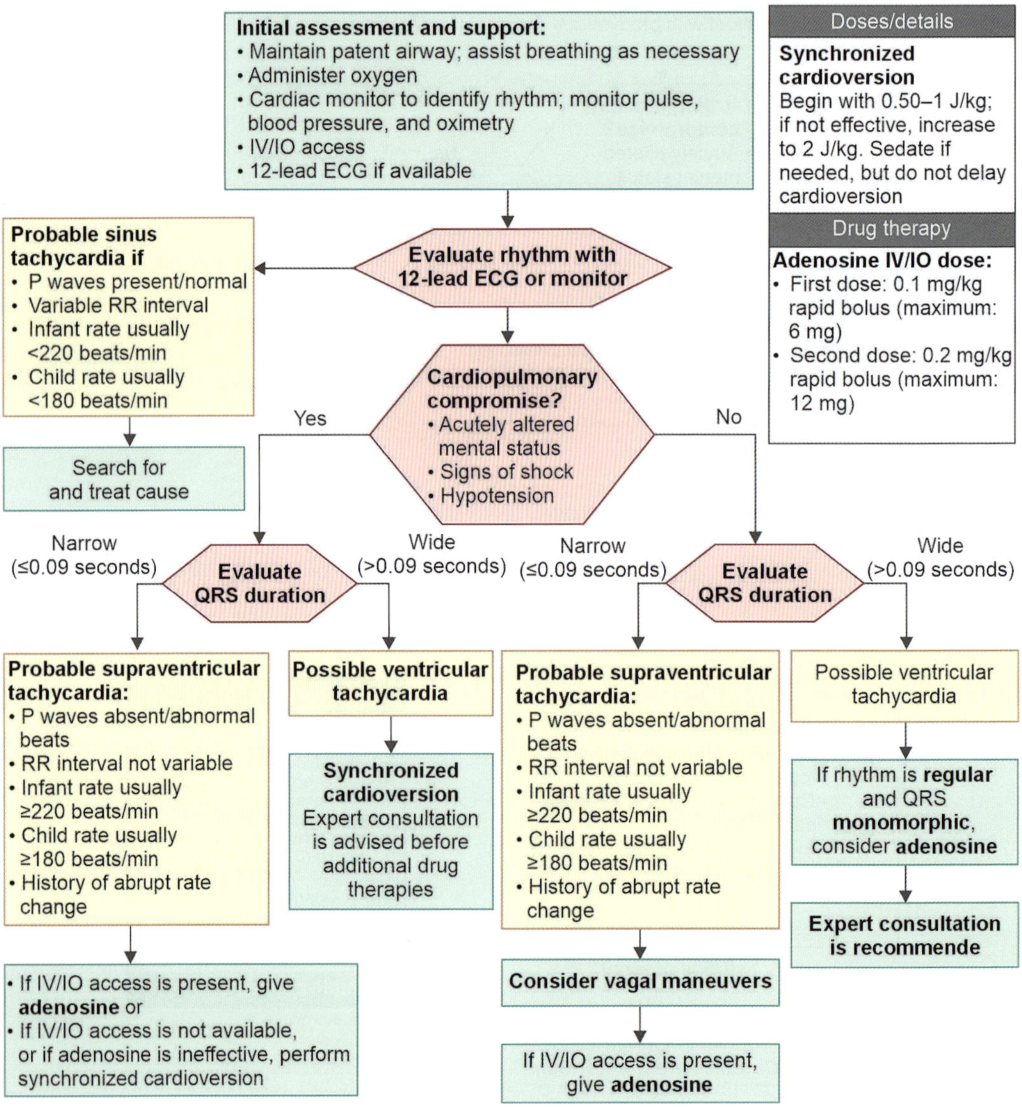

(ECG: electrocardiogram; IV/IO: intravenous/intraosseous)
Source: © 2020 American Heart Association.

SECTION 2

Medical Emergency Pathways

1. Emergency Preparedness in Pediatric Office Practice
2. Management of Croup in Children
3. Acute Asthma in Office Practice
4. Bronchiolitis and its Management
5. Nontraumatic Chest Pain in Children and Adolescents: Approach and Initial Management
6. Evaluation and Management of Syncope in Pediatric Patients
7. Brief Resolved Unexplained Events in Pediatric Emergency Management
8. Anaphylaxis and its Management Based on Current World Allergy Organization Guidelines
9. Emergency Management of the Pediatric Patient with Convulsive Status Epilepticus
10. Management of Mild Head Injury in Children
11. Emergency Department Approach to Nontraumatic Headache in Children
12. Excessive Crying in Infants and its Management
13. Management of a Febrile Infants below 3 Months of Age
14. Rabies Postexposure Prophylaxis Protocol in India
15. Management of Foreign Body Ingestion in Children
16. Common Household Poisoning

CHAPTER 1

Emergency Preparedness in Pediatric Office Practice

INTRODUCTION

Pediatric medical care requires a team approach, involving various health care and allied personnel. The continuum of care includes prevention, prehospital care, emergency room stabilization, inpatient treatment, rehabilitation, and counseling. Often, the entry point into the emergency care system is the pediatric physician's office. As the child's medical home, the pediatric clinic plays a crucial role in emergency care. Understanding the scope and limitations of one's setup is essential for providing the best chance of intact survival to vulnerable children.

It is not uncommon to encounter a pediatric emergency in a medical office, such as breathing difficulties, severe dehydration, trauma, poisoning, or seizures. Primary care physicians and their staff must be prepared to respond to these urgencies. It is our moral, social, ethical, professional, and possibly medicolegal responsibility to provide an initial response. A prompt and effective start can save a child's life, and the consequences of being unprepared can be severe.

What is a Pediatric Emergency?

A pediatric emergency is a medical condition that warrants immediate attention, where any delay may lead to loss of life or organ function.

The American Academy of Pediatrics (AAP) Committee on Pediatric Emergency Medicine issued a policy statement on "Preparation for Emergencies in the Offices of Pediatricians and Pediatric Primary Care Providers." The policy statement recommends a self-based assessment of office readiness for an emergency. Key self-assessment considerations include:

- Frequency and types of emergencies encountered
- Practice type and hours of operation
- Proximity to acute care facilities and availability of emergency medical response teams
- Care for children with special needs
- Written protocols for emergency response
- Availability and awareness of medical equipment and supplies
- Staff training in emergency recognition and response [e.g., basic life support (BLS) and advanced cardiovascular life support (ACLS)]
- Maintenance of skills and readiness through mock codes and training
- Documentation of events, parent education, and staff training
- Arrangements for safe transfer to definitive care

OFFICE PREPAREDNESS COMPONENTS

Office-based Assessment

Every clinic should conduct a thorough assessment of its readiness to handle emergencies. Essential personnel typically include a receptionist, a nurse practitioner or helper, housekeeping staff, and a physician. The receptionist, often the first point of contact, should be trained to identify urgent conditions using tools such as the Pediatric Assessment Triangle, which evaluates appearance, work of breathing, and circulation. Training should cover recognizing and responding to:

- Extremely labored breathing
- Cyanosis (blue or pale color)
- Noisy breathing (wheezing or stridor)
- Altered mental status
- Seizures
- Agitation (in the parent)
- Vomiting after a head injury
- Poisonings
- Uncontrolled bleeding

DEVELOPING AN EMERGENCY RESPONSE PLAN

Every clinic should develop a response plan to recognize, stabilize, and transfer sick children to appropriate acute care settings. This involves raising an alarm for help and activating emergency medical services (EMSs). Staff should initiate resuscitative measures and stabilize the child until EMS arrives or suitable transport is available. Regular mock codes and adherence to pediatric advanced life support (PALS)/advanced pediatric life support (APLS) algorithms are crucial. Staff should clearly communicate with the emergency medical team, providing information on the patient's condition, steps taken, and desired transport destination.

Training

Standard practice guidelines should be in place, and emergency equipment and drugs should be organized for easy access. Regular training, including mock codes and scavenger hunts, ensures staff readiness. Liaisoning with emergency medical teams can enhance coordination and preparedness. All team members should be aware of their roles and the sequence of role reversal during understaffing situations.

Triage

Clinic staff should be able to triage patients based on priority. Red flag signs of a child already in the office should prompt immediate evaluation by the clinician. Reception areas should be clearly visible, and receptionists should physically assess and inquire about the child's condition to prioritize care. Urgent cases should be directed to the nearest hospital if necessary.

Equipment and Medications (Box 1 and Tables 1 and 2)

A detailed list of required equipment and medications, categorized as mandatory or desired, should be maintained. Regular checks for expiry and functionality ensure preparedness. The appendix provides a comprehensive list of necessary items.

Transport

Each facility should identify an emergency transport service, local hospital emergency department (ED), local pediatric intensive care unit (PICU), and an emergency care physician. Contact information should be clearly displayed and known to all clinic staff. Proper communication with EMS is essential for successful handover and continued care.

Documentation

Proper documentation is critical and should include:

- Clinic preparedness details

BOX 1: Emergency office equipment (M—mandatory and D—desirable).

Airway management:
- Oxygen-delivery system (M)
- Bag-valve-mask (450 and 1,000 mL) (M)
- Clear oxygen masks with reservoirs (M)
- Suction device, bulb syringe, and mucous trap (M)
- Nebulizer or metered-dose inhaler (MDI) with spacer/mask (M)
- Oropharyngeal airways (sizes 00–5) (M)
- Pulse oximeter (M)
- Nasopharyngeal airways (sizes 12–30F) (D)
- Magill forceps (pediatric and adult) (D)
- Suction catheters (sizes 5–16F) and Yankauer suction tip (D)
- Nasogastric tubes (sizes 6–14F) (D)
- Laryngoscope handle (pediatric and adult) with extra batteries and bulbs (D)
- Laryngoscope blades (0–2 straight and 2–3 curved) (D)
- Endotracheal tubes (uncuffed 2.5–5.5; cuffed 6.0–8.0) (D)
- Stylets (pediatric and adult) (D)
- Esophageal intubation detector or end-tidal carbon dioxide detector (D)

Vascular access and fluid management:
- Catheter-over-needle device (14–24 gauge) (D)
- Arm boards, tape, and tourniquet (D)
- Intraosseous needles (16 and 18 gauge) (D)
- Intravenous tubing and microdrip (D)

Miscellaneous equipment and supplies:
- Color-coded tape or preprinted drug doses (M)
- Cardiac arrest board/backboard (M)
- Sphygmomanometer (infant, child, adult, and thigh cuffs) (M)
- Splints and sterile dressings (M)
- Automated external defibrillator with pediatric capabilities (D)
- Spot glucose test (D)
- Stiff neck collars (small/large) (D)
- Heating source (overhead warmer/infrared lamp) (D)

TABLE 1: Emergency use drugs (M—mandatory and D—desirable).

Oxygen (M)	***Corticosteroids (parenteral/oral) (D)***
Epinephrine (1:1,000) (M)	Activated charcoal (D)
Epinephrine (1:10,000) (M)	Antibiotics (D)
Salbutamol for inhalation (M)	Dextrose (25%) (D)
Diphenhydramine (parenteral, 50 mg/mL) (D)	Anticonvulsant agents (midazolam and lorazepam) (M)
Atropine sulfate (0.1 mg/mL) (D)	Naloxone (0.4 mg/mL) (D)
Normal saline solution or lactated Ringer's solution (500-mL bags) (D)	5% Dextrose 0.45 normal saline (500-mL bags)

TABLE 2: Important telephone numbers.

(Fill and display as applicable to your setting)	
Poison Control Center	1800-116-117
Poison Control Center	1800-425-1213
National Emergency Number	112
National Ambulance	102
National Fire	101
Child Helpline	1098
Ambulance Transport Services	
Pediatric Transport Team	
Referral hospital pediatric intensive care unit (PICU)	
Local emergency care physician	
Local police	

- Equipment and drug inventory
- Training logs
- Initial assessment and emergency response
- Communication with EMS
- Interventions and outcomes
- Parental communication

CONCLUSION

Being unprepared for emergencies can have serious consequences. Initial treatment provided in the office can mean the difference between life and death. Stabilizing pediatric emergencies and timely transfer for definitive care are responsibilities of every medical practitioner who cares for children.

FURTHER READING

1. American Academy of Pediatrics. Pediatric Preparedness Resource Kit. American Academy of Pediatrics, 2012.
2. Committee on Pediatric Emergency Medicine. Preparation for Emergencies in the Offices of Pediatricians and Pediatric Primary Care Providers. Pediatrics. 2007; 120(1):200-12.
3. Fuchs S. Pediatric office emergencies. Pediatr Clin North Am. 2013;60(5):1153-61.
4. Gausche-Hill M, Schmitz C, Lewis RJ. Pediatric preparedness of US emergency departments: a 2003 survey. Pediatrics. 2007; 120(6):1229-37.
5. Jesse Hackell; Preparedness for Emergencies in the Pediatric Office. Pediatrics September 2021;148(3):e2021051830.
6. Kalidindi S, Lacy TA. Primary Care Office Preparedness for Pediatric Emergencies. Pediatr Ann. 2018;47(3):e93-e96.
7. Yuknis ML, Abulebda K, Whitfill T, Pearson KJ, Montgomery EE, Auerbach MA; Improving Pediatric Acute Care Through Simulation (ImPACTS). Improving Emergency Preparedness in Pediatric Primary Care Offices: A Simulation-Based Interventional Study. Acad Pediatr. 2022;22(7):1167-74.

CHAPTER 2

Management of Croup in Children

INTRODUCTION

Croup is a common respiratory emergency in pediatric practice, characterized by its distinctive barking cough and stridor. While most cases are mild and self-limiting, the potential for rapid progression demands prompt recognition and appropriate intervention. This chapter outlines a systematic approach to diagnosis, severity assessment, and evidence-based management of croup, enabling healthcare providers to deliver optimal care across various clinical settings.

ETIOLOGY

Croup, also known as laryngotracheobronchitis, is a respiratory illness primarily affecting the larynx and subglottic airway, leading to characteristic inspiratory stridor, a barking cough, and hoarseness. It is usually caused by viral infections, with parainfluenza virus type 1 being the most common pathogen. Other viruses include rhinovirus, respiratory syncytial virus (RSV), and adenoviruses. While secondary bacterial infections can occur, they are relatively uncommon.

EPIDEMIOLOGY

Croup is among the most prevalent respiratory illnesses in young children, particularly affecting those ≤6 years old, with peak incidence between 6 months and 3 years. In temperate climates, croup cases predominantly occur in the fall and early winter. Host factors, such as a functional or anatomic susceptibility to upper airway narrowing, can contribute to the development of croup.

CLINICAL PRESENTATION

The symptoms of croup typically begin with nasal discharge and congestion, progressing over 12–48 hours to include fever, hoarseness, a barking cough, and inspiratory stridor. If the airway obstruction worsens, severe respiratory distress can develop. Croup is generally a self-limited illness, resolving within 3 days, although the cough may persist for up to a week.

Rapid Assessment

The rapid assessment of a child with croup aims to evaluate the severity of the illness and exclude other causes of upper airway obstruction. This includes assessing general appearance, vital signs, pulse oximetry, airway stability, and mental status to identify children with severe respiratory distress or impending respiratory failure.

Diagnosis

Croup is diagnosed clinically based on the characteristic barking cough and stridor. Radiographs or laboratory tests are not necessary for diagnosis but may be useful in select cases to exclude other causes. The characteristic radiographic finding in croup is subglottic narrowing, known as the "steeple sign."

DIFFERENTIAL DIAGNOSIS

The differential diagnosis of croup includes other causes of stridor and/or respiratory distress. Important considerations include:

- Acute epiglottitis
- Peritonsillar abscess
- Retropharyngeal abscess
- Foreign body aspiration
- Acute angioedema
- Upper airway injury (e.g., from caustic ingestion)
- Congenital abnormalities of the upper airway

If a child presents with recurrent episodes of croup-like symptoms that are atypical for simple croup, such as severe or prolonged symptoms or occurrences outside the typical age range, other underlying conditions should be suspected. Conditions such as congenital airway abnormalities, gastroesophageal reflux, or atopic conditions should be considered, and the child should be referred to an otolaryngologist for further evaluation.

SEVERITY ASSESSMENT

Management of croup begins with an assessment of severity, which can be done through telephone triage or by examining the child in an office or emergency department (ED) setting. Indicators for immediate medical evaluation include stridor at rest, underlying airway abnormalities, previous episodes of moderate-to-severe croup, and inability to tolerate fluids.

Mild croup:

- Barky cough and hoarse voice
- No stridor at rest
- Mild coarse stridor only during agitation or activity
- No or mild work of breathing

Moderate croup:

- Stridor at rest
- Tachypnea
- Moderate work of breathing
- Anxiety, agitation, or restlessness
- Difficulty talking or feeding

Severe croup:

- Stridor at rest
- Severe work of breathing or respiratory fatigue
- Self-positioning (e.g., tripoding and neck extension)
- Decreased level of consciousness (LOC)
- Inability to talk or feed
- Impending respiratory failure
- Stridor may be present or decreased
- Severe work of breathing
- Bradypnea or poor respiratory effort
- Cyanosis/hypoxemia despite supplemental oxygen
- Hypercarbia
- Listless or decreased LOC

MANAGEMENT (FIG. 1)

Home Treatment for Mild Croup

Children with mild symptoms (no stridor at rest and no respiratory distress) can be managed at home with supportive care, such as fever reduction and encouraging fluid intake. Parents should be instructed on indications to seek medical attention.

Outpatient Treatment for Mild Croup

For children with mild croup seen in an office or ED setting, a single dose of dexamethasone (0.15–0.6 mg/kg, maximum 16 mg) or prednisolone (1 mg/kg) is suggested over supportive care alone.

Management of Moderate-to-Severe Croup

Children with moderate croup (stridor at rest with mild-to-moderate retractions) should be evaluated in the office or ED, while those

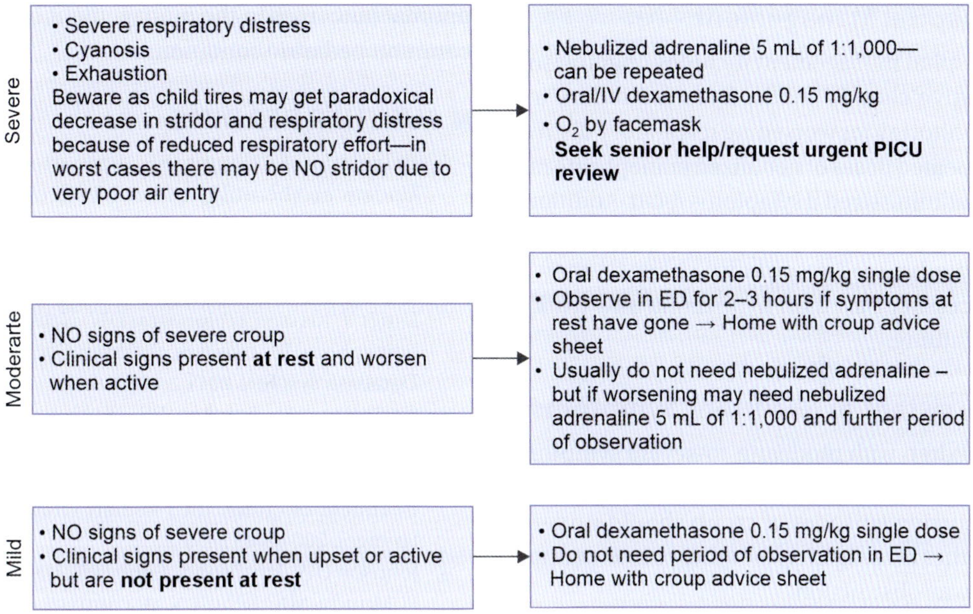

Fig. 1: Croup management in children. (ED: emergency department; IV: intravenous)
Source: Adapted from NHS. NHSGGC Paediatrics for Health Professionals. [online] Available from https://www.clinicalguidelines.scot.nhs.uk/nhsggc-guidelines/ [Last accessed August, 2024].

with severe croup (stridor at rest with marked retractions and significant distress) should be evaluated in the ED. Initial treatment with nebulized epinephrine and a single dose of glucocorticoid is recommended.

Dexamethasone

Dexamethasone is preferred for its long-acting effects and extensive study in croup treatment. It is given at 0.6 mg/kg (maximum 16 mg) orally, intravenously, or intramuscularly.

Nebulized Epinephrine

Dosing depends on the product used:

- *Racemic epinephrine:* 0.05 mL/kg per dose (maximum 0.5 mL) of a 2.25% solution diluted to 3 mL total volume with normal saline
- *L-epinephrine:* 0.5 mL/kg per dose (maximum 5 mL) of a 1 mg/mL solution
- Both are administered via nebulizer over 15 minutes and can be repeated every 15–20 minutes. Close cardiac monitoring is recommended if three or more doses are administered within a 2- to 3-hour period.

Supportive Care

Supportive care includes antipyretics, fluids [oral, if possible, intravenous (IV) if necessary], and oxygen or humidified air as needed.

OBSERVATION AND DISPOSITION

Children should be observed for 3–4 hours after nebulized epinephrine. Those who improve can be discharged home, while those with persistent or worsening symptoms after one to two doses of nebulized epinephrine should be admitted to the hospital.

Hospital Management

Hospital management includes ongoing supportive care, IV fluids, fever reduction, and monitoring for worsening respiratory distress. Repeated doses of nebulized epinephrine may be administered if symptoms recur. Additional respiratory support (humidified air, oxygen, and advanced respiratory support) may be necessary based on hypoxemia and work of breathing.

Persistent or Recurrent Symptoms

Children with moderate-to-severe symptoms that persist for more than a few days or recurring episodes of croup should undergo further investigation for other causes of upper airway obstruction.

Follow-up

Most children with croup recover uneventfully. Follow-up should be scheduled within 24 hours of discharge or as soon as possible for children who received nebulized epinephrine, had prolonged outpatient visits, or were admitted to the hospital.

CONCLUSION

Effective management of croup hinges on accurate severity assessment and timely intervention with proven therapies. While most cases can be managed in the outpatient setting, recognizing indicators for escalation of care remains crucial. This structured approach, combined with appropriate follow-up and family education, ensures optimal outcomes in the management of this common pediatric condition.

FURTHER READING

1. Beigelman A, Chipps BE, Bacharier LB. Update on the utility of corticosteroids in acute pediatric respiratory disorders. Allergy Asthma Proc. 2015;36:332-8.
2. Bjornson C, Russell KF, Vandermeer B, Durec T, Klassen TP, Johnson DW. Nebulized epinephrine for croup in children. Cochrane Database Syst Rev. 2011;2:006619.
3. Cetinkaya F, Tufekci BS, Kutluk G. A comparison of nebulized budesonide, and intramuscular, and oral dexamethasone for treatment of croup. Int J Pediatr Otorhinolaryngol. 2004;68(4):453-6.
4. Johnson DW, Jacobson S, Edney PC, Hadfield P, Mundy ME, Schuh S. A comparison of nebulized budesonide, intramuscular dexamethasone, and placebo for moderately severe croup. N Engl J Med. 1998;339:498-503.
5. Mandal A, Kabra SK, Lodha R. Upper Airway Obstruction in Children. Indian J Pediatr. 2015;82(8):737-44.
6. Petrocheilou A, Tanou K, Kalampouka E, Malakasioti G, Giannios C, Kaditis AG. Viral croup: Diagnosis and a treatment algorithm. Pediatr Pulmonol. 2014;49:421-9.
7. Russel KF, Liang Y, O'Gorman K, Johnson DW, Klassen TP. Glucocorticoids for croup. Cochrane Database Syst Rev. 2011(1):001955.
8. Taketomo CK, Hodding JH, Kraus DM. Pediatric & Neonatal Dosage Handbook: A Universal Resource for Clinicians Treating Pediatric and Neonatal Patients, 21st edition. Hudson, OH: Lexi-Comp; 2014.

CHAPTER 3

Acute Asthma in Office Practice

INTRODUCTION

The effective management of asthma exacerbations is built upon four key principles: Early recognition, assessment of attack severity, timely intervention, and continuous reassessment. The treatment approach must be tailored to the specific circumstances of each patient, taking into account the setting [home, outpatient, or emergency department (ED)], the medications and equipment available, and the clinical expertise of the healthcare provider.

EDUCATION AND ASTHMA ACTION PLAN

A critical aspect of managing asthma exacerbations is the education of patients and their caregivers. Each patient should receive an individualized, written asthma action plan. This plan must provide clear instructions on how to detect and respond to changes in symptoms, ensuring that both patients and caregivers understand the appropriate steps to take when asthma symptoms worsen.

Asthma Action Plan

- The action plan should detail daily management strategies, how to adjust medications in response to symptoms or peak flow readings, and when to seek urgent medical attention.
- It should be personalized to fit the patient's age, severity of asthma, and individual triggers.

Patient and Caregiver Education

- Education should include training on the correct use of inhalers and other medications, recognizing early signs of exacerbations, and understanding the importance of adherence to the action plan.
- Regular reviews and updates of the action plan should be conducted during clinical visits to ensure it remains relevant and understood.

ASSESSMENT

In clinical settings such as an office or urgent care, assessing the severity of an asthma exacerbation involves a comprehensive evaluation of symptoms, physical examination findings, and pulse oximetry readings.

- *Symptom evaluation:*
  - Key symptoms include breathlessness, wheezing, chest tightness, and coughing. The presence and severity of these symptoms help determine the level of exacerbation.
  - The ability to speak in full sentences versus short phrases or words can indicate the severity of breathlessness.
- *Physical examination:*
  - Healthcare providers should look for signs of respiratory distress, such

as the use of accessory muscles for breathing, retractions, and nasal flaring.
  - Auscultation of the lungs may reveal wheezing, reduced air entry, or silent chest in severe cases.
- *Pulse oximetry:*
  - Pulse oximetry is used to measure oxygen saturation levels, providing an objective metric to guide treatment decisions.
  - Normal oxygen saturation is generally above 95%. Levels below this threshold may indicate a need for more intensive treatment.

TREATMENT APPROACH (FLOWCHART 1)

Home Management

Home management of asthma exacerbations primarily involves the use of a rapid-onset beta agonist. Patients and caregivers should be instructed to administer up to three doses within 1 hour, with reassessment after each dose.

Short-acting Beta Agonists

- Short-acting beta agonists (SABAs) such as albuterol (salbutamol) or levalbuterol are the first line of treatment. Patients typically use a metered-dose inhaler (MDI) with a spacer, or a nebulizer for younger children or those with severe symptoms.
- *The action plan should specify the dosage:* Usually 2–4 puffs of an MDI or 1.25–2.5 mg via nebulizer for children under 4 years old and and 2.5–5 mg for older children.

Monitoring and Follow-up

- Patients should monitor their symptoms and peak flow readings. If symptoms persist or worsen despite initial treatment, they should seek medical attention immediately.
- Regular follow-up appointments with a healthcare provider are crucial to adjust the asthma management plan as needed.

Office/Outpatient Management

For mild-to-moderate exacerbations managed in an office or outpatient setting, the approach is similar to that used in EDs.

Initial therapy:
- Rapid-onset beta agonists are administered, with doses often higher than those used at home: albuterol 4–8 puffs via MDI or 2.5–5 mg via nebulizer.
- Ipratropium bromide may be added for patients with moderate-to-severe symptoms.

Systemic glucocorticoids:
- For severe symptoms or those with risk factors for fatal asthma, systemic glucocorticoids should be started immediately. Oral corticosteroids such as prednisone, prednisolone, or dexamethasone are commonly used.
- Glucocorticoids help to reduce airway inflammation and improve symptoms more rapidly than beta agonists alone.

Emergency Department Management

For severe exacerbations, immediate and aggressive treatment is required.

Systemic glucocorticoids:
- These should be given as soon as possible to reduce inflammation and prevent further deterioration. Intravenous options include methylprednisolone.
- Patients with risk factors for fatal asthma should receive systemic glucocorticoids as part of their initial therapy.

Flowchart 1: Acute asthma in primary care (children above 6 years and adults).

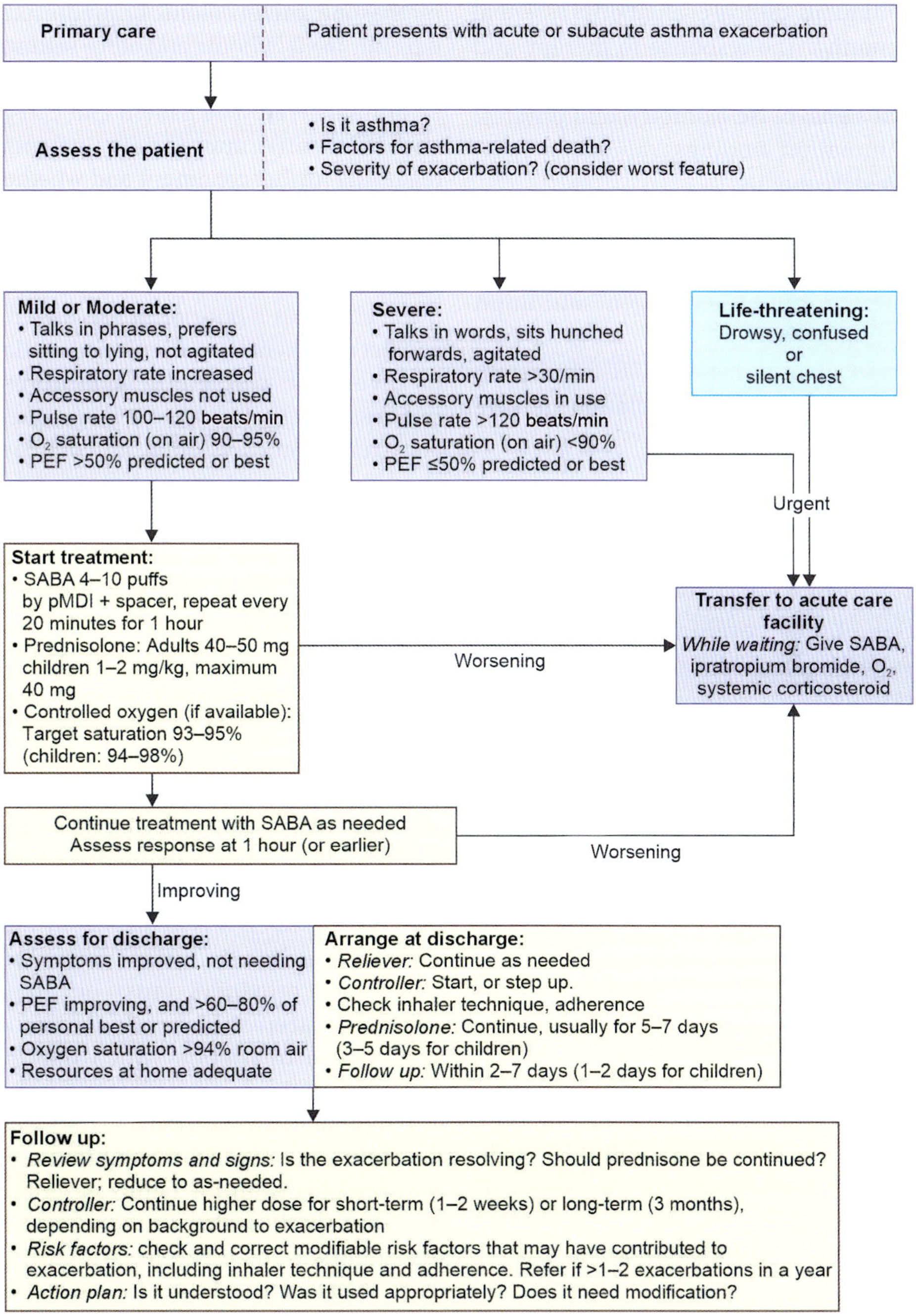

(PEF: peak expiratory flow; pMDI: pressurized metered-dose inhaler; SABA: short-acting beta agonist)
Source: Adapted from Global Initiative for Asthma. (2023). GINA Report, Global Strategy for Asthma Management and Prevention. [online] Available from https://www.knowledge-action-portal.com/en/content/global-strategy-asthma-management-and-prevention-0 [Last accessed August, 2024].

Frequent reassessment:

- Continuous clinical evaluation is essential to monitor the response to therapy and decide on the need for hospital admission.
- Vital signs, pulse oximetry, and physical examination findings should be reassessed frequently.

Oxygen therapy:

- Supplemental oxygen should be administered to maintain oxygen saturation levels above 92%.
- In cases of severe hypoxemia or respiratory failure, mechanical ventilation may be necessary.

SUBSEQUENT THERAPY AND DISPOSITION

Frequent Reassessment

Regular clinical evaluation is essential during the management of an acute asthma exacerbation to monitor the response to therapy and determine the need for ED transfer or admission. Patients who are moderately to severely ill on arrival and show little improvement after initial therapy with inhaled beta agonists and systemic glucocorticoids should be transferred to the ED.

Good Response

If signs and symptoms improve after one to two beta agonist treatments and do not return within 4 hours, the patient may continue at-home treatment with a rapid-onset beta agonist every 4–6 hours as needed. Follow-up should be arranged with the child's primary care clinician or asthma specialist.

Incomplete Response

If the child has an incomplete response with mild symptoms after two beta agonist treatments, systemic glucocorticoids should be initiated. Oral agents such as dexamethasone, prednisolone, or prednisone are typically used in home and office settings. An additional dose of beta agonist should also be administered. The patient and caregivers should receive appropriate instructions regarding further treatment and whether the child should be seen in the office or ED.

Poor Response

If the child has a poor response to two beta agonist treatments (i.e., continued moderate-to-severe or worsening symptoms, or recurrence of symptoms <2 hours after the last treatment), systemic glucocorticoids should be started immediately. Another dose of beta agonist should also be given and arrangements made for transport to the ED.

CONCLUSION

The management of acute asthma exacerbations in office practice requires a comprehensive, patient-centered approach. The critical components of effective asthma care are early recognition, accurate assessment, prompt intervention, and continuous re-evaluation. The individualized asthma action plans and patient education empower patients and caregivers to manage symptoms effectively at home. In the clinical setting, healthcare providers must be adept at assessing exacerbation severity and initiating appropriate treatment, which may range from inhaled beta-agonists to systemic glucocorticoids. Ultimately, successful management of acute asthma in office practice hinges on the clinician's ability to make timely decisions regarding treatment escalation and potential referral to emergency care. By following evidence-based guidelines and maintaining a high index of suspicion for severe exacerbations, healthcare providers can significantly improve outcomes for patients with acute asthma.

FURTHER READING

1. British Thoracic Society (BTS). BTS/SIGN British Guideline on the Management of Asthma. [online] Available from https://www.brit-thoracic.org.uk/quality-improvement/guidelines/asthma/ [Last accessed August, 2024].
2. Castro-Rodriguez JA, Beckhaus AA, Forno E. Efficacy of oral corticosteroids in the treatment of acute wheezing episodes in asthmatic preschoolers: Systematic review with meta-analysis. Pediatr Pulmonol. 2016; 51:868.
3. Global Initiative for Asthma (GINA). (2024). Global Strategy for Asthma Management and Prevention. [online] Available from https://ginasthma.org/2024-report/#:~:text=The%202024%20update%20of%20the,on%20the%20GINA%20Science%20Committee. [Last access August, 2024].
4. National Heart, Lung, and Blood Institute (NHLBI). (2012). Asthma Care Quick Reference: Diagnosing and Managing Asthma. [online] Available from https://www.nhlbi.nih.gov/resources/asthma-care-quick-reference-diagnosing-and-managing-asthma. [Last accessed August, 2024].
5. Rubilar L, Castro-Rodriguez JA, Girardi G. Randomized trial of salbutamol via metered-dose inhaler with spacer versus nebulizer for acute wheezing in children less than 2 years of age. Pediatr Pulmonol. 2000;29:264.

CHAPTER 4

Bronchiolitis and its Management

INTRODUCTION

Bronchiolitis is a common respiratory infection predominantly affecting infants and young children under the age of 2 years. Characterized by acute inflammation of the bronchioles, it is primarily caused by respiratory syncytial virus (RSV). The condition results in significant morbidity and is a leading cause of hospitalization in infants, particularly during the winter months. This chapter provides an overview of the pathophysiology, clinical presentation, diagnosis, and management strategies for bronchiolitis, along with a detailed management algorithm.

PATHOPHYSIOLOGY

Bronchiolitis begins with the infection of the upper respiratory tract, followed by a progression to the lower respiratory tract. The bronchioles, the small airways in the lungs, become inflamed and swollen, and their lumens are filled with mucus. This results in obstruction of airflow and impaired gas exchange. RSV, the most common causative agent, triggers an immune response, leading to epithelial cell necrosis and increased mucus production.

Other viral agents, such as human rhinovirus, parainfluenza virus, adenovirus, and metapneumovirus, can also cause bronchiolitis. The immune response to these infections includes the release of inflammatory cytokines and chemokines, contributing to airway hyperreactivity and edema.

CLINICAL PRESENTATION

The clinical presentation of bronchiolitis varies but typically includes:

- *Initial symptoms:* Rhinorrhea, cough, and low-grade fever
- *Progressive symptoms:* Tachypnea, wheezing, nasal flaring, retractions, and difficulty feeding
- *Severe symptoms:* Cyanosis, apnea (especially in preterm infants), and respiratory failure
- Physical examination findings may include diffuse wheezing and crackles on auscultation. The severity of symptoms can range from mild, self-limiting illness to severe respiratory distress, requiring hospitalization.

DIAGNOSIS

The diagnosis of bronchiolitis is primarily clinical, based on history and physical examination. Laboratory tests and imaging are not routinely required but may be considered in certain cases to rule out other conditions.

- *Clinical criteria:* History of upper respiratory symptoms followed by lower respiratory signs in a young child during the peak season for RSV
- *Laboratory tests:* Nasopharyngeal swab for viral testing can confirm the presence

of RSV or other viruses but is not essential for diagnosis.

- *Imaging:* Chest X-rays are not routinely indicated but may be used to exclude other diagnoses such as pneumonia or foreign body aspiration.

MANAGEMENT (FLOWCHART 1)

Management of bronchiolitis is largely supportive, as there are no specific antiviral treatments for most cases. The primary goals are to maintain adequate oxygenation, hydration, and nutrition.

Supportive Care

- *Oxygen therapy:* It is indicated for children with hypoxemia (oxygen saturation <90%). Options include nasal cannula, face mask, or high-flow nasal cannula (HFNC) in more severe cases.

Flowchart 1: Algorithm for managing bronchiolitis in infants.

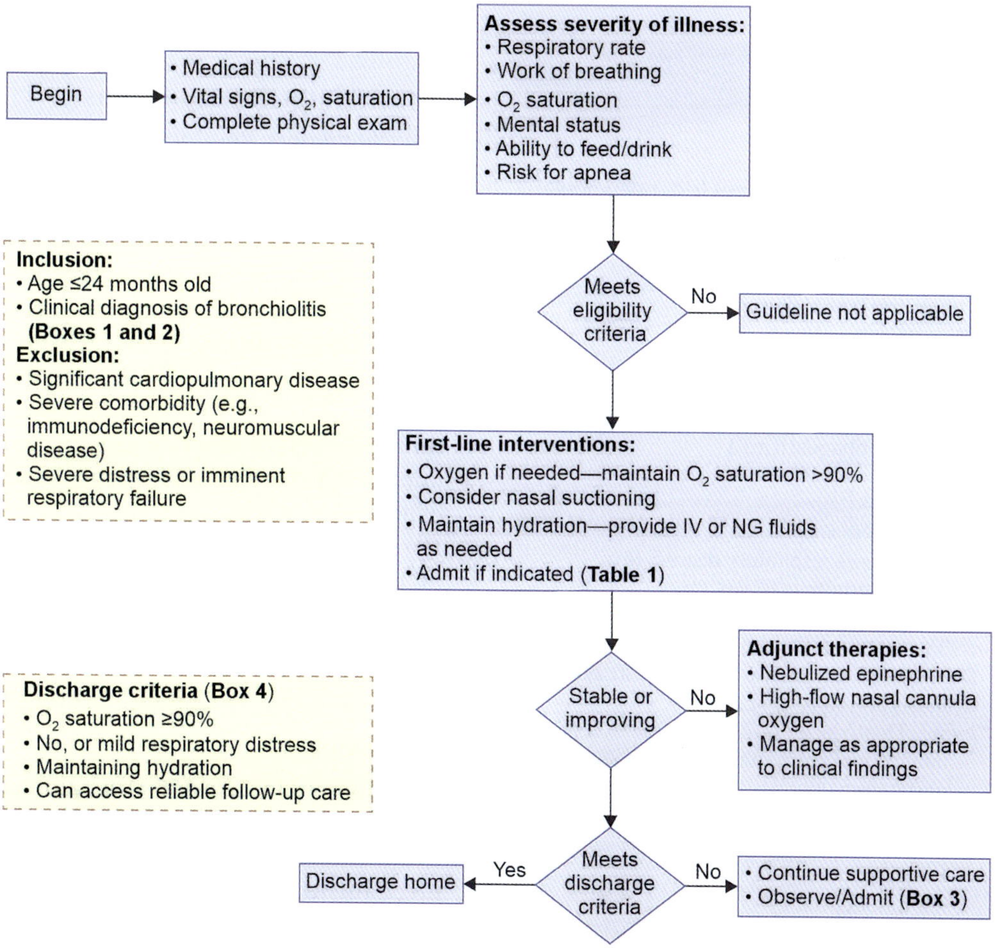

(IV: intravenous; NG: nasogastric)

Source: Adapted from: Bronchiolitis: Recommendations for diagnosis, monitoring and management of children one to 24 months of age: https://cps.ca/documents/position/bronchiolitis#Table%207

BOX 1: *Diagnosis:* History, symptoms, and signs of viral bronchiolitis.

- Preceding viral upper respiratory tract infection, cough and/or rhinorrhea
- Exposure to an individual with viral upper respiratory tract infection
- *Signs of respiratory illness may also include:*
  - Tachypnea
  - Intercostal and/or subcostal retractions
  - Accessory muscle use
  - Nasal flaring
  - Grunting
  - Color change or apnea
  - Wheezing or crackles
  - Lower O_2 saturations

BOX 2: Differential diagnosis for wheezing in young children.

- Viral bronchiolitis
- Asthma
- Other pulmonary infections (e.g., pneumonia)
- Laryngotracheomalacia
- Foreign body aspiration
- Gastroesophageal reflux
- Congestive heart failure
- Vascular ring
- Allergic reaction
- Cystic fibrosis
- Mediastinal mass
- Tracheoesophageal fistula

BOX 3: Guidelines for admission may include.

- Signs of severe respiratory distress (e.g., indrawing, grunting, RR >60/min)
- Supplemental O_2 required to keep saturations >90%
- Dehydration or history of poor fluid intake
- Cyanosis or history of apnea
- *Infant at high risk for severe disease:*
  - Infants born prematurely (<35 weeks' gestation)
  - <3 months of age at presentation
  - Hemodynamically significant cardiopulmonary disease
  - Immunodeficiency
- Family unable to cope

- *Hydration:* Ensuring adequate fluid intake is crucial. Intravenous fluids may be required for children who cannot maintain hydration orally.
- *Nutritional support:* Nasogastric or orogastric feeding may be necessary for infants with severe respiratory distress who cannot feed adequately.

BOX 4: Discharge from hospital.

- Tachypnea and work of breathing improved
- Maintain O_2 saturations >90% without supplemental oxygen OR stable for home oxygen therapy
- Adequate oral feeding
- Education provided and appropriate follow-up arranged

Pharmacologic Interventions

- *Bronchodilators:* Routine use of bronchodilators like albuterol is not recommended, as evidence suggests limited efficacy. A trial may be considered in severe cases to assess the response.
- *Corticosteroids:* Not routinely recommended due to lack of consistent benefit
- *Antibiotics:* Not indicated unless there is a coexisting bacterial infection
- *Antiviral therapy:* Ribavirin is rarely used due to limited evidence and potential side effects.
- *Hypertonic saline nebulization:* The role of hypertonic saline in bronchiolitis management has been a topic of interest and research.

Role of Hypertonic Saline Nebulization

- Hypertonic saline (3% or 5%) nebulization has been investigated as a potential treatment for bronchiolitis. The proposed mechanism involves reducing airway edema and improving mucus clearance through osmotic effects. Several studies and systematic reviews have evaluated its efficacy.

- *Mechanism of action:* Hypertonic saline is thought to draw water into the airway lumen, thinning mucus and facilitating its clearance. This can potentially reduce airway obstruction and improve breathing.
- *Evidence of efficacy:* The evidence on the use of hypertonic saline nebulization in bronchiolitis is mixed. Some studies have shown modest improvements in clinical scores and reduced length of hospital stay, while others have found no significant benefit. The American Academy of Pediatrics (AAP) suggests that hypertonic saline nebulization may be considered in hospitalized patients but does not recommend its routine use in emergency department or outpatient settings due to inconsistent results.
- *Clinical practice:* When used, hypertonic saline nebulization is typically administered 2–3 times a day. It may be combined with a bronchodilator to minimize potential bronchospasm. Clinical judgment is essential in determining its use on a case-by-case basis, considering potential benefits and the individual patient's response.

Nonpharmacologic Interventions

- *Chest physiotherapy:* It is not recommended routinely as it does not improve outcomes
- *Humidified air:* It can be beneficial in maintaining airway moisture, but evidence is mixed on its efficacy.

PREVENTION

Preventive measures include:

- *Palivizumab prophylaxis:* It is recommended for high-risk infants (e.g., premature infants, those with chronic lung disease or congenital heart disease) to prevent RSV infection.
- *Hand hygiene:* Emphasizing handwashing and hygiene practices to reduce viral transmission
- *Avoiding exposure:* Keeping infants away from sick contacts, especially during the RSV season

CONCLUSION

Bronchiolitis remains a significant health concern for infants and young children, primarily due to its potential for severe respiratory distress and hospitalization. Understanding the pathophysiology, recognizing the clinical presentation, and implementing evidence-based management strategies are crucial for optimizing patient outcomes. While supportive care remains the cornerstone of treatment, ongoing research into preventive and therapeutic options continues to evolve, offering hope for improved management of this common pediatric illness.

FURTHER READING

1. American Academy of Pediatrics Subcommittee on Diagnosis and Management of Bronchiolitis. Diagnosis and Management of Bronchiolitis. Pediatrics. 2006;118(4):1774-93.
2. Florin TA, Plint AC, Zorc JJ. Viral Bronchiolitis. The Lancet. 2017;389(10065):211-24.
3. Hall CB, Weinberg GA, Iwane MK, Blumkin AK, Edwards KM, Staat MA, et al. The Burden of Respiratory Syncytial Virus Infection in Young Children. New Engl J Med. 2009;360(6):588-98.
4. Ralston SL, Lieberthal AS, Meissner HC, Alverson BK, Baley JE, Anne MG, et al. Clinical practice guideline: The diagnosis, management, and prevention of bronchiolitis. Pediatrics. 2014;134(5):e1474-502.
5. Zhang L, Mendoza-Sassi RA, Wainwright C, Klassen TP. Nebulized Hypertonic Saline Solution for Acute Bronchiolitis in Infants. Cochrane Database Syst Rev. 2017;12(12):CD006458.

CHAPTER 5

Nontraumatic Chest Pain in Children and Adolescents: Approach and Initial Management

INTRODUCTION

Nontraumatic chest pain is a common concern in children and adolescents, frequently leading to medical consultations. Though typically benign, it can cause significant anxiety and activity limitations. A detailed history and physical examination are essential for identifying the cause and determining the need for further intervention. Laboratory testing is seldom required unless specific concerning symptoms are present.

EVALUATION

History

A detailed history is critical for identifying serious causes of chest pain. Important factors include:

- *Pain description:*
  - Substernal, crushing pain with radiation and associated symptoms (anginal pain)
  - Severe, tearing pain radiating to the back (aortic dissection)
  - Pleuritic pain with difficulty breathing (pneumonia, pneumothorax, and pulmonary embolus)
  - Sharp, retrosternal pain exacerbated by lying down, often with fever (pericarditis)
  - Drug-related pain from substances such as cocaine or amphetamines
- *Associated symptoms:*
  - Exertional syncope or dizziness (suggests cardiac anomalies or cardiomyopathy)
  - Palpitations
  - Difficulty breathing, fever, history of heart disease, recent COVID-19 vaccination, or conditions predisposing to pericarditis
- *Family history:*
  - Sudden death or hypertrophic cardiomyopathy in relatives
  - Genetic conditions associated with heart disease or aortic dissection
- *Temporal elements:*
  - Chronic pain often indicates a musculoskeletal, psychogenic, or idiopathic cause.
  - Acute pain suggests a medical condition such as asthma, pneumothorax, or pulmonary embolism.
- *Quality:*
  - Sharp, localized pain typically indicates a musculoskeletal origin.
  - Diffuse, radiating pain may suggest ischemia or other serious conditions.
- *Precipitating factors:*
  - Pain with deep breathing, swallowing, or exertion may indicate musculoskeletal, esophageal, or cardiac issues.

Physical Examination

A comprehensive physical examination can identify or rule out serious conditions.

- *Vital signs:*
  - Fever may indicate infections or inflammatory conditions.
  - Tachycardia and tachypnea suggest cardiac or respiratory issues.

    - Hypertension or hypotension can signal serious cardiac conditions.
    - Hypoxia needs urgent attention.
- *Chest wall*:
    - Tenderness often indicates a musculoskeletal cause.
    - Deformities or asymmetries might suggest underlying conditions such as pneumothorax.
- *Lungs:*
    - Diminished breath sounds, wheezing, or rales indicate respiratory conditions.
    - Crepitus can suggest pneumomediastinum or esophageal rupture.
- *Heart:*
    - Abnormal heart sounds can indicate serious cardiac issues such as hypertrophic cardiomyopathy, pericarditis, or myocarditis.
    - Specific murmurs and abnormal rhythms warrant further investigation and specialist consultation.

Ancillary Studies

Most children with chest pain do not need extensive testing. However, diagnostic studies are essential for those with concerning symptoms.

- *Electrocardiogram (ECG):*
    - It is recommended, if the cardiac disease is suspected or a noncardiac cause is not evident.
    - It can identify arrhythmias, hypertrophic cardiomyopathy, or ischemia.
- *Chest radiograph:*
    - Useful for suspected cardiac or pulmonary disorders, or esophageal foreign bodies
    - Can reveal heart enlargement, pulmonary hypertension, or infiltrates
- *Echocardiogram:*
    - Indicated for respiratory distress, abnormal heart sounds, exertional symptoms, or a history suggesting cardiac risk.
- *Other tests:*
    - Cardiac troponin testing for suspected myocardial injury
    - Ambulatory cardiac rhythm monitoring for recurrent palpitations or syncope

APPROACH AND INITIAL MANAGEMENT (FLOWCHART 1)

Unstable Patients

Immediate supportive care is necessary for patients with severe symptoms, following pediatric advanced life support (PALS) principles. Conditions such as airway obstruction, pneumothorax, status asthmaticus, pulmonary embolism, myocardial infarction, and heart failure require urgent intervention.

ACUTE CHEST PAIN WITH CONCERNING FINDINGS

Patients with potential cardiac issues need an ECG and possibly a chest radiograph. Those with abnormal findings should be referred to a pediatric cardiologist for further evaluation.

Common Findings

Most pediatric chest pain is benign. Key management strategies include:

- *Chest wall pain:* Often responds to analgesics and rest
- *Psychogenic pain:* Reassurance and counseling for stress-related or hyperventilation-induced pain
- *Respiratory conditions:* Appropriate treatment for conditions such as asthma or pneumonia
- *Gastrointestinal issues:* Management of gastroesophageal reflux disease or pill esophagitis

Flowchart 1: Management of chest pain in children.

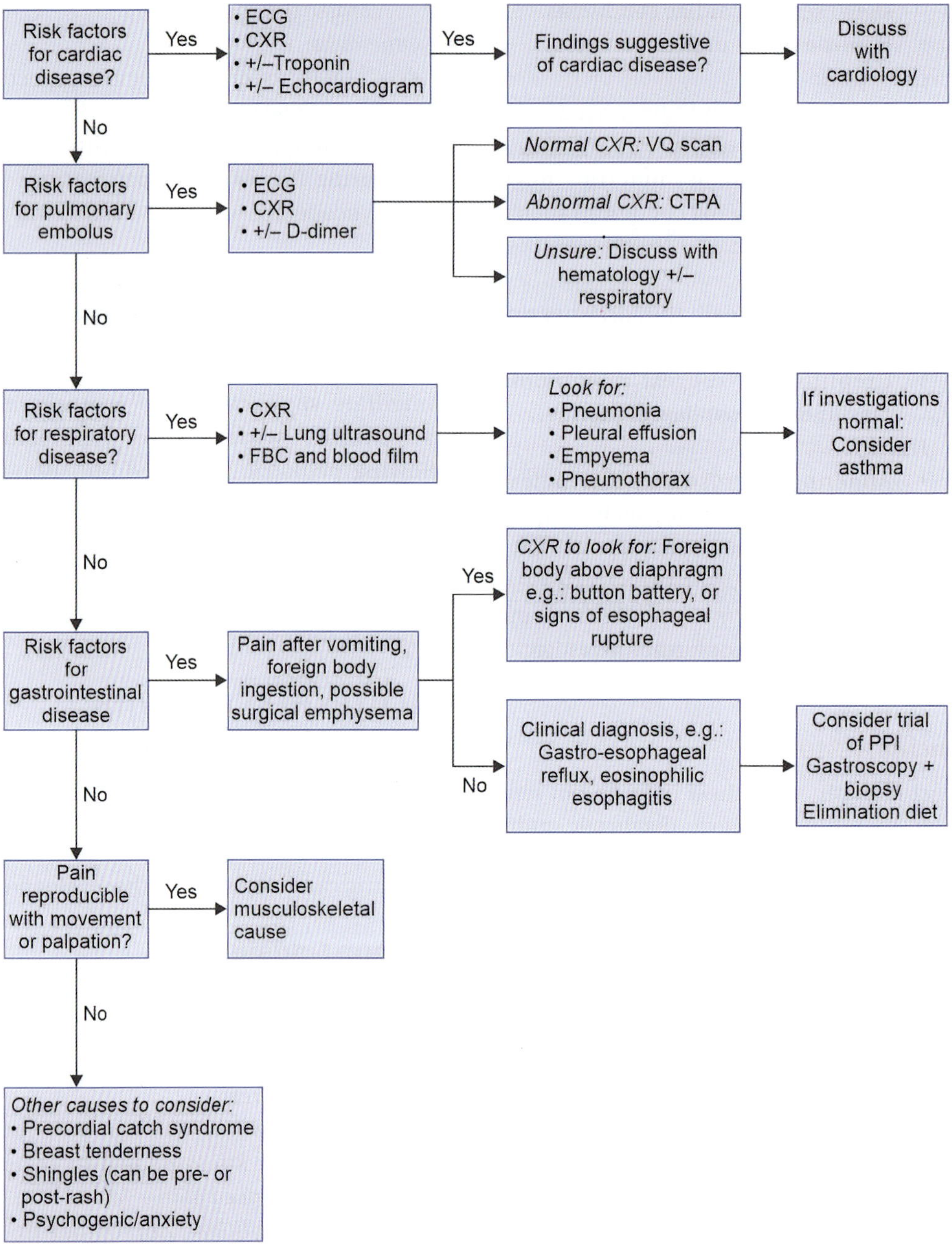

(CTPA: computed tomography pulmonary angiography; CXR: chest X-ray; ECG: electrocardiogram; FBC: full blood count; PPI: proton-pump inhibitor; VQ: ventilation-perfusion)

Source: Adapted from The Royal Children's Hospital Melbourne. (2023). Clinical Practice Guidelines. Chest Pain. [online] Available from https://www.rch.org.au/clinicalguide/guideline_index/chest_pain/ [Last accessed August, 2024].

Indications for Pediatric Subspecialty Consultation or Referral

Children with known heart disease or findings suggestive of a cardiac cause should see a pediatric cardiologist. Other referrals may be necessary for conditions such as recurrent pneumothorax, aortic dissection, pulmonary embolism, sickle cell disease, or serious emotional disturbances.

Disposition

- *Unstable patients:* Require hospitalization with intensive care capabilities
- *Stable patients with concerning findings:* May need hospitalization for further testing
- *Stable patients with benign findings:* Can be managed with follow-up care as appropriate for the underlying etiology

CONCLUSION

Chest pain in children and adolescents is usually benign but requires careful evaluation to rule out serious conditions. A thorough history and physical examination guide the need for further testing and specialist consultation. Most cases can be managed with reassurance and follow-up, while those with concerning findings warrant prompt specialist referral.

FURTHER READING

1. Alsabri M, Elshanbary AA, Nourelden AZ, Fathallah AH, Zaazouee MS, Pincay J, et al. Chest pain in pediatric patients in the emergency department- Presentation, risk factors and outcomes-A systematic review and meta-analysis. PLoS One. 2024;19(4):e0294461.
2. Atmanli A, Yen K, Zhou AZ. Diagnostic testing for chest pain in a pediatric emergency department and rates of cardiac disease before and during the COVID-19 pandemic: a retrospective study. Front. Pediatr. 2024; 12:1366953.
3. Collins SA, Griksaitis MJ, Legg JP. 15-minute consultation: a structured approach to the assessment of chest pain in a child. Arch Dis Child Educ Pract Ed. 2014;99:122.
4. Friedman KG, Alexander ME. Chest pain and syncope in children: a practical approach to the diagnosis of cardiac disease. J Pediatr. 2013;163:896.
5. Kapur N, Watson M, Kennedy A. Management of non-traumatic chest pain in children in primary care: An evidence-based review. Br J Gen Pract. 2023;73(718):181-8.
6. Pomerantz WJ, Bhagat MK, Sabin ML. Pediatric chest pain: Diagnostic approach and management. Pediatr Emerg Med Pract. 2022;19(8):1-24.
7. Selbst SM, Ruddy RM, Clark BJ, Henretig FM, Santulli T Jr. Pediatric chest pain: a prospective study. Pediatrics. 1988;82: 319-23.
8. Son MB, Sundel RP. Musculoskeletal causes of pediatric chest pain. Pediatr Clin North Am. 2010;57(6):1385-95.

CHAPTER 6

Evaluation and Management of Syncope in Pediatric Patients

INTRODUCTION

This chapter provides a detailed guide on the evaluation and diagnostic approach for syncope in children and adolescents. While syncope is often benign in pediatric patients, it can sometimes indicate a more serious underlying condition. This guide aims to help clinicians identify the cause of syncope and determine appropriate management and follow-up.

DEFINITION AND CAUSES

Syncope is defined as a sudden, brief loss of consciousness and postural tone, with spontaneous recovery. Approximately 15% of children experience at least one syncopal episode by the end of adolescence.

The causes of syncope can be categorized as autonomic (e.g., vasovagal, situational, and orthostatic), cardiac, metabolic, or conditions that mimic syncope. In pediatric emergency settings, autonomic forms constitute up to 80% of cases. Neurological causes, including seizures or migraines, account for up to 20% of cases. Although life-threatening conditions such as hypoglycemia, heat illness, anaphylaxis, cardiac arrhythmia, or structural cardiac disease are rare, they are significant enough to require careful diagnostic consideration.

EVALUATION

History

A thorough history is essential for identifying the cause of syncope and guiding further evaluation. Key elements to explore include the following described further.

Preceding Events or Triggers

Identifying the circumstances leading up to the syncopal event can provide critical clues. Considerations include:

- *Exercise:* Syncope during physical exertion raises concern for cardiac causes but can also be due to vasovagal syncope.
- *Acute arousal or loud noise:* Triggers such as sudden loud noises may indicate primary electrical disturbances such as long QT syndrome.
- *Postural changes:* Syncope following prolonged standing or a quick change in position often suggests a vasovagal cause.
- *Pain or emotional stress:* Painful stimuli or emotional stress can trigger vasovagal syncope. However, familial catecholaminergic polymorphic ventricular tachycardia can also present with arrhythmias under stress.

Description of the Event

Gather detailed descriptions from the child and any witnesses. Important aspects include:

- *Palpitations or chest pain:* These symptoms prior to or during syncope raise concerns for a cardiac etiology.
- *Loss of consciousness with abnormal motor activity:* Brief motor activity following syncope usually correlates with

neurocardiac syncope, while prolonged motor activity suggests a seizure.

- *Orthostatic symptoms:* Recurrence of symptoms upon sitting up after the event indicates orthostatic hypotension or vasovagal syncope.

Physical Examination

A comprehensive physical examination should include vital signs and a detailed cardiac and neurologic evaluation:

- *Vital signs:* Check for orthostatic hypotension by measuring blood pressure and heart rate changes from sitting to standing.
- *Cardiac examination:* Assess for murmurs, gallops, rubs, and signs of structural heart disease.
- *Neurologic examination:* Identify any focal deficits that might suggest a neurological cause.

Ancillary Studies

Guided by the history and physical examination, ancillary studies can help confirm the diagnosis.

Electrocardiogram

An electrocardiogram (ECG) is crucial in the syncope work-up, despite its low diagnostic yield. A normal ECG significantly lowers the likelihood of a cardiac cause. Look for:

- *Prolonged QT interval:* It suggests congenital or acquired long QT syndrome.
- *Short QT interval:* It suggests short QT syndrome
- *Brugada syndrome indicators:* Pseudo-right bundle branch block and persistent ST elevation in leads V1–V3
- *Preexcitation syndromes:* These are the indicators of Wolff–Parkinson–White syndrome.
- *Hypertrophic cardiomyopathy:* Signs of left ventricular hypertrophy and abnormal Q waves

Laboratory Tests

These tests may be useful in certain cases:

- *Blood glucose:* Especially if the patient presents immediately after the episode
- *Hematocrit:* For patients at risk of anemia
- *Pregnancy test:* For postmenarchal females
- *Toxicology screen:* If there is a suspicion of substance abuse

Diagnostic Approach (Flowchart 1)

A systematic approach, including a focused history, careful cardiac and neurologic evaluations, and selected ancillary studies, usually identifies the cause of syncope in most children.

Prolonged Loss of Consciousness

Evaluate for a neurological disorder, such as a seizure or migraine syndrome, if unconsciousness lasts more than a few seconds.

Transient Loss of Consciousness

Careful history, physical examination, and limited ancillary studies typically suffice to identify the underlying cause.

Abnormal Cardiac Evaluation

Most children with a cardiac cause of syncope can be identified by historical features, physical examination, and ECG findings.

Normal Cardiac Examination

Children with a normal ECG and cardiac examination are unlikely to have a cardiac cause for their syncope. However, further evaluation by a pediatric cardiologist is

Flowchart 1: Management of syncope in children.

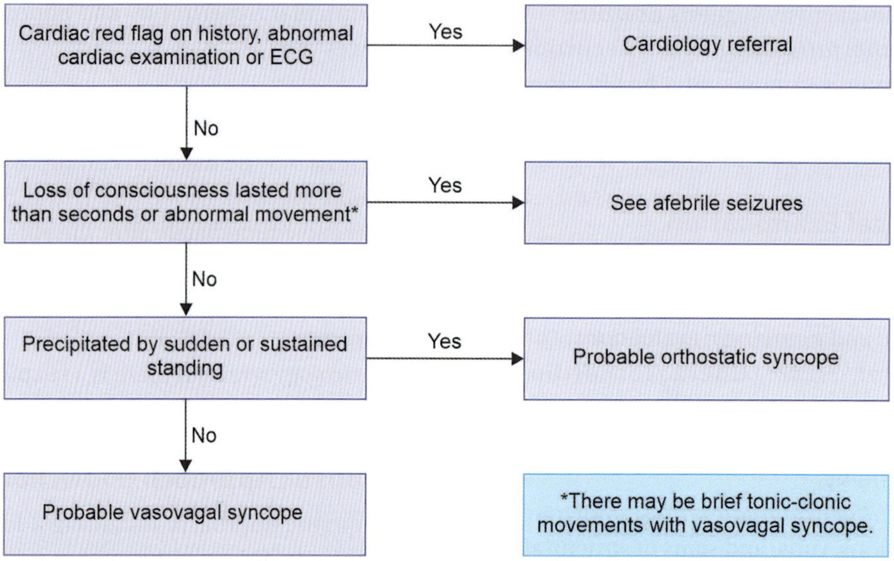

Note: Cardiogenic Syncope Red Flag: Syncope during exercise, usually no prodrome, however, may have chest pain or palpitations, past cardiac history, family history of early cardiac death, arrhythmia, or sudden death.

Source: Adapted from The Royal Children's Hospital Melbourne. (2023). Clinical Practice Guidelines. [online] Available from https://www.rch.org.au/clinicalguide/guideline_index/Syncope/ [Last accessed August, 2024].

warranted, if there are concerning historical features.

INDICATIONS FOR REFERRAL OR ADMISSION

Outpatient Follow-up

Most children who fully recover from a syncopal event and have no red flags for cardiac syncope can be followed as outpatients. Persistent syncope despite nonpharmacologic management may warrant a pediatric cardiology consultation.

Urgent Consultation

Urgent referral to a pediatric cardiologist is necessary, if there is suspicion of cardiac syncope based on history, physical examination, or ECG findings.

Hospital Admission

Hospital admission for further evaluation and observation may be required for patients with:

- *Cardiovascular disease*: Evidence of heart failure, arrhythmia, or heart block
- *Neurologic findings:* Persistent abnormal neurologic signs
- *Orthostatic hypotension:* Continued postural syncope that does not resolve with fluid therapy

TREATMENT

Management of pediatric syncope involves addressing the underlying cause. For vasovagal (neurocardiogenic) syncope, the following steps are suggested:

- *Increase fluid intake:* Encourage oral intake of 30–50 mL/kg/day.

- *Add salty snacks:* Include items such as pretzels, pickles, or crackers in the diet.
- *Avoid caffeine:* Recommend avoiding caffeinated beverages.
- *Prevent venous pooling:* Teach techniques such as keeping knees slightly bent when standing, isometric muscle contractions, and leg crossing.

Most patients with vasovagal syncope improve with these nonpharmacologic measures. Persistent symptoms despite these interventions warrant referral to a pediatric cardiologist.

CONCLUSION

Syncope in children and adolescents is typically benign but can sometimes indicate a serious underlying condition. A thorough history and physical examination are crucial in identifying the cause and guiding further evaluation and management. Most cases can be managed with reassurance and lifestyle modifications, while those with concerning features require a specialist referral and possibly further testing.

FURTHER READING

1. Bo I, Carano N, Agnetti A, Tchana B, Allegri V, Sommi Marcello, et al. Syncope in children and adolescents: a two-year experience at the Department of Paediatrics in Parma. Acta Biomed. 2009;80:36-41.
2. Friedman KG, Alexander ME. Chest pain and syncope in children: a practical approach to the diagnosis of cardiac disease. J Pediatr. 2013;163:896.
3. Hurst D, Hirsh DA, Oster ME, Ehrlich A, Campbell R, Mahle WT, et al. Syncope in the Pediatric Emergency Department - Can We Predict Cardiac Disease Based on History Alone? J Emerg Med. 2015;49:1-7.
4. Kapoor WN. Syncope. N Engl J Med. 2000;343:1856.
5. Lewis DA, Dhala A. Syncope in the pediatric patient. The cardiologist's perspective. Pediatr Clin North Am. 1999;46:205.
6. Massin MM, Bourguignont A, Coremans C, Comté L, Lepage P, Gérard P. Syncope in pediatric patients presenting to an emergency department. J Pediatr. 2004;145:223-8.
7. Pratt JL, Fleisher GR. Syncope in children and adolescents. Pediatr Emerg Care. 1989;5:80.
8. Zhang Q, Du J, Wang C, Du Z, Wang Li, Tang C. The diagnostic protocol in children and adolescents with syncope: a multi-centre prospective study. Acta Paediatr. 2009;98:879.

CHAPTER 7

Brief Resolved Unexplained Events in Pediatric Emergency Management

INTRODUCTION

A brief resolved unexplained event (BRUE), previously known as apparent life-threatening event (ALTE), represents a critical yet often benign episode in infants that necessitates immediate medical evaluation. The American Academy of Pediatrics (AAP) defines a BRUE as an event in an infant younger than 1 year, characterized by a sudden, brief, and resolved episode involving one or more of the following:

- Cyanosis or pallor
- Absent, decreased, or irregular breathing
- Marked change in muscle tone (hyper- or hypotonia)
- Altered level of responsiveness

This new terminology highlights the transient nature of these events and aims to reduce unnecessary anxiety and interventions when no serious underlying condition is found. This chapter delves into the clinical presentation, assessment, risk stratification, management strategies, and follow-up care for BRUE in the pediatric emergency context.

CLINICAL PRESENTATION

A BRUE typically presents as a sudden and alarming episode, often observed by a caregiver. Key features include:

- *Cyanosis or pallor:* The infant may exhibit a blue or very pale complexion.
- *Breathing changes:* Noticeable absence, decrease, or irregularity in breathing patterns
- *Muscle tone:* Either an increase (stiffness) or decrease (floppiness) in muscle tone
- *Responsiveness:* The infant might appear unresponsive or less responsive than usual.

These episodes are generally brief, lasting less than a minute, and resolve spontaneously, with the infant returning to their baseline state without intervention.

ASSESSMENT (FLOWCHART 1)

When a BRUE is reported, a comprehensive history and physical examination are essential to identify any potential underlying causes. Key components of the assessment include:

- *Detailed history:*
  - Obtain a thorough description of the event from the observer, including the duration, symptoms, and any resuscitative efforts.
  - Review the infant's medical history, including any previous similar events, prenatal and birth history, and family history of sudden infant death syndrome (SIDS) or genetic disorders.
  - Inquire about environmental factors, such as recent infections, exposure to smoke, or any new medications.
- *Physical examination:*
  - Conduct a detailed physical examination, focusing on signs of trauma, infection, congenital anomalies, and neurological abnormalities.

Flowchart 1: Assessment/risk stratification of BRUE presentation.

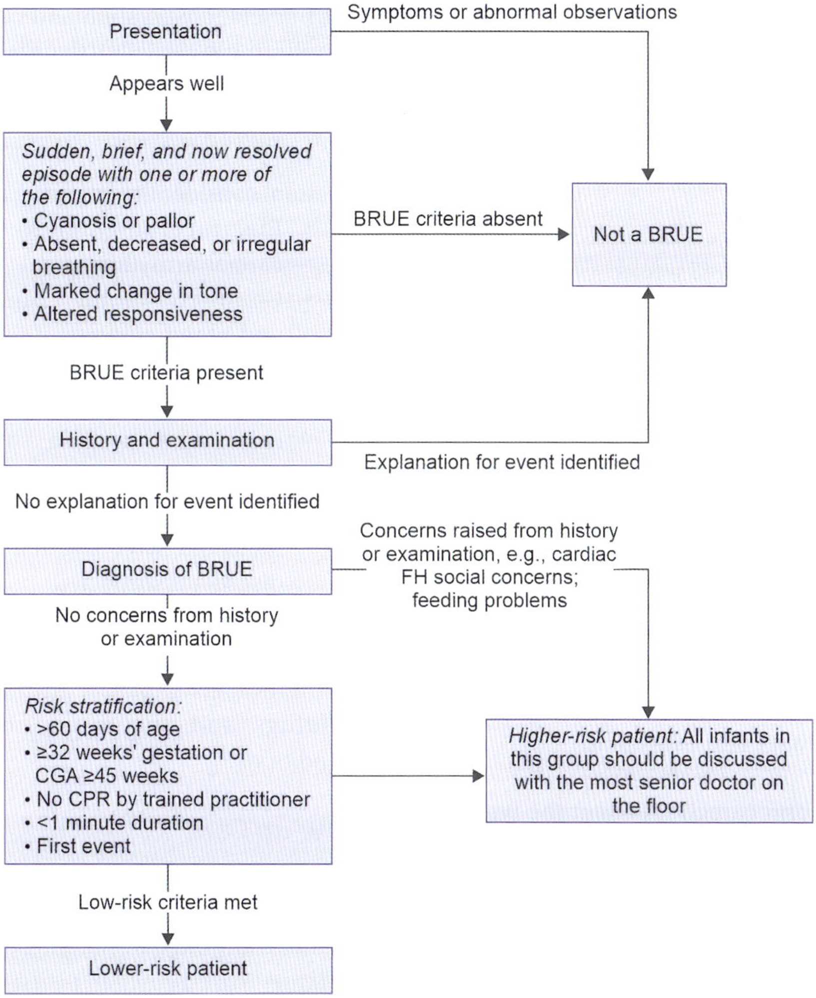

(BRUE: brief resolved unexplained event; CGA: corrected gestational age; CPR: cardiopulmonary resuscitation; FH: family history)

Source: Adapted from Tieder JS, Bonkowsky JL, Etzel RA, Franklin WH, Gremse DA, Herman B, et al.; American Academy of Pediatrics. Brief resolved unexplained events (formerly Apparent life-threatening events) and evaluation of lower risk infants. Pediatrics. 2016;137(5):e20160590.

- Pay particular attention to the cardiovascular, respiratory, and neurological systems.
- *Diagnostic testing:*
  - Routine extensive testing is not recommended for low-risk BRUE.
  - If the history or physical examination suggests a specific cause, targeted testing [e.g., electrocardiogram (ECG) for arrhythmias and blood cultures for infection] may be appropriate.
  - For high-risk cases, consider a broader range of diagnostic tests, including metabolic screening and neuroimaging.

RISK STRATIFICATION

The AAP guidelines recommend categorizing BRUE into low-risk and high-risk groups based on specific criteria. An infant is considered low risk if all the following criteria are met:

- Age >60 days
- Gestational age ≥32 weeks and postconceptional age ≥45 weeks
- No cardiopulmonary resuscitation (CPR) by a trained medical provider was required.
- Event duration <1 minute
- First occurrence of the event
- No concerning historical features or physical examination findings

MANAGEMENT STRATEGIES

Low-risk BRUE

For infants classified as low-risk, management involves minimal intervention and focuses on reassurance and education:

- *Education and reassurance:*
  - Inform caregivers about the typically benign nature of BRUE and the low likelihood of recurrence or serious underlying pathology.
  - Emphasize the importance of normal monitoring and adherence to safe sleep practices to reduce the risk of SIDS.
- *Observation:* Brief observation in the emergency department (ED) may be warranted to ensure the infant remains stable.
- *Follow-up:* Schedule follow-up visits with the primary care provider (PCP) within 24–48 hours to reassess the infant and address any caregiver concerns.

High-risk BRUE

Infants who do not meet the low-risk criteria require more comprehensive evaluation and potentially inpatient observation:

- *Inpatient monitoring:* Admit the infant for hospital observation and continuous monitoring, especially if there is a concern for serious underlying conditions.
- *Targeted diagnostic testing:*
  - Depending on the clinical presentation, consider the following tests:
    - Electrocardiogram to rule out cardiac arrhythmias
    - Complete blood count (CBC) and blood cultures, if infection is suspected
    - Neuroimaging [e.g., magnetic resonance imaging (MRI) and computed tomography (CT) scan), if there are neurological concerns
    - Metabolic screening, if a metabolic disorder is suspected
- *Consultations:* Involve relevant specialists, such as cardiologists, neurologists, or pulmonologists, based on the clinical findings and suspected underlying conditions.

Follow-up Care

Regardless of the risk stratification, follow-up care is crucial to ensure the infant's well-being and address any ongoing parental concerns:

- *Primary care provider visits:* Ensure a follow-up appointment with the infant's PCP within 24–48 hours postdischarge to review the event, re-examine the infant, and determine, if further evaluations or referrals are needed.
- *Parent education:*
  - Continually educate caregivers on recognizing potential warning signs and the importance of safe sleep practices.
  - Provide resources and support to help manage anxiety related to the BRUE incident.

CONCLUSION

A BRUE represents a common yet challenging condition in pediatric emergency medicine, necessitating a balanced approach of careful evaluation and appropriate reassurance. Effective management involves identifying low-risk versus high-risk infants, providing suitable follow-up care, and supporting anxious caregivers. Adhering to current guidelines ensures that infants receive optimal care while minimizing unnecessary interventions and anxiety for families.

FURTHER READING

1. American Academy of Pediatrics. (2022). Guidelines for the Management of Brief Resolved Unexplained Events (BRUE). [online] Available from https://publications.aap.org/pediatriccare/article-abstract/doi/10.1542/aap.ppcqr.396132/1576/Brief-Resolved-Unexplained-Event-BRUE?redirectedFrom=fulltext [Last accessed August, 2024].
2. Ramgopal S, Colgan JY, Roland D, Pitetti RD, Katsogridakis Y. Brief resolved unexplained events: a new diagnosis, with implications for evaluation and management. Eur J Pediatr. 2022;181(2):463-470.
3. Saseen JJ, Grizzle AJ. Evaluation and Management of Brief Resolved Unexplained Events (BRUE) in Infants. Am Fam Physician. 2018;98(3):171-5.
4. Tieder JS, Bonkowsky JL, Etzel RA, Franklin WH, Gremse DA, Herman B, et al. Brief Resolved Unexplained Events (Formerly Apparent Life-Threatening Events) and Evaluation of Lower-Risk Infants. Pediatrics. 2016;137(5):e20160590.

CHAPTER 8

Anaphylaxis and its Management Based on Current World Allergy Organization Guidelines

INTRODUCTION

Anaphylaxis is a severe, potentially life-threatening systemic hypersensitivity reaction characterized by rapid onset and the involvement of multiple organ systems. Prompt recognition and immediate management are critical to preventing morbidity and mortality. This chapter discusses the pathophysiology, clinical presentation, and current management guidelines for anaphylaxis, based on the recommendations of the World Allergy Organization (WAO).

UNDERSTANDING ANAPHYLAXIS

Definition

The WAO defines anaphylaxis as a serious allergic reaction that is rapid in onset and may cause death. It typically involves multiple organ systems, including the skin, respiratory, cardiovascular, and gastrointestinal systems.

Pathophysiology

Anaphylaxis results from the release of mediators from mast cells and basophils, often triggered by immunoglobulin E (IgE)-mediated hypersensitivity reactions. Common triggers include:

- Foods (e.g., peanuts, tree nuts, and shellfish)
- Insect stings (e.g., bees and wasps)
- Medications (e.g., antibiotics and non-steroidal anti-inflammatory drugs)
- Latex
- Physical factors (e.g., exercise-induced anaphylaxis)

Clinical Presentation

Anaphylaxis presents with a wide range of symptoms that can vary in severity. These symptoms typically occur within minutes to hours of exposure to the allergen and may include:

- *Skin and mucosa:* Urticaria, angioedema, flushing, and pruritus
- *Respiratory:* Dyspnea, wheezing, stridor, cough, and nasal congestion
- *Cardiovascular:* Hypotension, tachycardia, syncope, and shock
- *Gastrointestinal:* Nausea, vomiting, diarrhea, and abdominal pain
- *Neurological:* Dizziness, confusion, and loss of consciousness

DIAGNOSIS

Criteria for Diagnosis

The WAO suggests that anaphylaxis can be diagnosed based on any one of the following three criteria:

1. Acute onset of an illness (minutes to several hours) with involvement of the skin, mucosal tissue, or both, and at least one of the following:
   a. Respiratory compromise
   b. Reduced blood pressure or associated symptoms of end-organ dysfunction

2. Two or more of the following that occur rapidly after exposure to a likely allergen:
   a. Involvement of the skin or mucosal tissue
   b. Respiratory compromise
   c. Reduced blood pressure or associated symptoms
   d. Persistent gastrointestinal symptoms
3. Reduced blood pressure after exposure to a known allergen:
   a. *Infants and children:* Low systolic blood pressure (age-specific) or greater than 30% decrease from baseline
   b. *Adults:* Systolic blood pressure <90 mm Hg or >30% decrease from baseline

MANAGEMENT (FLOWCHART 1)

Immediate Management

- *Epinephrine administration:*
  - *First-line treatment:* Intramuscular (IM) epinephrine (0.01 mg/kg, maximum dose 0.5 mg) should be administered into the mid-outer thigh as soon as anaphylaxis is suspected. This is the most critical intervention and can be lifesaving.
  - *Repeat dosing:* If symptoms persist or worsen, additional doses can be administered every 5–15 minutes.
- *Positioning:*
  - *Supine position:* The patient should be placed in a supine position with legs elevated unless there is respiratory distress, in which case they should be positioned to comfort (e.g., sitting up).
- *Oxygen and airway management:*
  - *Oxygen therapy:* Administer high-flow oxygen via mask or nasal cannula.
  - *Airway management:* Be prepared for advanced airway interventions, if there is airway compromise or severe respiratory distress.
- *Intravenous (IV) access and fluids:*
  - *Intravenous access:* Establish IV access for administration of medications and fluids.
  - *Fluid resuscitation:* Administer isotonic crystalloids (e.g., normal saline) rapidly, if there is hypotension or shock.

Adjunctive Therapies

- *Antihistamines:*
  - *H1 antagonists:* Diphenhydramine or cetirizine can be administered for cutaneous symptoms. However, they should not delay the administration of epinephrine.
  - *H2 antagonists:* Ranitidine may be used as an adjunctive treatment.
- *Corticosteroids:*
  - *Administration:* Corticosteroids (e.g., prednisone or methylprednisolone) may help prevent protracted or biphasic reactions, although they do not have immediate effects.
- *Bronchodilators:*
  - *Beta-agonists:* Nebulized albuterol can be administered for bronchospasm that does not respond to epinephrine.

Monitoring and Further Management

- *Observation:*
  - *Monitoring:* Patients should be monitored for at least 4–6 hours after symptoms resolve due to the risk of biphasic reactions.
  - *Discharge:* Patients should be stable, and vital signs should be normal before discharge. Those with severe reactions may require longer observation or hospital admission.

Flowchart 1: Anaphylaxis management.

Anaphylaxis?

↓

A = Airway B = Breathing C = Circulation D = Disability E = Exposure

↓

Diagnosis – look for:
- Sudden onset of airway and/or breathing and/or circulation problems
- And usually skin changes (e.g., itchy rash)

↓

Call for HELP
Call resuscitation team or ambulance

↓

- Remove trigger if possible (e.g., stop any infusion)
- Lie patient flat (with or without legs elevated)
  - A sitting position may make breathing easier
  - If pregnant, lie on left side

→ 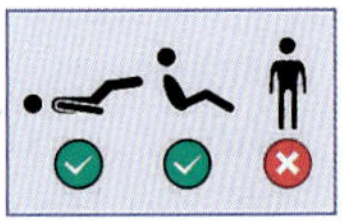

↓

Give intramuscular (IM) adrenaline[2]

← **Inject at anterolateral aspect –** middle third of the thigh

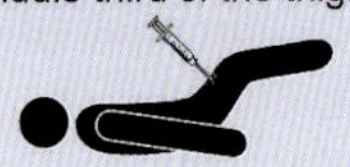

↓

- Establish airway
- Give high flow oxygen
- Apply monitoring, pulse oximetry, ECG, blood pressure

↓

If no response:
- Repeat IM adrenaline after 5 minutes
- IV fluid bolus[3]

↓

If no improvement in breathing or circulation problems[1] **despite TWO doses of IM adrenaline:**
- Confirm resuscitation team or ambulance has been called
- Follow refractory anaphylaxis algorithm

1. Life-threatening problems

Airway
hoarse voice, stridor

Breathing
↑ work of breathing, wheeze, fatigue, cyanosis, SpO_2 <94%

Circulation
Low blood pressure, signs of shock, confusion, reduced consciousness

2. Intramuscular (IM) adrenaline

Use adrenaline at 1 mg/mL (1:1,000) concentration
Adult and child >12 years: 500 µg IM (0.5 mL)
Child 6–12 years: 300 µg IM (0.3 mL)
Child 6 months to 6 years: 150 µg IM (0.15 mL)
Child <6 months: 100–150 µg IM (0.1–0.15 mL)

The above doses are for IM injection **only**
intravenous adrenaline for anaphylaxis to be given **only by experienced specialists** in an appropriate setting

3. IV fluid challenge

Use crystalloid
Adults: 500–1,000 mL
Children: 10 mL/kg

(ECG: electrocardiogram; IV: intravenous; SpO_2: oxygen saturation)

Source: Adapted from Resuscitation Council UK. (2021). Emergency Treatment of Anaphylaxis. [online] Available from https://www.resus.org.uk/sites/default/files/2021-04/Anaphylaxis%20algorithm%202021.pdf

- *Patient education and discharge planning*:
  - *Epinephrine autoinjector:* Prescribe an epinephrine autoinjector and educate the patient and caregivers on its use.
  - *Allergy referral:* Refer the patient to an allergist for further evaluation and management, including identification and avoidance of triggers.
  - *Action plan:* Provide a written emergency action plan outlining steps to take in case of future anaphylactic reactions.

Prevention and Long-term Management

Avoidance of Triggers

- *Identification:* Identify and avoid known allergens.
- *Label reading:* Educate patients and caregivers on reading food labels and recognizing potential allergens in foods and medications.

Immunotherapy

Allergen immunotherapy: Consider allergen-specific immunotherapy for certain triggers (e.g., insect stings) to reduce the risk of future anaphylactic reactions.

Medical Alert Identification

Wearable identification: Recommend that patients wear medical alert bracelets or carry identification that details their allergies and anaphylaxis action plan.

SPECIAL CONSIDERATIONS

Pediatric Considerations

- *Dosing:* Ensure appropriate dosing of epinephrine and other medications based on the child's weight.
- *Education:* Educate caregivers and school personnel on recognizing and managing anaphylaxis in children.

Elderly Considerations

- *Comorbidities:* Consider the presence of comorbid conditions that may complicate the management of anaphylaxis.
- *Polypharmacy:* Be aware of potential interactions with other medications the patient may be taking.

Pregnancy

- *Maternal and fetal safety:* Manage anaphylaxis aggressively to ensure the safety of both mother and fetus.
- *Medications:* Use medications that are safe for use during pregnancy.

CONCLUSION

Anaphylaxis is a medical emergency that requires immediate recognition and prompt management to prevent serious outcomes. The WAO guidelines provide a comprehensive framework for the diagnosis, treatment, and prevention of anaphylactic reactions. By adhering to these guidelines, healthcare providers can ensure that patients receive the best possible care and are equipped to manage future anaphylactic episodes effectively.

FURTHER READING

1. Lieberman P, Nicklas RA, Randolph C, Oppenheimer J, Bernstein D, Bernstein J, et al; World Allergy Organization. Anaphylaxis—a practice parameter update 2015. Ann Allergy Asthma Immunol. 2015;115(5):341-84.
2. Muraro A, Roberts G, Worm M, Bilò MB, Brockow K, Fernández Rivas M, et al. Anaphylaxis: guidelines from the

European Academy of Allergy and Clinical Immunology. Allergy. 2014;69(8):1026-45.
3. Sicherer SH, Simons FE. Section on Allergy and Immunology. Epinephrine for first-aid management of anaphylaxis. Pediatrics. 2017;139(3):e20164006.
4. Simons FE, Ardusso LR, Bilò MB, El-Gamal YM, Ledford DK, Ring J, et al; World Allergy Organization. World Allergy Organization anaphylaxis guidelines: summary. J Allergy Clin Immunol. 2011;127(3):587-93. e1-22.
5. Turner PJ, Jerschow E, Umasunthar T, Lin R, Campbell DE, Boyle RJ. Fatal anaphylaxis: mortality rate and risk factors. J Allergy Clin Immunol Pract. 2017;5(5):1164-70.

CHAPTER 9

Emergency Management of the Pediatric Patient with Convulsive Status Epilepticus

INTRODUCTION

Convulsive status epilepticus (CSE) is a critical medical emergency characterized by prolonged or repeated convulsive seizures without regaining consciousness between episodes. This chapter outlines a comprehensive approach to the emergency management of CSE in pediatric patients, highlighting the importance of timely intervention, accurate diagnosis, and effective treatment strategies.

UNDERSTANDING CONVULSIVE STATUS EPILEPTICUS

Definition and Epidemiology

Convulsive status epilepticus is defined as continuous generalized tonic-clonic seizure activity with loss of consciousness, lasting longer than 30 minutes, or two or more discrete seizures without a return to baseline mental status. Early or impending status epilepticus refers to seizures, lasting longer than 5 minutes without full recovery of consciousness between them. Prompt treatment is crucial, as delays increase morbidity and mortality.

The incidence of CSE in children ranges from 10 to 73 episodes per 100,000 children annually, with the highest rates observed in children under 2 years old. Mortality rates are between 2.7 and 8%, while morbidity, including neurological deficits and cognitive impairment, affects 10–20% of cases.

Common Etiologies

The causes of CSE can be broadly categorized into acute symptomatic, remote symptomatic, and idiopathic or cryptogenic origins. Common acute causes include central nervous system (CNS) infections (e.g., meningitis and encephalitis), metabolic derangements (e.g., hypoglycemia and hyponatremia), traumatic injury, and drug-related issues (e.g., antiepileptic drug noncompliance or overdose). Remote causes include cerebral dysgenesis, perinatal hypoxic-ischemic encephalopathy, and prior brain injuries. Idiopathic causes remain unknown despite extensive investigation.

EMERGENCY MANAGEMENT PROTOCOLS (FLOWCHART 1)

Initial Assessment and Stabilization

The primary objectives in managing CSE are maintaining airway, breathing, and circulation (ABC), terminating the seizure, and addressing the underlying cause.

Airway Management

- *Positioning:* Place the child on their side to prevent aspiration and suction any accessible secretions. Avoid prying the mouth open.
- *Airway support:* Administer 100% oxygen by face mask. If respiratory depression or low oxygen saturation persists, consider assisted ventilation or intubation.

Flowchart 1: Management of convulsing child.

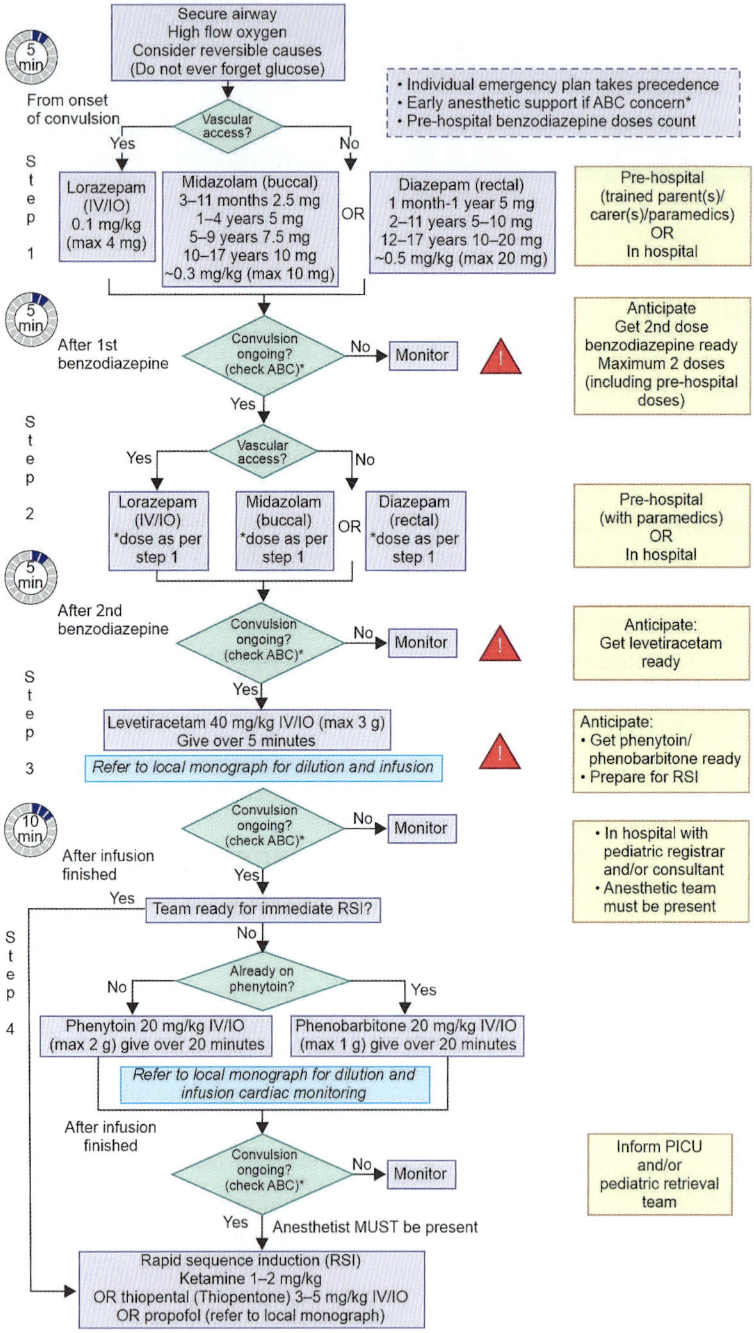

(ABC: airway, breathing, and circulation; IO: intraosseous; IV: intravenous; PICU: pediatric intensive care unit)
Source: Adapted from NEW Advanced Paediatric Life Support (APLS) algorithm on management of the convulsing child 2021. https://www.clinicalguidelines.scot.nhs.uk/nhsggc-guidelines/nhsggc-guidelines/emergency-medicine/status-epilepticus-management/.

- *Monitoring:* Use cardiorespiratory and oxygen saturation monitors continuously. Intravenous (IV) access should be established promptly.

Circulatory Support

Vital signs: Monitor heart rate and blood pressure (BP). Increased heart rate and BP are common during convulsions but should normalize postseizure. Bradycardia, hypotension, and poor perfusion are critical signs, requiring immediate intervention.

Blood Glucose

Hypoglycemia management: Measure bedside blood glucose. If ≤2.6 mmol/L, administer a dextrose bolus (0.5 g/kg). Recheck glucose levels 3–5 minutes postbolus and repeat if necessary.

SEIZURE TERMINATION

First-line Treatment

Benzodiazepines are the first-line treatment for CSE. Administer these medications promptly, regardless of IV access status.

- *Prehospital:* Options include intramuscular (IM), intranasal, or buccal midazolam; buccal lorazepam; or rectal diazepam. Midazolam is preferred for its efficacy and ease of administration.
- *In-hospital:* IV lorazepam or midazolam are equally effective. If IV access is delayed, use buccal, nasal, or IM routes.

If seizures persist after two doses of benzodiazepines, initiate second-line medications.

Second-line Treatment (Table 1)

Second-line medications include fosphenytoin, phenytoin, levetiracetam, and valproate.

- *Fosphenytoin/phenytoin:* It is effective in 50–80% of cases but requires monitoring for cardiac arrhythmias and hypotension.
- *Levetiracetam*: It has similar efficacy with fewer respiratory and cardiovascular side effects. It is useful in children with respiratory depression or hemodynamic compromise.
- *Valproate:* It is effective but requires caution in patients with liver disease or suspected mitochondrial disorders.

TABLE 1: Anticonvulsant drug therapies for CSE.

Drug	*Route*	*Dose*	*Max*	*Repeat/risks/comments*
Midazolam	IV, IO	0.1 mg/kg	5 mg	May repeat once after 5 minutes, if still seizing hypotension, respiratory depression, and sedation
	IM	0.2 mg/kg	10 mg	
	Buccal	0.5 mg/kg	10 mg	
	Intranasal	0.2 mg/kg	10 mg (5 mg per nostril)	
Lorazepam	IV, IO, buccal	0.1 mg/kg	4 mg	• Hypotension, respiratory depression, and sedation • Use sublingual tablets for buccal route
Diazepam	IV, IO	0.3 mg/kg	• 5 mg (<5 years) 10 mg • (≥5 years)	Hypotension, respiratory depression, and sedation
	PR	0.5 mg/kg	20 mg	

(CSE: convulsive status epilepticus; IO: intraosseous; IM: intramuscular; IV: intravenous; PR: per rectum)

Refractory Status Epilepticus (RSE)

If seizures persist despite first- and second-line treatments, consider RSE. Management may involve continuous midazolam infusion, pentobarbital, high-dose phenobarbital, or propofol. These require intensive care unit (ICU) management due to significant risks, including respiratory suppression and hypotension.

DIAGNOSTIC APPROACH

Initial Investigations

Perform investigations based on clinical presentation and history.

- *Blood tests:* Electrolytes, glucose, complete blood count, cultures (if sepsis is suspected), and blood gas analysis
- *Anticonvulsant levels:* Measure levels in patients on long-term anticonvulsant therapy.
- *Toxicology screening:* Urine and blood tests for potential toxins
- *Additional tests:* Serum calcium, blood urea nitrogen, magnesium, liver enzymes, lactate, and ammonia as indicated.

Imaging and Lumbar Puncture

- *Head CT scan:* It is indicated for trauma history, increased intracranial pressure (ICP), focal neurological signs, or unexplained loss of consciousness.
- *Magnetic resonance imaging (MRI):* It is considered when CT is inconclusive or for detailed brain imaging.
- *Lumbar puncture:* It is deferred until stable vitals and seizure cessation. Perform if CNS infection is suspected.

Management of Specific Conditions

Hypoglycemia

Administer dextrose bolus and recheck glucose levels, repeating as necessary.

Central Nervous System Infections

Administer IV antibiotics and antivirals urgently without delaying for culture results.

Raised Intracranial Pressure

Treat clinical signs of raised ICP or herniation immediately. Defer lumbar puncture in such cases.

Intoxication

Consider activated charcoal administration postseizure, if intoxication is suspected.

Nonconvulsive Status Epilepticus

If consciousness does not return postseizure or with neuromuscular paralysis, perform an electroencephalogram (EEG) to exclude non-CSE. Consult neurology for empirical treatment, if EEG is unavailable.

CONCLUSION

Effective management of CSE involves prompt assessment and stabilization, timely administration of appropriate medications, and thorough investigation to address underlying causes. Adhering to evidence-based protocols ensures better outcomes and minimizes the risk of long-term complications. All healthcare professionals involved in pediatric emergency care must be equipped with the knowledge and skills to manage CSE effectively.

FURTHER READING

1. Appleton R, Choonara I, Martland T, Phillips B, Scott R, Whitehouse W. The treatment of convulsive status epilepticus in children. The Status Epilepticus Working Party, Members of the Status Epilepticus Working Party. Arch Dis Child. 2000;83(5):415-9.
2. Friedman JN; Canadian Paediatric Society, Acute Care Committee. Emergency management of the paediatric patient with generalized

convulsive status epilepticus. Paediatr Child Health. 2011;16(2):91-104.

3. Gaínza-Lein M, Fernandez IS, Jackson M, Abend NS, Arya R, Brenton JN, et al. Association of time to treatment with short-term outcomes for pediatric patients with refractory convulsive status epilepticus. JAMA Neurol. 2018;75(4):410-8.
4. Kälviäinen R. Status epilepticus treatment guidelines. Epilepsia. 2007;48(Suppl 8): 99-102.
5. Riviello JJ, Ashwal S, Hirtz D, Glauser T, Ballaban-Gil K, Kelley K, et al.; American Academy of Neurology Subcommittee; Practice Committee of the Child Neurology Society. Practice parameter: Diagnostic assessment of the child with status epilepticus (an evidence-based review); Report of the Quality Standards Subcommittee of the American Academy of Neurology and the Practice Committee of the Child Neurology Society. Neurology. 2006;67(9):1542-50.
6. Singh RK, Gaillard WD. Status epilepticus in children. Curr Neurol Neurosci Rep. 2009;9(2):137-44.
7. Sofou K, Kristjánsdóttir R, Papachatzakis NE, Ahmadzadeh A, Uvebrant P. Management of prolonged seizures and status epilepticus in childhood: A systematic review. J Child Neurol. 2009;24(8):918-26.
8. Yoong M, Chin RF, Scott RC. Management of convulsive status epilepticus in children. Arch Dis Child Educ Pract Ed. 2009;94(1):1-9.

CHAPTER 10

Management of Mild Head Injury in Children

INTRODUCTION

Mild head injuries in children are a common occurrence and can range from minor bumps and bruises to more concerning symptoms. Proper management is crucial to ensure that serious conditions such as intracranial hemorrhage are not overlooked. The Pediatric Emergency Care Applied Research Network (PECARN) has developed guidelines to help clinicians determine when imaging, specifically computed tomography (CT) scans, is necessary and when observation is appropriate. This chapter will explore the PECARN guidelines and their application in the management of mild head injuries in children.

UNDERSTANDING MILD HEAD INJURY

Definition and Epidemiology

A mild head injury, often referred to as a concussion or minor traumatic brain injury (mTBI), is typically defined by a Glasgow Coma Scale (GCS) score of 13–15, brief or no loss of consciousness, and no focal neurological deficits. It is estimated that over half a million children visit emergency departments annually in the United States due to head injuries. Although most of these injuries are mild, a small percentage may lead to significant complications.

Symptoms of Mild Head Injury

Common symptoms include:

- Headache
- Nausea or vomiting
- Dizziness or balance problems
- Sensitivity to light or noise
- Irritability or behavioral changes
- Difficulty concentrating or remembering

Initial Assessment

The initial assessment of a child with a head injury involves a thorough history and physical examination. Key elements include:

- Mechanism of injury
- Loss of consciousness (duration and timing)
- Seizures postinjury
- Vomiting (frequency and timing)
- Amnesia or confusion
- Physical signs of trauma, such as scalp hematoma, especially in infants

PECARN GUIDELINES (FLOWCHARTS 1A AND B)

Overview

The PECARN guidelines provide a decision-making framework to identify children at low risk of clinically important traumatic brain injuries (ciTBI), who may not need a CT scan. This minimizes radiation exposure while ensuring high-risk children receive appropriate care.

Age-based Criteria

The PECARN provides separate criteria for two age groups: Children younger than

Flowcharts 1A and B: PECARN CT algorithm.

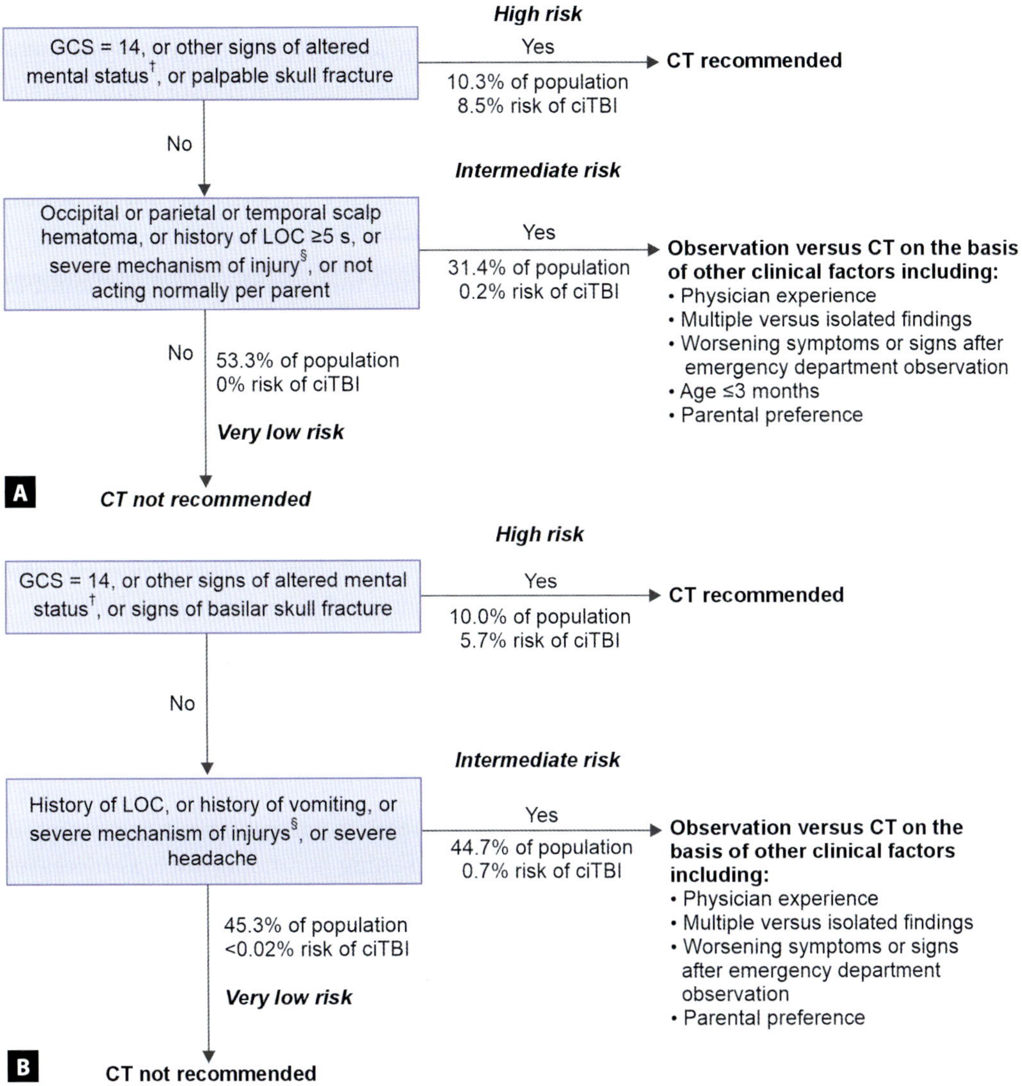

Note: PECARN CT algorithm for children younger than 2 years (A) and those aged 2 years and above (B).

†Signs of altered mental status: Agitation, somnolence, repetitive questioning, or slow response to verbal communication.

§Severe mechanism of injury: Motor vehicle collision with patient ejection, death of another passenger, or rollover; pedestrian or bicyclist without helmet struck by motorized vehicle; falls of >0.9 m (or >1.5 m for B); or head struck by high-impact object.

(ciTBI: clinically important traumatic brain injury; CT: computed tomography; GCS: Glasgow Coma Scale; LOC: loss of consciousness; PECARN: Pediatric Emergency Care Applied Research Network)

Source: Adapted from Bressan S, Eapen N, Phillips N, Gilhotra Y, Kochar A, Dalton S, et al.; Paediatric Research in Emergency Departments International Collaborative (PREDICT). PECARN algorithms for minor head trauma: Risk stratification estimates from a prospective PREDICT cohort study. Acad Emerg Med. 2021;28:1124-33.

2 years and those aged 2 years and older. This distinction is crucial due to differences in anatomy, physiology, and injury mechanisms.

Children Younger than 2 Years

For children under 2, the following factors are considered:

- Normal mental status
- No scalp hematoma (except frontal)
- No loss of consciousness or loss of consciousness less than 5 seconds
- Nonsevere mechanism of injury
- No palpable skull fracture
- Acting normally according to parents

If all these criteria are met, the risk of ciTBI is very low, and observation is typically sufficient. If any criteria are not met, the decision to perform a CT scan depends on clinical judgment, considering factors such as the severity of symptoms and parental concern.

Children Aged 2 Years and Older

For children aged 2 years and older, the guidelines consider:

- Normal mental status
- No loss of consciousness
- No vomiting
- Nonsevere mechanism of injury
- No signs of basilar skull fracture
- No severe headache

Meeting all these criteria suggests a low risk of ciTBI. If any criteria are not met, further evaluation, including possible CT imaging, should be considered based on clinical judgment.

MANAGEMENT STRATEGIES

Observation versus Imaging

The decision to observe or perform a CT scan is influenced by the PECARN criteria. Observation may be appropriate in the following scenarios:

- The child meets all PECARN criteria for low risk.
- There is reliable follow-up available, either through outpatient visits or reliable parents who can monitor the child at home.
- The child can be closely observed in the emergency department for a period, typically 4–6 hours.

Computed tomography imaging should be considered when:

- The child does not meet PECARN low-risk criteria.
- There are symptoms suggestive of more serious injury, such as prolonged loss of consciousness, worsening headache, or repeated vomiting.
- There are physical signs of possible skull fracture or focal neurological deficits.

FOLLOW-UP CARE

Follow-up care is essential in the management of mild head injuries. Key components include:

- Educating parents about symptoms of worsening condition, such as increased drowsiness, persistent vomiting, severe headache, or confusion
- Providing written discharge instructions
- Scheduling a follow-up visit within 24–48 hours
- Advising on gradual return to normal activities, including school and sports, following a stepwise approach

Return to Play

Returning to play or physical activity should be carefully managed to prevent complications such as second-impact syndrome. The following steps are recommended:

- Complete physical and cognitive rest until symptoms resolve

- Gradual return to activity, beginning with light aerobic exercise
- Incremental increase in activity intensity, ensuring no return of symptoms at each step
- Clearance by a healthcare professional before full return to play

CONCLUSION

The management of mild head injuries in children requires a careful balance between avoiding unnecessary radiation exposure and identifying serious injuries. The PECARN guidelines provide a valuable tool for clinicians to assess the risk of ciTBI and make informed decisions about imaging and observation. Through a thorough assessment, appropriate use of CT scans, and diligent follow-up care, healthcare providers can ensure the best outcomes for children with mild head injuries.

FURTHER READING

1. Atabaki SM, Stiell IG, Bazarian JJ, Sadow KE, Vu TT, Camarca MA, et al. A clinical decision rule for cranial computed tomography in minor pediatric head trauma. Arch Pediatr Adolesc Med. 2008;162(5):439-45.
2. Dayan PS, Holmes JF, Atabaki SM, Hoyle JD, Tunik MG, Lichenstein R, et al. Association of traumatic brain injuries with vomiting in children with blunt head trauma. Ann Emerg Med. 2014;63(6):657-65.
3. Greenes DS, Schutzman SA. Clinical indicators of intracranial injury in head-injured infants. Pediatrics. 1999;104(4):861-7.
4. Kuppermann N, Holmes JF, Dayan PS, Hoyle JD, Atabaki SM, Holubkov R, et al.; PECARN Head Injury Study Group. Identification of children at very low risk of clinically-important brain injuries after head trauma: a prospective cohort study. Lancet. 2009;374(9696):1160-70.
5. Lyttle MD, Crowe L, Oakley E, Babl FE, Anderson V, Hearps SJ, et al.; Pediatric Emergency Research in the UK and Ireland (PERUKI) network. Validation of a decision rule for identifying children at low risk of brain injuries after head trauma: a multicentre observational study. Lancet Child Adolesc Health. 2018;2(5):304-13.
6. Nigrovic LE, Schunk JE, Foerster A, Hoyle JD, Dayan PS, Atabaki SM, et al. The effect of observation on cranial computed tomography utilization for children after blunt head trauma. Pediatrics. 2011;127(6):1067-73.
7. Osmond MH, Klassen TP, Wells GA, Correll R, Jarvis A, Joubert G, et al.; Pediatric Emergency Research Canada (PERC). CATCH: a clinical decision rule for the use of computed tomography in children with minor head injury. CMAJ. 2010;182(4):341-8.
8. Schutzman SA, Barnes P, Duhaime AC, Greenes DS, Homer CJ, Jaffe D. Evaluation and management of children younger than two years old with apparently minor head trauma: proposed guidelines. Pediatrics. 2001;107(5):983-93.

CHAPTER 11

Emergency Department Approach to Nontraumatic Headache in Children

INTRODUCTION

Headache is a prevalent neurological complaint among children and a common reason for visits to the emergency department (ED). While most headaches in children are benign, they can sometimes signal serious underlying conditions. Effective management requires a thorough evaluation to differentiate between primary and secondary headaches and to identify any potential life-threatening causes. This chapter will discuss the classification, causes, evaluation, and management of headaches in children, providing a comprehensive approach for healthcare providers.

EPIDEMIOLOGY

Headaches are increasingly common in the pediatric population, with a rising prevalence and increasing ED visits and hospitalizations. Nontraumatic headaches account for approximately 2.5% of pediatric ED visits. Children often present to the ED with severe headaches or those unresponsive to over-the-counter medications.

CLASSIFICATION

Headaches in children can be classified into two main categories:

1. *Primary headaches:* These include migraines, tension-type headaches, and cluster headaches, which comprise 90% of pediatric headaches.
2. *Secondary headaches:* These are due to identifiable underlying conditions, such as infections, brain tumors, intracranial hemorrhage, or severe hypertension. Though most secondary headaches in children are benign, identifying serious causes is crucial.

Common Primary Headaches

- *Migraine:*
    - *Location:* Typically bilateral in young children; becomes unilateral in 60–70% of adolescents and young adults
    - *Characteristics:* Gradual onset, throbbing pain, moderate to severe intensity, and aggravated by physical activity
    - *Duration:* 2–72 hours.
    - *Associated symptoms:* Nausea, vomiting, photophobia, phonophobia, and sometimes aura (visual or sensory disturbances).
- *Tension-type headache:*
    - *Location:* Bilateral
    - *Characteristics:* Pressure or tightness that waxes and wanes
    - *Duration:* Variable
    - *Associated symptoms:* Generally, none, but may include slight discomfort
- *Cluster headache:*
    - *Location:* Always unilateral, usually around the eye or temple
    - *Characteristics:* Rapid onset, severe and explosive pain

- *Duration:* 30 minutes to 3 hours
- *Associated symptoms:* Ipsilateral lacrimation, eye redness, stuffy nose, rhinorrhea, pallor, sweating, and Horner syndrome.

Life-threatening Conditions

- *Infections:*
  - Bacterial meningitis: It presents with fever, neck stiffness, altered mental status, and headache. Early diagnosis and treatment are critical.
  - Viral encephalitis: It is characterized by fever, headache, altered sensorium, and potential focal neurological signs.
- *Brain tumors:*
  - Present with progressive headaches, often worsening in the morning or causing nocturnal awakenings. Associated symptoms include vomiting, visual disturbances, and ataxia.
- *Intracranial hemorrhage:*
  - Sudden onset of severe headache, often described as a "thunderclap" headache. May present with focal neurological signs or altered mental status
- *Acute obstructive hydrocephalus:*
  - Characterized by a sudden increase in intracranial pressure, causing headache, vomiting, lethargy, and signs of brain herniation.

EVALUATION (FLOWCHART 1)

History and Physical Examination

- *Age of onset:* Headaches in children under age 6 years are more likely due to underlying conditions.
- *Headache characteristics:* Mode of onset, duration, severity, location, and associated symptoms help in diagnosing the type and cause of headache.
- *Associated symptoms:* Fever, neck stiffness, vomiting, visual disturbances, and behavioral changes may suggest specific diagnoses.

Neuroimaging

Indicated for children with red-flag findings such as focal neurological deficits, signs of increased intracranial pressure, or "thunderclap" headache. Magnetic resonance imaging (MRI) is preferred due to the lack of radiation, but computed tomography (CT) is used when MRI is unavailable or in unstable patients.

Lumbar Puncture

Necessary in cases of suspected meningitis, encephalitis, or subarachnoid hemorrhage, and to measure opening pressure for idiopathic intracranial hypertension.

MANAGEMENT

Primary Headaches

- *Migraines:* Treated with analgesics (acetaminophen and ibuprofen), antiemetics for nausea, and triptans for severe cases. Lifestyle modifications, such as regular sleep, hydration, and avoiding triggers, are recommended.
- *Tension-type headaches:* Managed with stress reduction techniques, analgesics, and addressing underlying causes such as oromandibular dysfunction.
- *Cluster headaches:* Acute management with oxygen therapy and triptans. Preventive treatment includes verapamil and corticosteroids.

Secondary Headaches

- *Infections:* Prompt antibiotic or antiviral therapy based on the causative pathogen.

Flowchart 1: Pediatric headache approach.

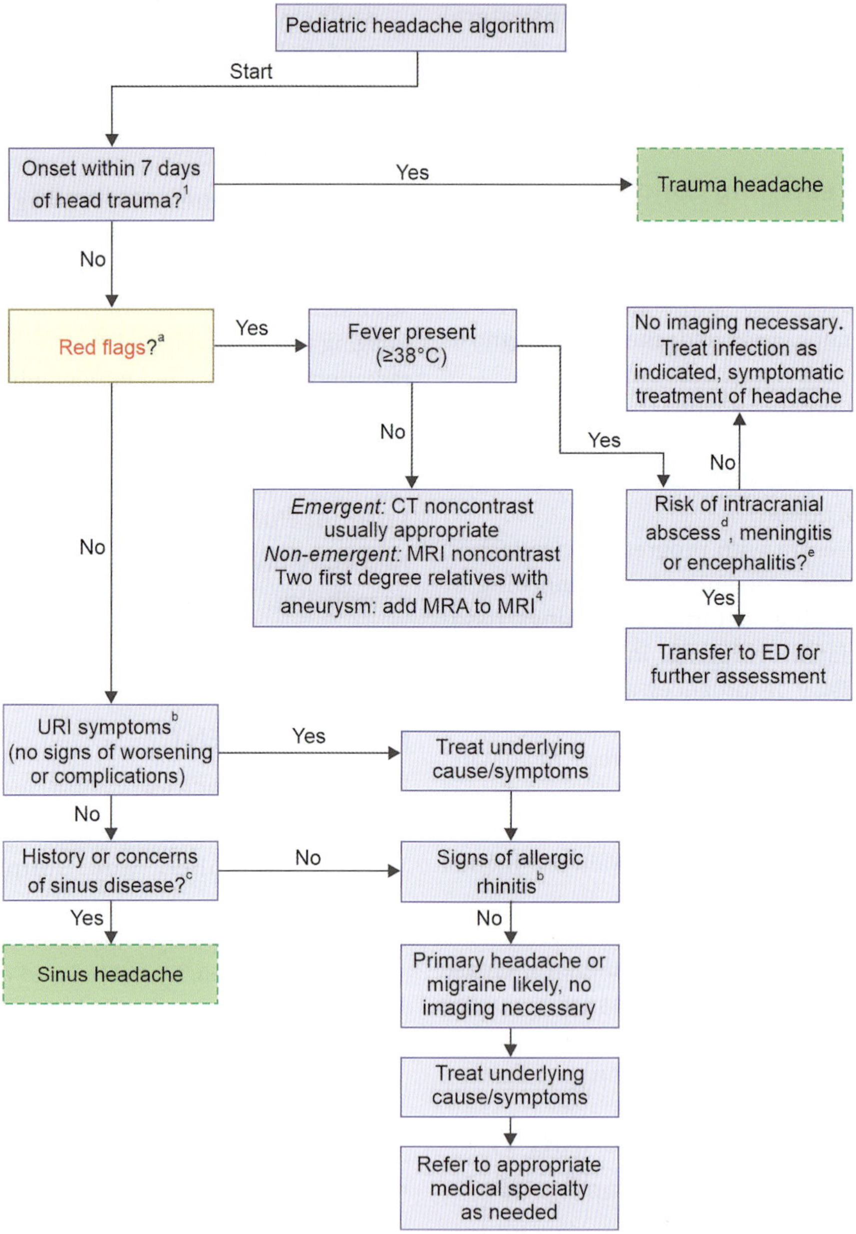

(CT: computed tomography; ED: emergency department; MRA: magnetic resonance angiography; MRI: magnetic resonance imaging)

Source: Adapted from Imaging for Pediatric Headache: Clinical Algorithms to Guide Imaging Decision Making. Developed and contributed by Emory University School of Medicine, Emory University Department of Radiology and Imaging Sciences, and Children's Healthcare of Atlanta (Egleston), Department of Radiology. [online] Available from https://www.acr.org/-/media/ACR/NOINDEX/RSCAN/Combined_PedsHeadache_Algorithms_PDF.pd. [Last accessed August, 2024.]

- *Brain tumors and hydrocephalus:* Require surgical intervention and management by specialists.
- *Intracranial hemorrhage:* Stabilization, neuroimaging, and possibly surgical intervention.

GENERAL RECOMMENDATIONS

- Maintain a headache diary to identify and manage triggers.
- Educate families on the importance of regular follow-ups and adherence to treatment plans.

FURTHER READING

1. Abu-Arafeh I, Razak S, Sivaraman B, Graham C. Prevalence of headache and migraine in children and adolescents: a systematic review of population-based studies. Dev Med Child Neurol. 2010;52:1088-97.
2. Gelfand AA, Goadsby PJ. Migraine in children: present and future directions. Curr Opin Neurol. 2012;25:289-95.
3. Hershey AD, Powers SW, Vockell AL, LeCates SL, Ellinor PL, Segers A, et al. Coenzyme Q10 deficiency and response to supplementation in pediatric and adolescent migraine. Headache. 2007;47:73-80.
4. Kabbouche MA, Linder SL, Rothner AD. The evaluation and management of headaches in children and adolescents. Semin Pediatr Neurol. 2010;17:93-100.
5. Landgraf MN, von Kries R, Heinen F, Straube A. Self-medication and medication prescribed by the physician in children and adolescents with headache. Cephalalgia. 2012;32:847-55.
6. Lewis DW, Ashwal S, Dahl G, Dorbad D, Hirtz D, Prensky A, et al. Practice parameter: evaluation of children and adolescents with recurrent headaches: report of the Quality Standards Subcommittee of the American Academy of Neurology and the Practice Committee of the Child Neurology Society. Neurology. 2002;59:490-8.
7. Lewis DW. Pediatric migraine. Neurol Clin. 2009;27:481-501.
8. Maytal J, Schechter A, Mahajerin A, Merritt JL. Paediatric headache in the emergency department: presentation, diagnosis, and management. Arch Dis Child. 2020;105:180-7.
9. Silberstein SD. Preventive migraine treatment. Continuum (Minneap Minn). 2015;21:973-89.
10. Unalp A, Dirik E, Kurul S. Clinical and demographic characteristics of pediatric headache: a retrospective review of 630 cases. Turk J Pediatr. 2007;49:145-9.
11. Viswanathan A, Bridges SJ. Evaluation of headache in children. Post TW, UpToDate. Waltham, MA: UpToDate Inc.
12. Winner P, Wasiewski W, Gladstein J, Linder S. Multicenter prospective evaluation of proposed pediatric migraine revisions to the IHS criteria. Headache. 2005;45:902-10.

CHAPTER 12

Excessive Crying in Infants and its Management

INTRODUCTION

Excessive crying in infants, often referred to as colic, presents a significant challenge for parents and healthcare providers. While colic is a benign and self-limited condition that typically resolves by the age of 3–4 months, it can cause considerable distress. Parents may interpret the crying as a sign of illness or an indication of their inadequacy in caregiving. This chapter provides an in-depth look at the definitions, epidemiology, differential diagnosis, clinical features, evaluation, diagnosis, potential sequelae, and management strategies for excessive crying in infants.

DEFINITIONS

Normal patterns of crying: During the first 3 months of life, infants cry more than at any other time. Studies have shown that the average duration of crying during this period ranges from 68 to 133 minutes per day. A comprehensive meta-analysis of 28 studies involving 8,690 infants documented that the mean duration of crying was between 117 and 133 minutes per day during the first 6 weeks, decreasing to 68 minutes per day by 10–12 weeks. However, these averages exhibit wide variability among individual infants.

Colic: Colic is broadly defined for clinical purposes as crying for no apparent reason that lasts for 3 or more hours per day, occurring on 3 or more days per week, in an otherwise healthy infant under 3 months of age. This broad definition accommodates the diverse experiences and thresholds of concern among parents, ultimately shaping their relationship with their child.

EPIDEMIOLOGY

Estimates of the prevalence of colic in infants range from 8 to 40%, influenced by varying diagnostic criteria, study designs, populations, and family perceptions of what constitutes excessive crying. A systematic review of parental diary studies found that colic was documented in 17–25% of infants aged less than 6 weeks, 11% of those aged 8–9 weeks, and 0.6% of those aged 10–12 weeks.

Colic does not appear to differ significantly among males and females, breast- and formula-fed infants, full-term and preterm infants, or first-born and subsequent-born children. However, it seems to be more prevalent in industrialized countries, among White infants, and in regions farther from the equator. There is also an association between colic and various psychosocial factors, such as dissatisfaction in the marital relationship, parental stress, and levels of family stress.

DIFFERENTIAL DIAGNOSIS OF EXCESSIVE CRYING IN INFANTS (FLOWCHART 1)

Effective management of excessive crying requires ruling out identifiable causes. These can be categorized into several conditions:

Flowchart 1: Excessive crying baby.

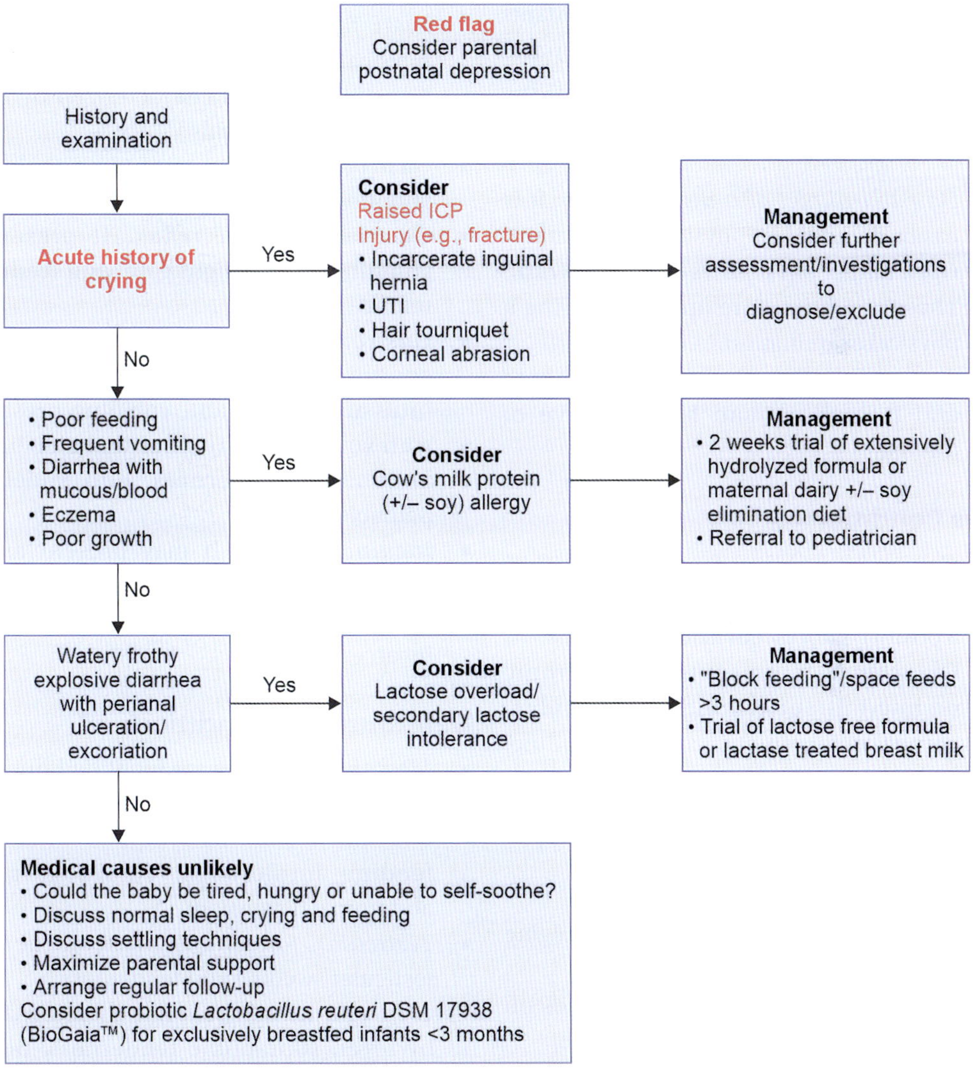

(DSM: Diagnostic and Statistical Manual of Mental Disorders; ICP: increased intracranial pressure; UTI: urinary tract infection)

Source: Adapted from The Royal Children's Hospital Melbourne. (2019). Clinical Practice Guidelines. Unsettled or crying babies. [online] Available from https://www.rch.org.au/clinicalguide/guideline_index/crying_baby_infant_distress/ [Last accessed August, 2024].

General Conditions

- *Drug ingestion or overdose:* History of medication administration, particularly pseudoephedrine, can cause excessive crying.
- *Hunger or inadequate feeding:* Signs of hypovolemia or undernutrition, such as a sunken fontanelle, dry mucous membranes, and decreased subcutaneous fat, may indicate insufficient feeding.

- *Neonatal abstinence syndrome:* This condition should be suspected in infants with a maternal history of prenatal substance use or a positive urine screen.

Skin Conditions

- *Hair tourniquet of a digit or penis:* It is easily identified on physical examination
- *Open diaper pin injuries and diaper rash:* These conditions are apparent during a physical examination.
- *Trauma (abusive or nonabusive):* Bruising and lacerations can be indicative of trauma.

Eye Conditions

- *Corneal abrasions or foreign bodies:* They may cause photophobia, detected through a positive fluorescein examination.
- *Glaucoma:* It presents with chronic or intermittent tearing, photophobia, corneal enlargement, corneal clouding, and optic nerve cupping.

Ear, Nose, and Oropharynx Conditions

- *Otitis media:* It is diagnosed by a bulging tympanic membrane.
- *Thrush:* It presents as white plaques on the buccal mucosa, tongue, or palate.

Cardiovascular Conditions

- *Anomalous origin of the left coronary artery:* It presents with cardiomegaly and heart failure.
- *Heart failure:* Its symptoms include feeding intolerance, tachycardia, poor perfusion, and tachypnea.
- *Supraventricular tachycardia:* It may be indicated by pallor, irritability, poor feeding, and cyanosis.

Gastrointestinal Conditions

- *Anal fissures:* They are apparent on physical examination.
- *Constipation*: It is characterized by the passage of hard stools.
- *Gastroenteritis:* Its symptoms include vomiting and diarrhea.
- *Gastroesophageal reflux:* It presents vomiting, poor weight gain, and feeding refusal.
- *Gastrointestinal obstructions:* Their conditions such as pyloric stenosis, intussusception, and volvulus present with vomiting, gastrointestinal bleeding, abdominal tenderness, and specific palpable masses.
- *Inguinal hernia:* It may present as a bulge in the groin area, with vomiting and abdominal distension indicating incarceration.

Genitourinary Conditions

- *Meatal ulcers:* They are identified during examination.
- *Ovarian torsion:* Its symptoms include feeding intolerance, vomiting, and abdominal distension.
- *Testicular torsion:* It presents acute testicular swelling and tenderness.
- *Urinary tract infection:* It is characterized by fever, suprapubic tenderness, poor feeding, and poor weight gain.
- *Urinary tract obstruction:* Its symptoms include abdominal distension, difficulty voiding, and poor urinary stream.

Skeletal Conditions

- *Fractures:* They present with decreased movement of the extremity, localized swelling, and increased pain response.
- *Osteomyelitis or septic arthritis:* Its symptoms include fever, decreased

movement of the extremity, and increased pain response with movement.

Neurologic Conditions

- *Abusive head trauma:* Its symptoms include seizures, respiratory difficulty, and retinal hemorrhages.
- *Meningitis:* It is characterized by fever, bulging fontanelle, and irritability.
- *Neuromuscular diseases, CNS disorders, and metabolic diseases:* They present with abnormal muscle tone and weakness.

CLINICAL FEATURES

Colic is distinguished by paroxysms of crying that start and stop without an obvious cause. The crying is typically louder, higher in pitch, and more turbulent than normal crying. Physical signs such as facial flushing, tense abdomen, and hypertonia are common. Infants with colic are often difficult to console, regardless of the parents' efforts.

EVALUATION

The evaluation for colic includes a thorough history and physical examination to identify potential causes of excessive crying. Laboratory and imaging studies are generally unnecessary unless specific indicators suggest otherwise.

History: Important aspects of the history include the infant's feeding, stooling, urination, and sleeping patterns, prenatal and perinatal history, and psychosocial factors. Specific questions about the timing, duration, and nature of the crying, as well as parental responses, provide valuable insights.

Examination: The physical examination should focus on observing the infant during a crying episode, assessing temperament and responsiveness, and checking for growth deviations. It also involves a thorough assessment of conditions that can cause prolonged crying.

DIAGNOSIS

A presumptive diagnosis of infantile colic is made in an otherwise healthy infant under 3 months of age who cries for at least 3 hours per day on 3 or more days per week, with other causes excluded by history and examination.

POTENTIAL SEQUELAE

While colic is not harmful to the infant in the short or long term, it can lead to serious consequences such as physical abuse, postpartum depression, and early cessation of breastfeeding. Observational studies suggest a significant impact on maternal mental health and breastfeeding practices.

MANAGEMENT

Caregiver support and education: Educating and supporting caregivers are crucial. Parents need reassurance that colic is a temporary and benign condition. Healthcare providers should emphasize the importance of self-care and taking breaks when necessary. Support groups or counseling may be beneficial for parents experiencing high levels of stress or anxiety.

Soothing techniques: Various soothing techniques can help reduce crying episodes:

- *Swaddling:* Wrapping the infant snugly in a blanket to provide a sense of security.
- *Side or stomach position:* Holding the baby on their side or stomach while awake.
- *Shushing sounds:* Creating white noise or using a fan to mimic the sounds of the womb.
- *Swinging:* Gently rocking the baby in a rhythmic motion.
- *Sucking:* Allowing the infant to suck on a pacifier or their thumb.

Feeding techniques: Modifications in feeding practices can help alleviate colic symptoms:

- *Frequent, smaller feedings:* To prevent overfeeding and reduce the likelihood of gas.
- *Upright positioning:* Keeping the baby upright during and after feeding to minimize reflux.
- *Burping:* Regularly burping the baby during and after feedings to expel swallowed air.

Dietary modifications: For breastfeeding mothers, eliminating certain foods from their diet, such as dairy, caffeine, and spicy foods, may reduce colic symptoms. For formula-fed infants, switching to a hypoallergenic formula might be beneficial.

Probiotics: Some studies suggest that probiotics, particularly *Lactobacillus reuteri*, may help reduce crying time in infants with colic. However, further research is needed to confirm their efficacy and safety.

Medical interventions: In rare cases, medical interventions may be necessary:

- *Simethicone drops*: These can help reduce gas and bloating.
- *Proton pump inhibitors (PPIs) or H_2-blockers:* They are used to treat gastroesophageal reflux disease (GERD) if it is contributing to colic symptoms.

CONCLUSION

Excessive crying in infants, or colic, presents a significant challenge in pediatric care, impacting both infant well-being and family dynamics. While typically benign and self-limiting, its management requires a comprehensive approach. This chapter has emphasized the importance of thorough differential diagnosis, highlighting the wide range of potential underlying causes and the critical role of detailed history-taking and physical examination. The multifaceted management strategy encompasses caregiver support and education, various soothing techniques, feeding modifications, and in some cases, dietary changes or probiotic use. Healthcare providers play a crucial role in ensuring infant safety, providing reassurance, and offering practical coping strategies to prevent potential long-term consequences such as physical abuse or postpartum depression. Ultimately, understanding colic as a developmental phase rather than a disease helps frame our interventions and guides our support for affected families through this challenging period.

FURTHER READING

1. St. James-Roberts I. Persistent infant crying. Arch Dis Child. 1991;66(5):653-5.
2. Sung V, St James-Roberts I. Infant colic. In Pediatric Neurogastroenterology: Gastrointestinal Motility and Functional Disorders in Children, 2nd edition, Springer International Publishing, 2017 Faure C, Thapar N, Di Lorenzo C (Eds). pp. 369-79.
3. Wessel MA, Cobb JC, Jackson EB, Harris Jr GS, Detwiler AC. Paroxysmal fussing in infancy, sometimes called colic. Pediatrics. 1954;14(5):421-35.
4. Wolke D, Bilgin A, Samara M. Systematic review and meta-analysis: Fussing and crying durations and prevalence of colic in infants. J Pediatr. 2017;185:55-61.
5. Zeevenhooven J, Koppen IJN, Benninga MA. The New Rome IV Criteria for Functional Gastrointestinal Disorders in Infants and Toddlers. Pediatric Gastroenterology, Hepatology & Nutrition. 2017;20(1):1-13.

CHAPTER 13

Management of a Febrile Infants below 3 Months of Age

INTRODUCTION

The management of febrile infants younger than 90 days of age is a critical aspect of pediatric care. Infants in this age group are at a higher risk for serious bacterial infections (SBIs), and the approach to their evaluation and treatment requires a careful balance between thoroughness and the avoidance of unnecessary interventions. This chapter outlines current guidelines and best practices for managing febrile infants less than 3 months old, focusing on the identification of invasive bacterial infections (IBIs), such as bacteremia and meningitis.

TERMINOLOGY AND DEFINITIONS

Fever

For infants younger than 3 months, a rectal temperature of ≥38°C (100.4°F) is considered a fever. This method of measurement is preferred due to its accuracy in this age group. Other methods of temperature measurement and caregiver reports of fever are less reliable and should be interpreted with caution.

Invasive Bacterial Infection

Invasive bacterial infection refers to the presence of bacteremia or meningitis. These conditions require prompt identification and treatment to prevent serious outcomes.

Well Appearing

The term "well appearing" refers to infants who do not display signs of severe illness. However, distinguishing between well and ill-appearing infants can be challenging, as their condition may deteriorate rapidly. Clinical guidelines should be adapted if an infant's appearance worsens during evaluation.

MANAGEMENT STRATEGIES

Age Stratification and Risk Assessment

Management of febrile infants is stratified by age and initial ancillary study results to assess the risk for IBI.

Infants 29–60 Days Old (Flowchart 1)

For well-appearing febrile infants in this age group without focal infection, management is guided by the 2021 American Academy of Pediatrics Clinical Practice Guideline (AAP CPG).

- *Increased risk for IBI:*
    - *Evaluation:* Full sepsis workup, including blood, urine, and cerebrospinal fluid (CSF) cultures
    - *Management:* Empiric antibiotics (e.g., ceftriaxone or cefotaxime). CSF should be obtained before antibiotic administration, but treatment should

Flowchart 1: Infants 29 days to 3 months corrected age.

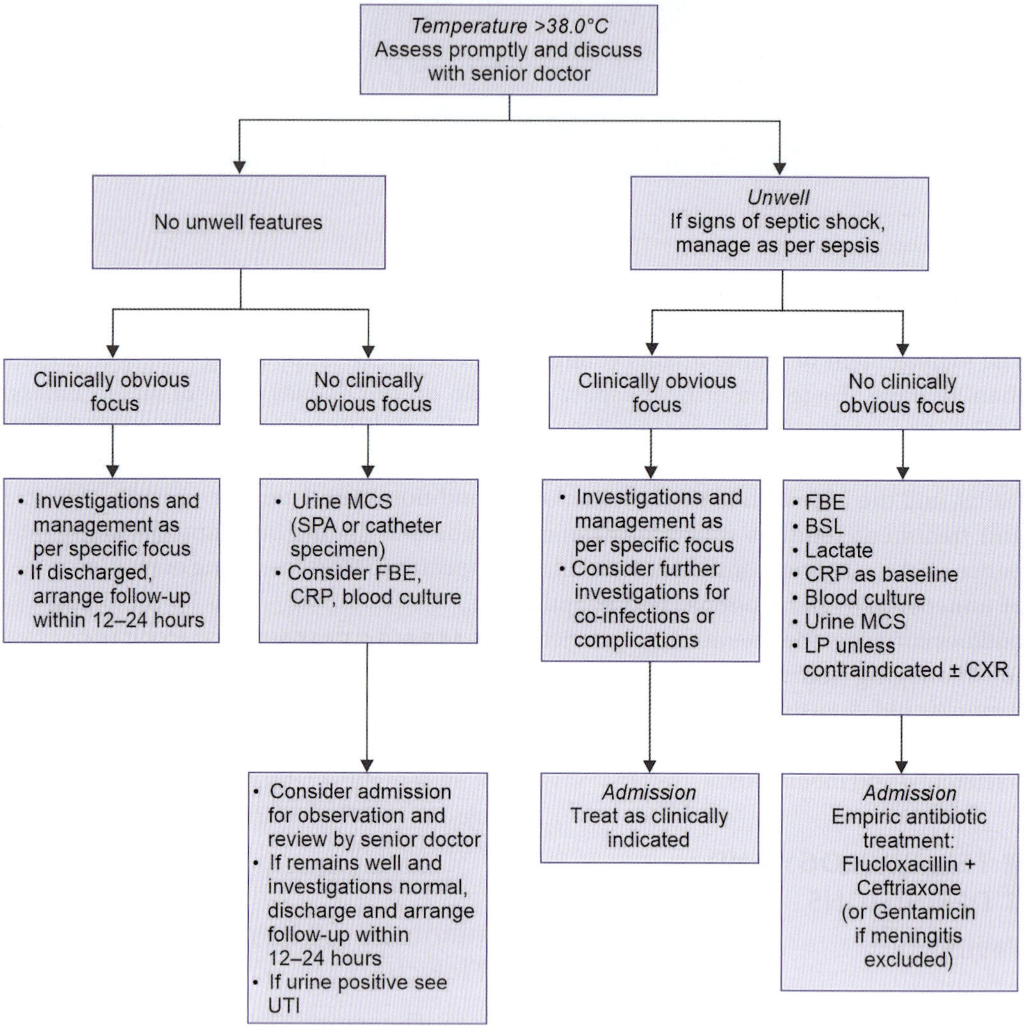

(BSL: blood sugar level; CRP: C-reactive protein; CXR: chest X-ray; FBE: full blood examination; LP: lumbar puncture; MCS: Microscopy, Culture & Sensitivity; SPA: suprapubic aspirate)

Source: Adapted from The Royal Children's Hospital Melbourne. (2022). Clinical Practice Guidelines. Febrile child. [online] Available from https://www.rch.org.au/clinicalguide/guideline_index/Febrile_child/ [Last accessed August, 2024].

not be delayed if lumbar puncture is not immediately possible.

- *Admission:* Infants with significant comorbidities, abnormal inflammatory markers, or signs suggestive of bacterial pneumonia require hospital admission.

- *CSF pleocytosis:*
  - *Treatment:* Empiric treatment for bacterial meningitis and admission. Antiviral therapy with acyclovir is added if there is a history of maternal genital herpes or signs of herpes infection.

- *Suspected urinary tract infection (UTI):*
  - *With risk factors for IBI:* Perform lumbar puncture, start empiric antibiotics, and admit to hospital.
  - *Without risk factors for IBI:* Oral antibiotics and close outpatient follow-up are recommended.

Infants 61–90 Days Old

Management for well-appearing infants in this age group without focal infection varies based on the presence of risk factors for IBI.

- *With risk factors for IBI:*
  - *Evaluation:* Urine testing, blood inflammatory markers, blood culture, and chest radiograph if respiratory symptoms are present.
  - *Management:* Empiric antibiotics and hospital admission if any blood inflammatory markers are abnormal.
- *Without risk factors for IBI:*
  - *Evaluation:* Urine dipstick or urinalysis and urine culture.
  - *Management:* Outpatient observation with close follow-up if initial urine tests are normal. Oral antibiotics if urine tests indicate UTI.

SPECIAL CONSIDERATIONS

Ill-Appearing Infants

Regardless of age, ill-appearing infants with fever are at a higher risk for IBI and other serious conditions such as sepsis and herpes simplex virus (HSV) infection. These infants require immediate and comprehensive evaluation and treatment.

- *Septic shock:* Follow resuscitation guidelines and administer broad-spectrum antibiotics.
- *Other causes of Ill appearance:* Evaluate for congenital heart disease, adrenal hyperplasia, metabolic disorders, and other potential causes.
- *Empiric antimicrobials:* Administer age-appropriate empiric antibiotic regimens. Add acyclovir if HSV infection is suspected.

Viral Infections

Certain viral infections can modify the approach to evaluation and management:

- *Herpes simplex virus:*
  - Febrile infants with signs of HSV infection or maternal history of genital herpes should undergo a full sepsis evaluation, receive empiric acyclovir and antibiotics, and be admitted to the hospital.
- *Respiratory syncytial virus (RSV) and influenza:*
  - Infants with RSV bronchiolitis or influenza have a reduced risk of IBI. They should be managed based on the severity of their viral illness and only require antibiotics if a bacterial infection is also suspected.
- *Coronavirus disease 2019 (COVID-19):*
  - Testing for severe acute respiratory syndrome coronavirus 2 (SARS-CoV-2) is warranted in hospitalized febrile infants to prevent transmission. Management of COVID-19 follows specific pediatric guidelines.

Outpatient Follow-up

For well-appearing infants who are discharged home, follow-up within 24 hours is essential. This visit should include a review of preliminary culture results and an assessment of the infant's clinical status. Any signs of deterioration warrant re-evaluation and possible hospital admission.

Discharge Criteria for Admitted Patients

Early discharge at 24–36 hours may be feasible in hospitals with continuous blood culture monitoring. Criteria for discharge include:

- *Afebrile and well-appearing:* Infants who remain well-appearing and afebrile can be discharged after 36 hours of negative cultures.
- *Febrile but well appearing:* Observation of antibiotics in the hospital is reasonable for infants who remain febrile but clinically improve. Any deterioration warrants further evaluation.

CLINICAL PRACTICE GUIDELINES

The 2021 AAP CPG for the evaluation and management of well-appearing febrile infants 8–60 days of age provides a framework based on evidence and expert consensus. These guidelines help standardize care and improve outcomes by ensuring consistent and thorough evaluation and treatment.

CONCLUSION

The management of febrile infants less than 3 months old requires careful evaluation to identify SBIs while minimizing unnecessary interventions. Adhering to current guidelines ensures that healthcare providers can provide effective and safe care for this vulnerable population. Continuous monitoring, appropriate use of antibiotics, and close follow-up are essential components in achieving positive outcomes for febrile infants.

FURTHER READING

1. American Academy of Pediatrics. Clinical Practice Guidelines for the Management of Febrile Infants. Pediatrics. 2021;148(2): e2021052228.
2. Aronson PL, Thurm C, Williams DJ, Alpern ER, McCulloh R, Nigrovic LE, et al. Association of clinical practice guidelines with emergency department management of febrile infants ≤56 days of age. JAMA Pediatrics. 2018;172(5):e181055.
3. Baskin MN, O'Rourke EJ, Fleisher GR. Outpatient management of febrile infants 28 to 89 days of age with intramuscular ceftriaxone and careful follow-up. Pediatrics. 1992;89(2):619-22.
4. Biondi EA, Byington CL, Goldman RD. Fever and serious bacterial infection in infants younger than 3 months: a systematic review. Arch Dis Child. 2014;99(1):61-7.
5. Cruz AT, Mahajan P. Febrile young infants: making rational choices in the era of shared decision-making. Pediatr Emergency Care. 2019;35(11):807-10.
6. Jain S, Cheng J, Alpern ER, Thurm C, Schroeder L, Black KM, et al. Management of febrile neonates in pediatric emergency departments. Pediatrics. 2014;33(2):187-95.
7. Kuppermann N, Holmes JF, Dayan PS, Hoyle JD, Atabaki SM, Holubkov R, et al.; PECARN Head Injury Study Group. Identification of children at very low risk of clinically-important brain injuries after head trauma: a prospective cohort study. Lancet. 2009;374(9696):1160-70.

CHAPTER 14

Rabies Postexposure Prophylaxis Protocol in India

INTRODUCTION

Rabies is a fatal viral disease that is preventable through prompt postexposure prophylaxis (PEP) after an animal bite. In India, the protocol for rabies PEP includes wound care, rabies immunoglobulin (RIG), and rabies vaccine. Here is a detailed overview.

IMMEDIATE WOUND CARE

- *Washing and cleaning:* The wound should be washed immediately and thoroughly with soap and water for at least 15 minutes. This reduces the viral load at the site of the bite.
- *Antiseptics:* After washing, apply antiseptics such as povidone-iodine or alcohol.

Rabies Immunoglobulin

Types of RIGs: There are two types of RIGs available:

1. Human rabies immunoglobulin (HRIG)
2. Equine rabies immunoglobulin (ERIG).

Administration: RIG should be infiltrated into and around the wound as much as anatomically feasible. The remaining dose, if any, should be administered intramuscularly at a site distant from the site of vaccine administration.

Rabishield (Monoclonal Antibodies)

Rabishield is a monoclonal antibody (mAb) preparation used for rabies PEP as an alternative to traditional RIG. It provides passive immunity by neutralizing the rabies virus at the site of infection.

Composition and Mechanism

- Rabishield consists of human mAbs, specifically targeting the rabies virus glycoprotein, which is essential for viral entry into host cells.
- These antibodies bind to the virus, neutralizing it and preventing infection from spreading.

Advantages over Traditional Rabies Immunoglobulin

- *Safety:* Rabishield is derived from human cells, reducing the risk of allergic reactions and serum sickness compared to ERIG.
- *Availability:* Being a laboratory-produced product, Rabishield offers a more consistent and reliable supply than HRIG, which is limited by donor availability.
- *Efficacy:* Studies have shown that Rabishield is effective in neutralizing the rabies virus and is a suitable alternative to RIG for PEP.

Administration

- Rabishield is administered similarly to RIG. It should be infiltrated into and around the wound site as much as anatomically feasible.

- The remaining dose, if any, should be given intramuscularly at a site distant from the rabies vaccine administration.

Rabies Vaccine

Vaccination Schedule

The vaccines used are either cell culture vaccines or embryonated egg vaccines. The common schedules are:

- *Intramuscular (IM) regimen:*
  - *The Essen regimen:* 0, 3, 7, 14, and 28 days
- *The Zagreb regimen:* 0, 7, and 21 days
- *Intradermal (ID) regimen:* The Updated Thai Red Cross (TRC) regimen: 2-2-2-0-2 on days 0, 3, 7, and 28
- *Site of administration:*
  - *IM:* Deltoid area for adults and anterolateral thigh for children
  - *ID:* Over the deltoid area or the suprascapular region.

Indications for PEP (Flowchart 1)

Category I Exposure

- Touching or feeding animals, licking on intact skin
- *Action:* No PEP required

Category II Exposure

- Nibbling of uncovered skin, minor scratches, or abrasions without bleeding
- *Action:* Immediate vaccination and local treatment of the wound.

Category III Exposure

- Single or multiple transdermal bites or scratches, licks on broken skin, contamination of mucous membrane with saliva (i.e., licks), and exposures to bats.
- *Action:* Immediate use of RIG and vaccination along with local treatment of the wound.

KEY POINTS

- *Timeliness:* PEP should be initiated as soon as possible after exposure.
- *Completion of course:* It is crucial to complete the full course of vaccination for effective protection.
- *Public health measures:* Education about avoiding animal bites and promoting vaccination of pets and stray animals.
- *Availability and access:*
  - Public health facilities: Rabies PEP is often available free of cost at government hospitals and primary health centers.
  - Private healthcare providers: PEP is also available in private hospitals and clinics, although it may be at a cost.

SPECIAL CONSIDERATIONS

- *Pregnancy and immunocompromised individuals:* Rabies PEP is safe and should be administered as per the standard schedule.
- *Follow-up:* Regular follow-up is necessary to ensure the completion of the vaccination schedule and monitor for any adverse reactions.

CONCLUSION

Rabies PEP in India involves a comprehensive approach including wound care, administration of RIG, and a structured vaccination regimen. Public awareness and prompt action are key to preventing rabies, a disease that is almost always fatal once clinical symptoms appear.

PRE-EXPOSURE PROPHYLAXIS

WHO SHOULD RECEIVE PRE-EXPOSURE PROPHYLAXIS (PREP)?

People at high risk of rabies exposure, including:

- Veterinarians and their assistants.
- Animal handlers and trainers.

Flowchart 1: Rabies postexposure prophylaxis guidelines.

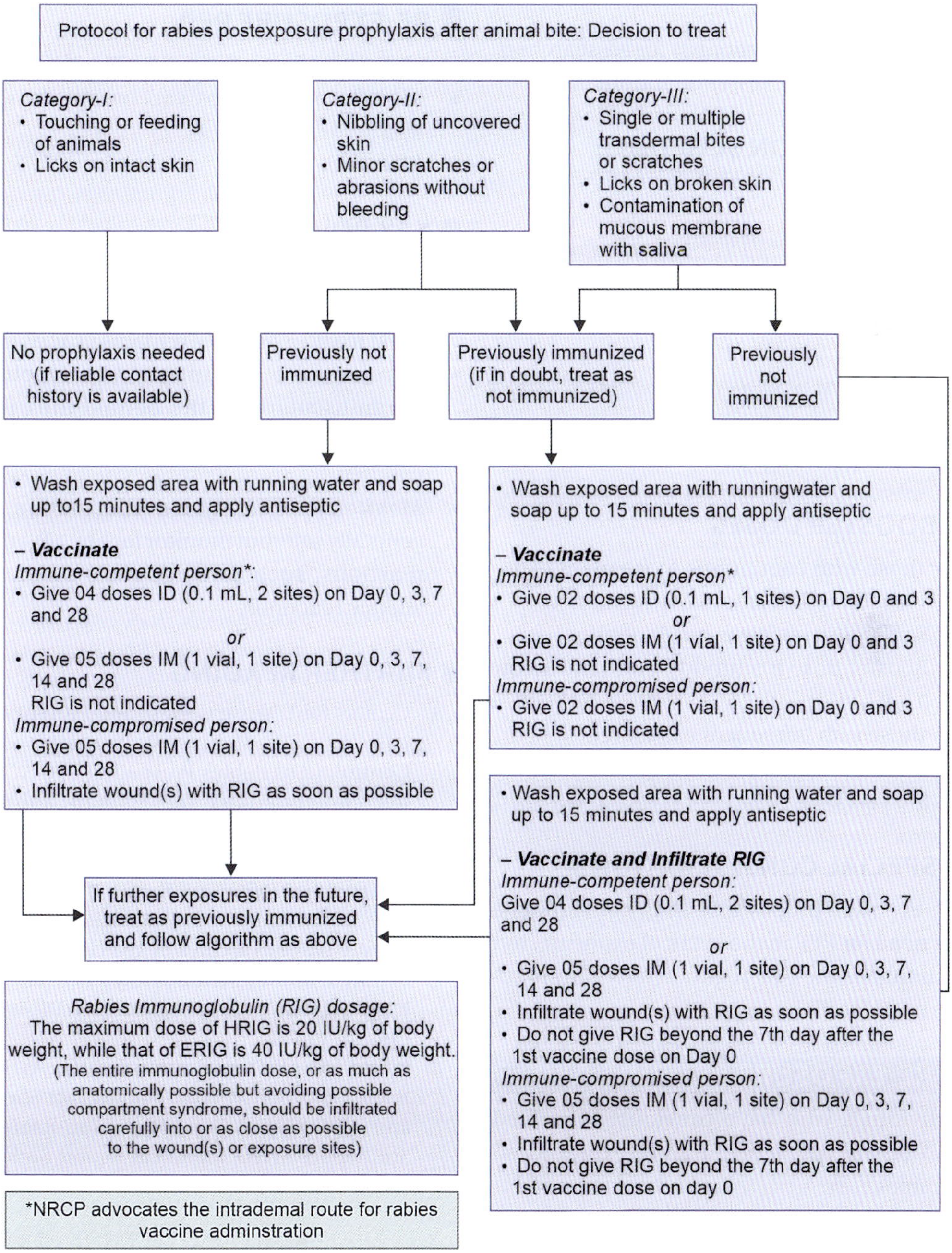

(ERIG: equine rabies immunoglobulin; HRIG: human rabies immunoglobulin; ID: intradermal; IM: intramuscular)

Source: Adapted from National Centre for Disease Control (NCDC). National Guidelines for Rabies Prophylaxis and Intra-dermal Rabies Vaccination. National Rabies Control Programme (NRCP), Government of India.

- Laboratory workers dealing with the rabies virus.
- Wildlife conservationists and researchers.
- Travelers to rabies-endemic areas.

VACCINATION SCHEDULE FOR PREP

- *Intramuscular regimen:*
    - *Days:* 0, 7, and 21 or 28
    - *Site:* Deltoid area in adults and anterolateral thigh in children
- *ID regimen:*
    - *Days:* 0, 7, and 21 or 28
    - *Site:* Over the deltoid area or suprascapular region.

BOOSTER DOSES

For those with continuous or frequent exposure to rabies (e.g., laboratory workers):

- Serological testing every 6 months
- Booster dose if antibody titer falls below 0.5 IU/mL

For those with infrequent exposure:

- Booster dose at 1 year, then every 3-5 years.

SPECIAL CONSIDERATIONS

Pre-exposure prophylaxis does not eliminate the need for PEP in the event of exposure, but it simplifies the PEP regimen and eliminates the need for RIG.

RE-EXPOSURE PROPHYLAXIS

Individuals who have previously received PrEP or a full course of PEP and are re-exposed to rabies.

VACCINATION SCHEDULE FOR RE-EXPOSURE PEP

For those who have received PrEP or full PEP:

- Two doses of rabies vaccine on days 0 and 3
- RIG is not required.

KEY POINTS

- *Wound care:* Immediate and thorough washing of the wound with soap and water for at least 15 minutes remains crucial.
- *Vaccination:* Administer the vaccine intramuscularly in the deltoid area for adults and in the anterolateral thigh for children.
- *Monitor for side effects:* Vaccination is generally safe, but monitor for any adverse reactions, such as fever, local pain, or allergic reactions.

FURTHER READING

1. Centers for Disease Control and Prevention (CDC): CDC Rabies Prevention and Control: CDC Rabies Prevention and ACIP Recommendations for Human Rabies Prevention: CDC MMWR Recommendations and Reports.
2. National Guidelines for Rabies Prophylaxis and Intradermal Administration of Cell Culture Rabies Vaccines by the Government of India: National Guidelines for Rabies Prophylaxis: National Centre for Disease Control, India.
3. World Health Organization (WHO): WHO Rabies Fact Sheet: WHO Rabies Fact Sheet and WHO Expert Consultation on Rabies, 3rd Report. WHO Technical Report Series, No. 1012. 2018.

CHAPTER 15

Management of Foreign Body Ingestion in Children

INTRODUCTION

Foreign body ingestion is a prevalent pediatric emergency, with children between 6 months and 6 years of age being particularly vulnerable due to their exploratory behavior. While most ingested objects traverse the gastrointestinal (GI) tract without incident, certain foreign bodies can cause significant complications, including obstruction, perforation, and infection. The management of foreign body ingestion in children necessitates a prompt, methodical approach encompassing clinical evaluation, diagnostic imaging, and when necessary, therapeutic intervention.

EPIDEMIOLOGY

The incidence of foreign body ingestion is highest in toddlers and young children. Commonly ingested items include coins, small toys, button batteries, magnets, and food items such as nuts and seeds. The risk of complications is contingent upon the object's size, shape, and chemical properties, as well as the anatomical location within the GI tract.

CLINICAL PRESENTATION

Asymptomatic: A significant proportion of children may remain asymptomatic, especially when the ingested object is small and smooth.

Symptomatic: Symptoms are largely dependent on the location of the foreign body and may include:

- *Esophageal:* Drooling, dysphagia, refusal to eat, retrosternal pain, vomiting, choking, or respiratory distress
- *Gastric and intestinal:* Abdominal pain, vomiting, hematemesis, melena, or signs indicative of bowel obstruction such as abdominal distention and constipation.

HISTORY AND EXAMINATION

- A meticulous history taking is imperative, focusing on the type of object ingested, the time of ingestion, any witnessed choking episodes, and the presence of preexisting conditions (e.g., congenital GI anomalies).
- Physical examination should assess for respiratory distress, signs of perforation (e.g., fever and acute abdomen), and GI obstruction.

DIAGNOSIS

Radiologic Evaluation

Plain radiographs: The initial diagnostic tool for radiopaque objects (e.g., coins, batteries, and some toys).

- *Esophageal:* Lateral neck, chest, and abdominal X-rays
- *GI tract:* Abdominal X-rays to monitor the progression of the object through the GI tract

Nonradiopaque objects: For objects not visible on plain radiographs, contrast studies or computed tomography (CT) scans may be employed, particularly if complications are suspected.

Endoscopy

Both diagnostic and therapeutic, endoscopy is indicated for nonradiopaque objects, objects causing symptoms, or those with a high risk of complications (e.g., batteries and sharp objects).

MANAGEMENT

General Principles

- *Airway and breathing:* Ensure that the child's airway is not compromised and provide immediate supportive care if respiratory distress is evident.
- *Monitoring:* Continuous monitoring for signs of complications, such as perforation or obstruction, is essential.

Specific Management

Coins (Table 1)

Esophageal:

- *Asymptomatic and small coins (<2 cm):* Observation for 24 hours is reasonable as spontaneous passage is common.
- *Symptomatic or large coins:* Immediate endoscopic removal is warranted.

Stomach and beyond: Most coins will pass spontaneously. Follow-up X-rays may be performed to confirm passage if symptoms develop.

TABLE 1: Management of coin and blunt object ingestion.

Scenario	*Procedure*
In the esophagus	• *Symptomatic:* Unable to tolerate secretions • Emergent endoscopy
	• *Asymptomatic:* Urgent endoscopy • Radiographs should be taken again before the endoscopy (it may have fallen into the stomach)
In the stomach	• It may be expected to pass • If it is not passed in the stool and if it is not symptomatic, it may be followed up with radiographs at 1–2 weeks intervals/laxative if necessary • Elective endoscopy, if it is not passed out within 2–4 weeks
In the small intestine	Clinical observation/if it becomes symptomatic, endoscopy or surgery

Source: Adapted from Demiroren K. Management of Gastrointestinal Foreign Bodies with Brief Review of the Guidelines. Pediatr Gastroenterol Hepatol Nutr. 2023;26(1):1-14.

Batteries (Table 2)

Esophageal: Immediate endoscopic removal is critical due to the risk of mucosal injury, perforation, and severe complications such as tracheoesophageal fistula.

Stomach and beyond: If asymptomatic and the battery is small (<2 cm), observation with serial X-rays is appropriate. Symptomatic batteries or those not progressing may require endoscopic or surgical removal.

Sharp Objects (Table 3)

Esophageal: Urgent endoscopic removal to prevent perforation.

Gastric and beyond: Observation may be sufficient for small, asymptomatic objects. However, removal is necessary if the object remains in the stomach or complications arise.

Magnets

Single magnet ingestion typically requires monitoring, whereas multiple magnet ingestions pose a high risk for bowel necrosis, perforation, and fistula formation,

TABLE 2: Management of battery ingestion.

Clinical scenario	***Procedure***
Button battery in the esophagus:	
The patient is stable	Emergent endoscopy
The patient is unstable or there is bleeding	Emergent endoscopy by a pediatric surgeon and a cardiovascular surgeon in the operating room
There is a suspicion of aortic injury (in the presence of bleeding, drop in hemoglobin, extensive and deep ulcer)	CT angiography or MRI
After battery removal	Treatment and follow-up in terms of corrosive injury and perforation (if symptomatic, CT/MRI scans)
Button battery in the stomach or below:	
Patient aged <5 years and battery ≥20 mm in size	Endoscopy within 24–48 hours
There is evidence of esophageal injury	Initial evaluation by CT
Patient aged >5 years and battery ≥20 mm in size	Endoscopy within 48 hours
Patient aged >5 years and battery <20 mm in size	Radiographic follow-up/endoscopy if not excreted on days 7–14
Symptomatic and/or there is a known anatomical pathology	Emergent endoscopy
Cylindrical batteries:	
In the esophagus	Urgent endoscopy
In any part of the gastrointestinal tract and symptomatic	Urgent endoscopy
In the stomach or below and asymptomatic	It can be monitored for 7–14 days
Multiple cylindrical batteries in the stomach	Urgent endoscopy

(CT: computed tomography; MRI: magnetic resonance imaging)

Source: Adapted from Demiroren K. Management of Gastrointestinal Foreign Bodies with Brief Review of the Guidelines. Pediatr Gastroenterol Hepatol Nutr. 2023;26(1):1-14.

necessitating urgent endoscopic or surgical intervention.

Food Impaction

It commonly affects the esophagus. If the child is symptomatic (e.g., drooling and dysphagia), endoscopic removal is indicated.

Postremoval Care

- Monitor for complications such as perforation, infection, or bleeding.
- Educate caregivers on preventive measures to avoid future incidents.

COMPLICATIONS

- *Perforation:* It may occur at any site along the GI tract, presenting with severe pain, fever, and signs of peritonitis.
- *Obstruction:* Its symptoms include vomiting, abdominal distention, and failure to pass stool or gas.
- *Infection:* It can arise secondary to perforation or a retained foreign body.

TABLE 3: Management of pointed object ingestion.

Clinical scenario	*Procedure*
Radiopaque:	
In the esophagus	Emergent/urgent endoscopy
In the stomach	Urgent/emergent endoscopy
In the small intestine	*Symptomatic*: Enteroscopy or surgery
	• *Asymptomatic*: Clinical follow-up with serial radiographs • Surgery if the patient becomes symptomatic or the object is not removed/passed out for more than 3 days
Radiolucent (foreign body thought to have been ingested by self-statement/witness statement)	
Symptomatic	Emergent endoscopy
Asymptomatic	Endoscopy if evidence of esophagogram or computed tomography (CT); clinical follow-up if there is no evidence of esophagogram or CT

Source: Adapted from Demiroren K. Management of Gastrointestinal Foreign Bodies with Brief Review of the Guidelines. Pediatr Gastroenterol Hepatol Nutr. 2023;26(1):1-14.

- *Stricture formation:* It may occur particularly with caustic or sharp objects.

PREVENTION

- *Education:* Inform parents and caregivers about the dangers of small objects and the importance of keeping hazardous items out of reach.
- *Safe toys:* Encourage the use of age-appropriate toys without small, detachable parts.
- *Supervision:* Close supervision of young children during play and feeding times.

CONCLUSION

The effective management of foreign body ingestion in children requires a systematic approach, encompassing initial assessment, appropriate diagnostic evaluation, and timely therapeutic intervention. Prompt recognition and treatment are paramount in preventing serious complications and ensuring favorable outcomes.

FURTHER READING

1. Conners GP, Mohseni M. Pediatric Foreign Body Ingestion. [Updated 2023 Jun 12]. In: StatPearls [Internet]. Treasure Island (FL): StatPearls Publishing; 2024 Jan-. Available from: https://www.ncbi.nlm.nih.gov/books/NBK430915/
2. Demiroren K. Management of Gastrointestinal Foreign Bodies with Brief Review of the Guidelines. Pediatr Gastroenterol Hepatol Nutr. 2023;26(1):1-14.
3. Ghosh A, Pal S, Das D, Debojyoti S, Rishavdeb P, Ruchirendu S. Management of foreign body ingestion in pediatric population: A single-center study. Annals of Medical Science and Research 2(2):98-103, May-August 2023.
4. Ikenberry SO, Jue TL, Anderson MA, Appalaneni V, Banerjee S, Ben-Menachem T; ASGE Standards of Practice Committee. Management of Ingested Foreign Bodies and Food Impactions. Gastrointest Endosc. 2011;73(6):1085-91.
5. Kramer RE, Lerner DG, Lin T, Manfredi M, Shah M, Stephen TC, et al. North American Society for Pediatric Gastroenterology, Hepatology, and Nutrition Endoscopy Committee. Management of ingested foreign bodies in children: a clinical report of the NASPGHAN Endoscopy Committee. J Pediatr Gastroenterol Nutr. 2015;60(4):562-74.

CHAPTER 16

Common Household Poisoning

INTRODUCTION

Poisoning is responsible for 2–3% of emergency room visits in various hospitals across the globe. It accounts for about 7–10% of accidents in children under 5 years of age. It is also implicated in about 2% of all injury deaths in children in developed countries and about 5% in developing countries. True incidence of accidental poisoning is difficult to assess in India, as most of the cases are not reported. But poisoning represents one of the most common medical emergencies encountered by young children and adolescents. Accidental poisoning is particularly common in young children aged 1–5 years who innocently ingest a small amount of a single substance like household products or drugs. Male gender, hyperactivity, and increased finger mouth activity or pica put these children at higher risk of poisoning. Environmental factors such as new baby in house, marital disharmony among parents, illness, and economic crisis add further risk. Pediatricians can play an important role in preventing poisoning in these children by providing anticipatory guidance. Most of the accidental poisoning occurs in home settings.

For convenience's sake, the accidental poisoning has been arbitrarily grouped in the following categories:

- Household products
- Pesticides
- Drugs
- Plants and fungi
- Miscellaneous
- Nontoxic ingestion

HOUSEHOLD PRODUCTS (TABLE 1)

Accidental exposure to substances other than drugs in the domestic environment is very common, particularly in children. As the number of household consumer products is increasing, so is the incidence of accidental poisoning related to these products. However, severe toxicity is relatively rare.

Hydrocarbons

Most of the hydrocarbons are petroleum distillates. The most common accidental poisoning in children particularly in rural area is kerosene poisoning. Other commonly encountered household hydrocarbons are paints and lubricant oils. Hydrocarbons defat mucous membranes and cause buccal and gastrointestinal irritation. Aspiration, however, is the main risk and may occur during ingestion, or if vomiting occurs subsequently. Any patient with respiratory symptoms or who has vomited following ingestion of a petroleum distillate should be referred for assessment of respiratory complications.

Antiseptics, Disinfectants, and Sterilants

A chemically diverse group of agents are used as antiseptics, disinfectants, and sterilants.

TABLE 1: Common household products and their effects.

Class	*Example*	*Toxicity*
Alcohols		
Acetone	Solvents and nail polish remover	Inebriation
Diethylene glycol and glycol ethers	Brake fluid	Ethylene glycol like
Ethanol	Mouthwash, perfume, video head cleaner, rubbing alcohol, and many liquid medications	Inebriation
Ethylene glycol	Radiator antifreeze de-ice	Acidosis/renal failure
Methanol	Gasoline antifreeze (dry gas), windshield wiper fluids, solvent, de-icer, and furniture stain remover	Acidosis/ocular toxicity
Isopropyl alcohol	Rubbing alcohol, de-icer, and pharmaceutical preparations	Inebriation
Caustics /corrosives		
Alkali	Oven cleaner, drain opener, hair relaxer, brass cleaner, and automatic dish detergent	Liquefaction necrosis
Acid	Toilet bowel cleaner and drain opener	Coagulation necrosis
Bleach	Hypochlorite (Clorox) and tile cleaner	Irritant and act as caustic at high concentration
H_2O_2	Hydrogen peroxide (3%)	Irritant and acts as caustic at high concentration
Hydrofluoric acid	Rust remover, glass-etching solution, and mag wheel cleaner	Hypocalcemia/CV
Ammonium bifluoride	Wheel cleaner	Hypocalcemia/CV
Calcium chloride	Ice melt	Irritant/caustic
Gas		
Chlorine (Cl_2)	Bleach + acid	Medium solubility irritant
Chloramine ($NHCl_2$ and NH_2Cl)	Bleach + ammonia	High solubility irritant
Hydrogen sulfide (H_2S)	Sewers	Cyanide-like, but reversible
Carbon monoxide (CO)	Furnace, fireplace, car exhaust, stove (burning), and alternative heaters	Binds hemoglobin and prevents O_2 binding and shifts dissociation curve
Radon	Leaches from ground	Pulmonary cancer
Heavy metals		
Asbestos	Insulation	
Cadmium	Batteries	Nephrotoxicity/GI caustic and obstruction

Contd...

Contd...

Class	*Example*	*Toxicity*
Lead	Pipes, soil, paint, and ceramics	Learning disability, motor palsy, and encephalopathy
Lithium	Batteries and medication	GI caustic/obstruction
Metals oxide fumes	Welding and smokescreens	Metal fume fever
Hydrocarbons		
Aliphatic	Furniture polish	Aspiration risk, pulmonary
CCl	Spot remover	Hepatic/cardiac/CNS
Gasoline	Fuels	Aspiration risk/pulmonary
Kerosene	Fuels	Aspiration risk/pulmonary
Methylene chloride	Furniture stripper	Cardiac/CNS
Mineral seal oil	Polishes	Aspiration risk/pulmonary
Pine oil	Furniture cleaners/polishes	Aspiration + CNS
Toluene	Glues and paints	CNS/renal
Trichloroethane and related	Correction fluid	CNS/renal cardiac
Teflon	Burning	Polymer fume fever
Baby products		
Talc	Baby powder	Pulmonary fibrosis
Benzocaine/lidocaine	Oral pain relievers	Methemoglobinemia
Infant formula	Concentrated overdiluted	Necrotizing enterocolitis and hyponatremia
Mothballs		
Camphor	Muscle rub (e.g., Icy-hot Bengay) and chest rub (e.g., Vicks VapoRub)	Seizures
Paradichlorobenzene	Mothballs, diaper pail deodorizer, and urinal cubes	Minimally toxic
Nail products/beauty aids		
Acetonitrile	Artificial nail remover	Cyanide-like
Toluene/acetone	Nail polish	Small quantity
Acetone	Nail polish remover	Inebriation
Hair colorants	p-phenylenediamine	Edema/renal
Cold wave neutralizers	Bromates and thioglycolates	Hearing loss/renal and alkali burns
Pest control		
DEET	Insect repellents	Seizures
Boric acid	• Medicinals • Roach killer	Nausea/vomiting, hypotension, and rash

Contd...

Contd...

Class	*Example*	*Toxicity*
Pyrethrins and pyrethroids	• Mosquito and cockroach repellants (Good Night and Lakshmanrekha) • Antilice and antiscabies treatment (Perlice and Permite)	• Anaphylaxis • In high doses can cause neurotoxicity
Long-acting anticoagulants	Rat and mouse poison (e.g., bromadiolone such as Mortien and Roban)	Delayed anticoagulation
Organophosphate/ carbamate	Insecticide (Finit and Baygon)	Cholinergic/nicotinic effects
Lindane	Antilice treatment and antiscabies treatment)	Seizures
Chlorophenoxy compounds	Herbicide	CNS/CV/respiratory
Metaldehyde	Snail and slug bail	Seizures and coma
Tooth care products		
Fluoride	Mouthwash and toothpaste gel	Hypocalcemia and hyperkalemia
Toys		
Cobalt	Chemistry kits and magnets	Cardiac and GI
Copper	Chemistry kits	Gastroenteritis
Nitrate and nitrites	Chemistry kits	Methemoglobinemia
Methylene blue	Chemistry kits	Methemoglobinemia
Over-the-counter		
Phosphate	Phospho-soda (e.g., fleet enema)	Hypocalcemia
Magnesium	Citrate of magnesia	Hypotension/CV and CNS
Hexachlorophene	Skin cleansers	CNS/CV
Imidazoline decongestants	Oxymetazoline (e.g., Afrin)	CNS depression/bradycardia
Nicotine	Cigarette, patch, and gum	Nicotinic symptoms
Potassium chlorate	Matches	Methemoglobinemia/hemolysis

(CCI: ceramic coating inc; CNS: central nervous system; CV: cardiovascular; DEET: N,N-diethyl-meta-toluamide; GI: gastrointestinal)

Many of the more toxic agents such as iodine, phenol, and chlorates, which were used as cleaning agents, are gradually disappearing but still may be available in some settings. Formaldehyde exposure, while also not very common, can also cause significant problems. Frequently employed antiseptics such as chlorhexidine and quaternary ammonium compounds have a relatively low toxicity. Ingestion of iodophor like Betadine does not usually cause significant toxicity, but absorption through other routes may still produce significant adverse effects. Ingestion of hydrogen peroxide, particularly the more concentrated formulations, may be problematic.

Detergents and Household Bleaches

Detergents are of low toxicity but irritant. Anionic and nonionic surfactants are less irritating than cationic surfactants. The main risk is aspiration of the foam produced during vomiting or when large volumes are ingested. This is a rare complication.

Household bleaches are commonly 5% sodium hypochlorite solutions and cause moderate mucosal irritation. Although alkaline, they do not tend to cause corrosive damage unless large quantities or concentrated solutions are ingested. Corrosive injury of the stomach and hypernatremia with hyperchloremic acidosis has been reported after ingestion of a large quantity. Hydrogen peroxide is used for bleaching hair, in some disinfectant solutions for contact lenses, in chlorine free “environmentally friendly” bleaches and some newer fabric stain removers/bleaches.

Higher concentration of hydrogen peroxide (35%) is used in industrial grade bleaches. In the presence of organic matter or if permitted to become alkaline, hydrogen peroxide vigorously decomposes to oxygen and water. Ingestion results in gastrointestinal irritation and sometimes burns, the severity of which depends on the concentration of the solution. There is also a risk of gas embolism, and deaths have been reported, but in most cases, concentrated solutions of 30–40% were involved. Usually, however, ingestion of hydrogen peroxide results in only mild effects. Any patient symptomatic after ingestion of hydrogen peroxide should be referred to the hospital.

Camphor and Moth Repellents

The most common component of mothballs has been camphor, naphthalene, and paradichlorobenzene. In most of the developed world, paradichlorobenzene has replaced the camphor and naphthalene as the most common component of mothballs and moth flakes, because it has minimal toxicity. But in India due to cost reasons, naphthalene and camphor both are used more commonly. Moreover, camphor is commonly used during various religious rituals. Both can cause life-threatening toxicity such as convulsions and status epilepticus. Naphthalene in addition may also cause methemoglobinemia and intravascular hemolysis particularly in glucose-6-phosphate dehydrogenase (G6PD)-deficient patients.

Corrosives

Corrosives such as alkalis (e.g., oven cleaners, dishwasher products, and drain cleaners) and acids (e.g., descalers and drain cleaners) may cause severe burns to the skin and, if ingested, to the gastrointestinal tract. Many people also store sulfuric acid as drain cleaner. It is an important cause of corrosive burns due to accidental ingestion in children. Dermal burns from alkalis are a particular problem as they may initially be painless and can progress over a period of hours. Any patient with alkali on the skin should have the area thoroughly irrigated immediately and be referred to hospital even if there is no visible injury. Ingestion of corrosive substances can result in severe gastrointestinal injury including perforation. Long-term complications include stricture and esophageal or gastric cancer. Neutralizing chemicals must never be given as neutralization produces heat, and this may exacerbate injury.

Essential Oils

Essential oils, such as clove and eucalyptus, may cause toxicity if ingested. Individual oils vary in toxicity. Essential oils may cause systemic toxicity with coma, respiratory depression, and convulsions. In some cases, hepatotoxicity and nephrotoxicity have also been reported. They may also be aspirated and cause respiratory complications.

Baking Soda

Baking soda (sodium bicarbonate) is commonly used as a home remedy for gastrointestinal symptoms. Acute ingestion following a large meal can rarely result in gastric rupture due to the formation of carbon dioxide gas from the reaction of bicarbonate and gastric acid. Chronic ingestion of baking soda can result in metabolic disturbances including hypochloremic metabolic alkalosis, hypernatremia, and hypokalemia.

Button Batteries

Children often ingest button batteries, such as those used in hearing aids and calculators. Sometimes adults may also ingest these in mistake for tablets. They may cause corrosive effects, and some also contain mercury salts, which can cause toxicity. Most batteries pass through the gut with no complications. However, it is recommended that their progress is monitored with repeat X-rays to determine the presence of leaking or stationary batteries, which may require surgical removal. Local corrosive damage may also occur from batteries inserted into the ear and nose. This can occur quickly and can result in scarring and long-term complications including perforation of the nasal septum or eardrum.

Cigarettes

Children frequently ingest cigarettes, but the majority suffers only mild effects. The clinical effects of nicotine toxicity are usually rapid in onset and develop within 15–90 minutes. Common effects are nausea, vomiting, salivation, and abdominal pain. In more severe cases, there may be respiratory depression, hypotension, arrhythmia, and convulsions.

PESTICIDES

A large number of pesticides are often found in a common Indian home, which are used for killing rats (rodenticide), mosquitoes (mosquito repellants), insects (insecticides), and unwanted vegetation (herbicide). These are very common causes of accidental poisoning in children.

Rodenticide

There are large numbers of chemicals used as rodenticides. The frequently used rodenticide in Indian urban homes is bromadiolone, a superwarfarin (Mortein rodenticide). It is an anticoagulant, which is 100 times more potent than warfarin, and the anticoagulant effects can last up to 6–7 weeks. Fortunately, most of the accidental poisonings are nontoxic if a small quantity is ingested. But suicidal or large accidental ingestion can cause bleeding tendencies lasting 6–7 weeks. Barium carbonate and zinc phosphide on the other hand are highly toxic compound, resulting into high morbidity and mortality. Barium carbonate particularly causes severe hyperkalemia and all kinds of arrhythmias. Zinc phosphide has toxicity similar to aluminum phosphide (Alphos).

Mosquito Repellents

The frequently used mosquito repellants are pyrethrins or pyrethroids (Good Night, All Out, and Mortein mosquito repellents). Toxicity of pyrethrins is further enhanced by combination piperonyl butoxide. It incapacitates and knocks down the insects quickly. Most mammal species are relatively resistant because they can rapidly metabolize and detoxify these. Generally, the toxicity associated with pyrethrins is the result of allergic reactions. The chemical used as mosquito repellent is N,N-diethyl-benzamide (12% in Odomos cream), which is similar to N,N-diethyl-meta-toluamide (DEET). It is safe when applies on skin. If ingested by mistake, toxicity appears to be minimal, suggesting a substantial margin of toxicity.

Insecticides

The three largest groups of chemicals, which are used as insecticide, are organophosphates, carbamates, and organochlorines. Organophosphate and carbamate cause prominent cholinergic, nicotinic, and central nervous system (CNS) toxicity. The common organochlorines stored in household are dichloro-diphenyl-trichloroethane (DDT) and Alderin. These have predominantly CNS excitatory effect, leading to convulsions and status epilepticus. Another insecticide, which can cause accidental poisoning, is Alphos. It is used as grain preservative in Indian rural regions, and its morbidity and mortality are very high.

DRUGS

Accidental drug overdose is fairly common, although severe cases are rare. In children, the most serious accidental poisoning occurs with iron, methadone, and tricyclic antidepressants, and death may result.

Sympathomimetics

The one of the most common accidental poisonings occurs due to cough syrups, containing phenyl propylamine, phenylamine, pseudoephedrine, or salbutamol. Generally, the margin of safety is high, and most of this accidental ingestion is trivial. But all these are well known to cause tachycardia, hypertension, and arrhythmia.

Paracetamol

One of the most common problems is inadvertent overdose with paracetamol, either by increased dosing or by taking it with a combination product also containing paracetamol. Since paracetamol overdose may not cause any features of toxicity in the early stages, the individual may not realize that a toxic dose has been taken until it is too late for effective treatment. The efficacy of antidotal therapy declines with time postingestion. Some people, such as alcoholics, malnourished individuals or anorexics, or those on enzyme-inducing drugs such as phenytoin, carbamazepine, and rifampicin, are more at risk from paracetamol toxicity. In healthy adults, a dose of 150 mg/kg or 12 g or more in total may be hepatotoxic. A dose of <125 mg/kg is unlikely to cause liver damage, but >350 mg/kg would be expected to cause severe damage in almost all cases. Peak hepatotoxicity occurs 72–96 hours postingestion. Children are known to be more tolerant of paracetamol in overdose. Any patient with a suspected paracetamol overdose should be referred to hospital immediately.

Thyroxin

Better screening program for hypothyroidism and increasing awareness of doctor regarding this problem have made tablet thyroxin a common drug being prescribed. So, it is becoming one of the most common drugs for accidental poisoning. Dose below 0.5 mg is generally asymptomatic, but a dose more than this can cause arrhythmia, particularly supraventricular tachycardia, diarrhea, sweating, etc. Symptoms are generally delayed for 3–4 days as thyroxin tablets have

T-4, which is converted to T-3 that is the active form.

Iron

Initial features of iron toxicity include vomiting, diarrhea, and abdominal pain. In severe cases, there may be drowsiness, convulsions, metabolic acidosis, shock, gastrointestinal hemorrhage, and hepatotoxicity. Iron poisoning is a particular risk in families with young children where the mother is (or has been) taking iron supplements, usually during or after pregnancy. There is also the problem that iron is widely perceived as beneficial, and many people do not realize that iron overdose is potentially serious. Referral to hospital for determination of serum iron concentration and gastric decontamination is required urgently, particularly in any child with CNS depression after ingestion of iron.

Tricyclic Antidepressants

Tricyclic antidepressant ingestion is also serious in children because a small amount can cause toxicity. The most common tricyclic antidepressants that cause serious toxicity in children are amitriptyline and imipramine. This may, in part, be because older siblings are given these drugs for nocturnal enuresis. Severe poisoning may result in coma, convulsions, hypotension, respiratory depression, and arrhythmias. Urgent referral to hospital is needed for gastric decontamination and cardiac monitoring. Newer antidepressants have wider margin of safety.

Other Drug

Almost every drug has been found to cause accidental poisoning in children at one or the other occasion. In Indian scenario, these include antitubercular drugs, antihypertensives, oral hypoglycemics, and antipsychiatric drugs.

Herbal Remedies

Herbal drugs and traditional remedies have also been a source of poisoning, usually when taken chronically. This may occur from toxicity of the individual ingredients or from contaminants such as mercury, lead, and arsenic. It is essential that patients with unexplained illness, who have been taking herbal or traditional drugs, are investigated for possible toxicity due to the medication. Toxicity may manifest as liver or kidney function abnormalities, gastrointestinal symptoms, skin reactions, and cardiac effects. One of the common acute ingestions is seen with tablet Parad. Parad is used as grain preservative. Generally, it is not associated with any significant toxicity.

PLANTS AND FUNGI

Severe poisoning from accidental ingestion of plants is uncommon. Most cases of plant ingestion involve children eating berries or houseplant material. Gastrointestinal irritation is usually all that occurs. Dhatura poisoning is more often used with deceitful intentions. Accidental poisoning can occur but not very common. This plant has anticholinergic effects. Severe fungal poisoning is also rare, since relatively few species are highly toxic, and most species do not contain toxic compounds. The most toxic species contain amatoxins such as death cap (Amanita phalloides); this species alone is responsible for about 90% of all mushroom-related deaths. There is a latent period of 6 hours or more between ingestion and the onset of clinical effects with these more toxic species. Therefore, any patient with delayed gastrointestinal effects thought to be due to ingestion of a mushroom should be referred immediately to hospital. In most cases, these are early onset gastrointestinal effects due to ingestion of mushrooms containing gastrointestinal irritants. Anyone who has collected wild mushrooms but is unsure of their identity or toxicity should not eat them.

MISCELLANEOUS

Paint

The toxicity of lead paint is a subject that has recently received some media attention. Absorption of lead may follow inhalation of fumes from heat treatment of lead-containing paint or from inhalation or ingestion of dust or flaky paint being sanded or decaying. Paint applied before 1960 is likely to contain a high percentage of lead. Young children, particularly those with pica (unusual cravings), are at risk of exposure if they repeatedly ingest paint particles. Clinical features of acute lead poisoning (plumbism) may include anorexia, constipation, abdominal pain, behavioral changes, vomiting, lethargy or hyperactivity, clumsiness, and ataxia. In severe cases, convulsions and coma can also occur. The clinical features of chronic lead poisoning may be rather nonspecific, including vague aches and pains, behavioral changes, nephritis, and peripheral neuropathy. Those affected should get the blood lead measurements done for proper management.

Carbon Monoxide

Carbon monoxide is not an uncommon cause of accidental poisoning. It particularly occurs in areas where people sleep while coal oven is put on during winter season and room is closed. It can be a result of fires, faulty gas appliances or if a child is left in car while engine is on. The primary effects are due to hypoxia. In mild-to-moderate exposures, clinical effects are nonspecific, including headache, weakness, and fatigue, often with nausea and vomiting, and are commonly mistaken for food poisoning or flu. In more severe cases, there may be coma with convulsions, hypotension, respiratory depression, arrhythmias, and cerebral edema. Patients recovering from carbon monoxide poisoning may suffer neurological sequelae including tremors, personality changes, memory impairment, visual loss, inability to concentrate, and Parkinsonism. Any illness affecting the whole family should be investigated. Methane (a natural gas) is a simple asphyxiant and is not a source of carbon monoxide unless it is burnt in faulty equipment with insufficient oxygen.

NONTOXIC ACCIDENTAL INGESTIONS

Many of the household products are nontoxic, which do not necessitate any kind of treatment **(Box 1)**. These children can be safely sent home after providing anticipatory poison prevention guidance.

BOX 1: Nontoxic substances.

- *Pharmaceuticals:* Antacids, antibiotics, contraceptives, corticosteroids, laxatives, mineral oil, vitamins (without iron), and zinc oxide
- *Cosmetics:* Baby products, cologne, deodorants, eye makeup, hand lotion, hair products, hydrogen peroxide (household, 3%), lipstick, and perfumes
- *Soaps and detergents:* Suntan lotion, soap, bath foam, bubble bath, fabric softener, hand and dish washing soap, laundry detergent, and shampoo
- *Household products:* Artificial sweeteners, lubricating oil, ballpoint pen ink, bath oil, matches, candles, crayons, dehumidifying packets, deodorizers, silica gel, household bleach, shaving cream, shoe polish, thermometers (mercury), and watercolors
- *Miscellaneous:* Chalk, cigarettes, clay, glues and paste, greases, pencil lead, and paint

The two common products in this group are silica gel and mercury in thermometer. Silica gel, a desiccant found in some tablet containers and new leather goods, is inert and not toxic despite "Do not eat" warnings. The mercury in thermometers is not toxic by ingestion (although it can cause poisoning if inhaled over a prolonged period). Oral contraceptives, if ingested in quantity, may cause gastrointestinal irritation, and in females of any age, there may be a withdrawal bleed a couple of days later.

CONCLUSION

Household poisoning in children is a serious concern, often resulting from accidental ingestion, inhalation, or skin contact with common household items like medicines, cleaning products, and alcohol. Most incidents occur in children under 5 years old due to their natural curiosity and tendency to explore by tasting and touching. Prevention is key, involving storing hazardous substances out of reach and educating caregivers about potential risks. Immediate action and contacting a poison control center can be crucial in managing such emergencies.

FURTHER READING

1. Academy of Pediatrics, India. Guidelines for Management of Poisoning in Children. Pediatr Today. 2017;8(1):12-24.
2. Indian Journal of Pediatrics. Accidental Poisoning in Indian Children. Indian J Pediatr. 2020;87(6):455-62.
3. Peshin SS, Gupta YK. Poisoning due to household products: a ten years retrospective analysis of telephone calls to the National Poisons Information Centre, All India Institute of Medical Sciences, New Delhi, India, J Forensic Leg Med. 2018;58: 205-11.
4. Srivastava A, Peshin SS, Thomas K, Gupta SK. An epidemiological study of poisoning cases reported to the National Poisons Information Centre, All India Institute of Medical Sciences, New Delhi. Human & Experimental Toxicology. 2005;24(6): 279-85.
5. Sharma S, Singh M. Pediatric Emergencies in India: A Practical Guide. Jaypee Brothers Medical Publishers; 2015.
6. World Health Organization (WHO). (2018). Lead poisoning and health. [online] Available from https://www.who.int/news-room/fact-sheets/detail/lead-poisoning-and-health [Last accessed August, 2024].

SECTION 3

Pediatric Office Emergency Procedures

Part 1: Eye and ENT

1. Management of Nasal Foreign Body in Children
2. Procedure for Management of Epistaxis in Children
3. Procedure for Management of Nasal Injury in Children
4. Procedure for Management of Foreign Body in Ear in Children
5. Procedure for Management of Cerumen Impaction in Children
6. Procedure for Management of Ocular Foreign Body in Children
7. Procedure for Eye Drop Administration in Children

Part 2: GIT and Genitourinary

8. Procedure for Management of Paraphimosis in Children
9. Procedure for Zipper Injury in Children
10. Procedure for Detorsion of Testes in Children
11. Manual Reduction of Obstructed Inguinal Hernia
12. Procedure for Rectal Prolapse Reduction in Children
13. Management of Constipated Stool Impaction in Children
14. Procedure for Umbilical Granuloma in Children

Part 3: Minor Surgical Emergencies

15. Procedure for Ring Removal in Children
16. Procedure for Subungual Hematoma in Children
17. Procedure for Management of Paronychia in Children
18. Management of Ingrowing Toenail in Children
19. Procedure for Management of Fingernail and Toenail Avulsion in Children
20. Procedure for Fishhook Removal in Children
21. Procedure for Management of Hair Tourniquets in Children
22. Superficial Splinter Removal in Children
23. Management of Warts and Calluses in Children
24. Management of Simple Lacerations in Children
25. Management of Simple Tongue and Lip Lacerations in Children

26. Procedure for Management of Pencil Point Puncture in Children

Part 4: Trauma and Orthopedic

27. First Aid Splint for Children with Fracture
28. Procedure for Management of Pulled Elbow in Children
29. Procedure for Management of Clavicle Fracture in Children
30. Procedure for Management of Ankle Sprain in Children
31. Procedure for Management of Avulsed Tooth in Children

Part 5: Poisoning and More

32. Administration of Activated Charcoal in Children
33. Gastric Lavage for Poisoning in Children
34. Management of Hymenoptera and Bee Stings in Children
35. Procedure for Rabies Immune Globulin Administration in Children
36. Intranasal Administration of Midazolam and Fentanyl in Children
37. Buccal Drug Administration in Children
38. Making Intramuscular Injections Pain Free in Children
39. Rectal Drug Administration in Children

CHAPTER 1

Management of Nasal Foreign Body in Children

INTRODUCTION

Nasal foreign body insertion is a common occurrence in children, often resulting from curiosity or accidental insertion during play. Prompt and appropriate management is crucial to prevent complications such as infection, aspiration, or nasal obstruction.

INDICATIONS

- Observation or suspicion of a foreign body in the nasal cavity
- Symptoms such as unilateral nasal discharge, foul odor, nasal obstruction, or bleeding.

CONTRAINDICATIONS

- Severe trauma to the nasal passage, requiring surgical intervention
- Suspected button battery or high-risk object that needs immediate specialized care
- Patient uncooperativeness, requiring sedation or general anesthesia.

EQUIPMENT AND SUPPLIES

- Sterile gloves
- Nasal speculum
- Bright light source or headlamp
- Suction device (if available)
- Cotton-tipped applicators
- Alligator forceps or bayonet forceps
- Right-angle hook or cerumen loop
- Nasal decongestant spray (e.g., oxymetazoline)
- Topical anesthetic (e.g., lidocaine spray)
- Magnifying glass or loupe (optional)
- Balloon catheter (optional)
- Irrigation syringe with saline (for certain types of foreign bodies)
- Personal protective equipment (PPE)

PREPARATION

- *Explain the procedure:*
  - Inform the child (if age-appropriate) and caregivers about the situation, the procedure, its purpose, and what to expect.
  - Obtain informed consent from the caregivers.
- *Positioning:* Position the child sitting upright or slightly reclined with the head supported. Use an assistant if necessary to help hold the child still.

PROCEDURE STEPS

1. *Initial assessment:*
   a. Conduct a thorough history and physical examination to determine the type and location of the foreign body.
   b. Inspect the nasal cavity using a nasal speculum and a bright light source to visualize the foreign body.
2. *Preparation:*
   a. Apply a nasal decongestant spray to reduce mucosal swelling and improve visualization.

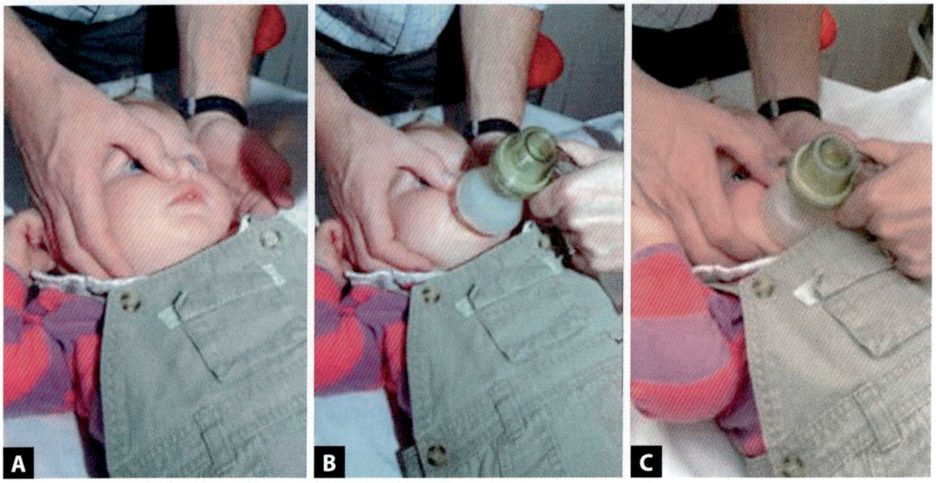

Figs. 1A to C: Nasal foreign body removal by AMBU bag.

b. Administer a topical anesthetic to minimize discomfort during the procedure.

3. *Removal techniques:*
   a. *Positive pressure technique* ***(Figs. 1A to C)****:*
      i. *Indications:* Effective for small, nonobstructing foreign bodies.
      ii. *Procedure:*
         - Close the unaffected nostril by pressing it shut.
         - Healthcare providers give a quick, forceful puff of air with an AMBU bag with baby mask into the child's mouth while keeping the unaffected nostril closed. The positive pressure may expel the foreign body.
   b. *Parent's Kiss method* ***(Fig. 2)****:*
      i. *Indications:* Suitable for cooperative children with nonobstructing foreign bodies.
      ii. *Procedure:*
         - Instruct the caregiver to place their mouth over the child's mouth, forming a seal.

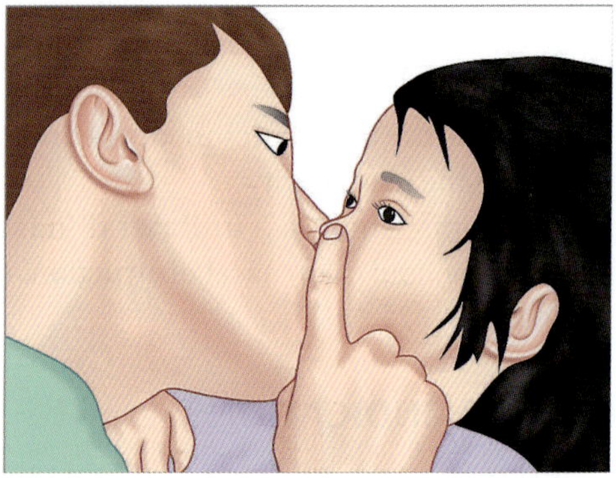

Fig. 2: Nasal foreign body removal by Parent's Kiss method.

         - The caregiver gives a sharp puff of air while closing the unaffected nostril with a finger. This positive pressure can help expel the foreign body.
   c. *Instrumental removal:*
      i. *Preparation:* Ensure adequate visualization of the foreign body using a nasal speculum and a bright light source.
      ii. *Procedure:*
         - Using appropriate tools (alligator forceps, bayonet forceps,

right-angle hook, or cerumen loop), carefully grasp or hook the foreign body.
- Gently extract the foreign body, ensuring not to push it further into the nasal cavity.
- If the foreign body is impacted or difficult to grasp, a balloon catheter can be inserted past the object, inflated, and then gently pulled out to extract the foreign body.

d. *Irrigation method:*
   i. *Indications:* Suitable for small, nonabsorbent objects
   ii. *Procedure:*
   - Fill an irrigation syringe with saline solution.
   - Tilt the child's head slightly forward to avoid aspiration.
   - Gently irrigate the nasal cavity to flush out the foreign body. Avoid excessive force to prevent aspiration.

4. *Postprocedure care:*
   a. *Inspection:* Re-examine the nasal cavity to ensure complete removal of the foreign body.
   b. *Observation:* Monitor the child for any signs of distress, bleeding, or complications.
   c. *Wound care:* If there is minor bleeding or irritation, apply antibiotic ointment to the nasal mucosa.

AFTERCARE

- *Monitoring:*
  - Observe the child for signs of nasal obstruction, bleeding, or infection postremoval.
  - Provide instructions to caregivers on monitoring for any delayed complications.
- *Follow-up:*
  - Schedule a follow-up appointment with a healthcare provider to ensure complete resolution and healing of the nasal mucosa.
  - Further evaluation may be necessary if there are recurrent episodes of foreign body insertion.
- *Education:*
  - Educate caregivers and children about the risks of inserting objects into the nose.
  - Encourage supervision and safe play practices to prevent future incidents.

COMPLICATIONS

- *Infection:* Secondary infection due to retained foreign body or trauma during removal
- *Epistaxis:* Nasal bleeding, which is usually minor but may require further intervention if severe
- *Aspiration:* Rare but serious risk if the foreign body is pushed into the airway
- *Mucosal damage:* Trauma to the nasal mucosa can occur during removal.

PREVENTION

- *Supervision:* Close supervision of young children during playtime.
- *Education:* Teach children about the dangers of inserting objects into their nose or other body orifices.
- *Safe toys:* Provide age-appropriate toys that do not have small detachable parts.

CONCLUSION

The management of nasal foreign bodies in children involves prompt and careful removal to prevent complications. Proper technique, adequate aftercare, and education are crucial for successful outcomes and preventing recurrence.

FURTHER READING

1. Baranowski K, Al Aaraj MS, Sinha V. Nasal Foreign Body. [Updated 2023 Jul 3]. In: StatPearls [Internet]. Treasure Island (FL): StatPearls Publishing; 2024 January. Available from: https://www.ncbi.nlm.nih.gov/books/NBK459279/
2. Guidera AK, Stegehuis HR. Button batteries: the worst case scenario in nasal foreign bodies. N Z Med J. 2010;123:68-73.
3. Patil PM, Anand R. Nasal foreign bodies: a review of management strategies and a clinical scenario presentation. Craniomaxillofac Trauma Reconstr. 2011;4(1):53-8.
4. Shaffer AD, Jacobs IN, Derkay CS, Goldstein NA, Giordano T, Ho S, et al. Management and outcomes of button batteries in the aerodigestive tract: A multi-institutional study. Laryngoscope 2021;131(1):E298-E306.
5. Zavdy O, Viner I, London N, Menzely T, Hod R, Raveh E, Gilony D. Intranasal foreign bodies: A 10-year analysis of a large cohort, in a tertiary medical center. Am J Emerg Med. 2021;50:356-9.

CHAPTER 2

Procedure for Management of Epistaxis in Children

INTRODUCTION

Epistaxis, or nosebleed, is a common occurrence in children and can range from a minor nuisance to a significant medical concern. While most cases are benign and self-limiting, prompt and appropriate management is essential to control bleeding, prevent recurrence, and address any underlying causes.

INDICATIONS

- Active nasal bleeding that does not stop with initial first aid measures
- Recurrent episodes of epistaxis
- Significant blood loss or signs of anemia
- Bleeding associated with trauma, underlying medical conditions, or foreign body insertion

CONTRAINDICATIONS

- Severe facial trauma with suspected nasal fracture or skull base fracture
- Suspected coagulopathy or bleeding disorder, requiring specialist management

EQUIPMENT AND SUPPLIES

- Sterile gloves
- Nasal speculum
- Bright light source or headlamp
- Suction device (if available)
- Gauze pads or cotton balls
- Vasoconstrictive agents (e.g., oxymetazoline spray)
- Topical anesthetic (e.g., lidocaine with epinephrine)
- Silver nitrate sticks
- Nasal-packing materials (e.g., absorbable hemostatic gauze and nasal tampons)
- Antibiotic ointment (optional)
- Nasal balloon catheter (if necessary)
- Analgesics
- Hemostatic agents (e.g., tranexamic acid, if available)
- Personal protective equipment (PPE)

PREPARATION

- *Explain the procedure:*
    - Inform the child (if age-appropriate) and caregivers about the condition, the procedure, its purpose, and what to expect.
    - Obtain informed consent from the caregivers.
- *Positioning:*
    - Position the child sitting up with the head slightly forward to prevent blood from flowing down the throat.
    - Encourage the child to breathe through their mouth and avoid swallowing blood.

PROCEDURE STEPS

1. *Initial first aid measures* ***(Fig. 1)****:*
    a. *Pinch the nose:* Instruct the child or caregiver to pinch the soft part of the nose firmly for 5–10 minutes without releasing.

b. *Apply a cold compress:* Place a cold compress or ice pack on the nasal bridge to help constrict blood vessels and reduce bleeding.

2. *Examination and assessment:*
   a. *Visual inspection:* Using a nasal speculum and a bright light source, inspect the nasal cavity to identify the source of bleeding. Anterior bleeds are more common and easier to manage.
   b. *Suction:* Use a suction device if necessary to clear blood and visualize the bleeding site.

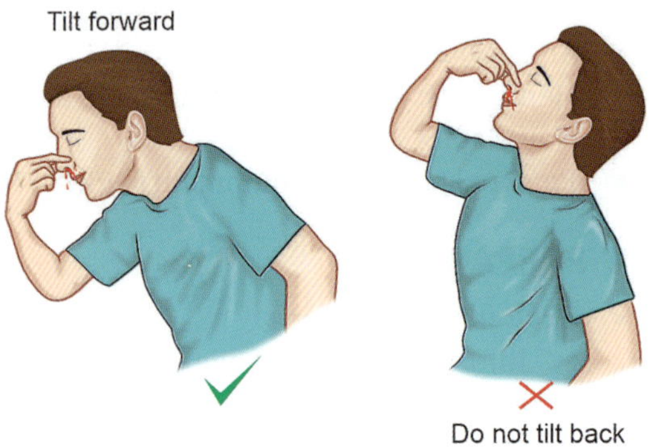

Fig. 1: Epistaxis first aid pinch the nose.

3. *Topical vasoconstriction and anesthesia:*
   a. *Vasoconstrictive agent:* Apply a vasoconstrictive agent (e.g., oxymetazoline spray) to the affected nostril to reduce bleeding.
   b. *Topical anesthetic:* Apply a topical anesthetic (e.g., lidocaine with epinephrine) to the nasal mucosa to facilitate further management and reduce discomfort.
4. *Chemical cautery:*
   a. *Preparation:* If the bleeding site is visible and accessible, prepare a silver nitrate stick.
   b. *Application:* Gently apply the silver nitrate stick to the bleeding site for a few seconds until hemostasis is achieved. Be careful to avoid excessive application, which can cause tissue necrosis.
5. *Nasal packing* ***(Fig. 2)****:*
   a. *Preparation:* If chemical cautery is unsuccessful or not feasible, prepare nasal-packing materials.
   b. *Insertion:*
      i. Insert absorbable hemostatic gauze or a nasal tampon into the bleeding

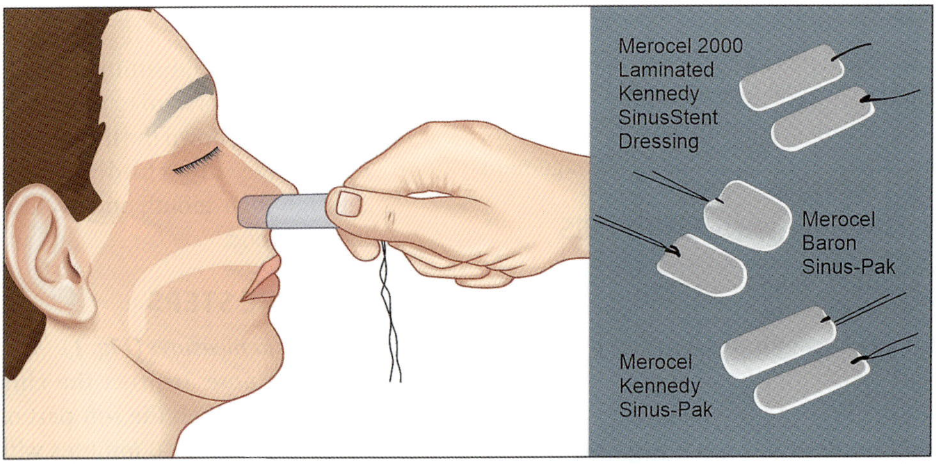

Fig. 2: Epistaxis management—nasal tampon.

nostril. Ensure it is positioned to apply pressure to the bleeding site.

ii. *Technique:* Ensure you have the appropriate size Merocele tampon. Have the patient seated upright with their head tilted slightly forward. Apply a water-based lubricant to the Merocele tampon to ease insertion. Gently insert the tampon horizontally along the floor of the nasal cavity. Use bayonet forceps or your fingers to guide the tampon. Advance it until fully inserted, typically about 4–5 cm into the nasal passage. Once in place, apply saline solution to the exposed end of the tampon. This will cause the Merocele to expand and fill the nasal cavity. For securing, ensure the string or tail of the tampon is visible outside the nostril. This will facilitate easier removal later. Advise the patient not to blow their nose or manipulate the tampon. Explain when and how the tampon will be removed (typically after 24–72 hours)

iii. For posterior bleeds or if anterior packing is insufficient, consider using a nasal balloon catheter.

6. *Postprocedure care:*
   a. *Observation:* Monitor the child for continued bleeding and signs of respiratory distress.
   b. *Analgesia:* Administer appropriate analgesics to manage discomfort.
   c. *Antibiotic ointment:* Apply antibiotic ointment to the nasal mucosa if there is significant mucosal damage or risk of infection.

AFTERCARE

- *Monitoring:* Observe the child for signs of continued bleeding, infection, or adverse reactions to the treatment.
- *Follow-up:* Schedule a follow-up appointment with a healthcare provider to reassess the nasal mucosa, remove any nonabsorbable packing, and evaluate for underlying causes of recurrent epistaxis.
- *Education:*
  - Educate caregivers on preventive measures such as humidifying the air, using saline nasal sprays, and avoiding nose picking or excessive nasal trauma.
  - Advise on the importance of maintaining proper nasal hygiene and monitoring for signs of recurrent bleeding.
- *Activity modification:* Recommend avoiding strenuous activities, bending over, or blowing the nose vigorously for a few days to allow the nasal mucosa to heal.

COMPLICATIONS

- *Recurrent bleeding:* Recurrence of epistaxis may require further evaluation and management.
- *Infection:* Nasal packing can increase the risk of infection; appropriate follow-up and prophylactic antibiotics may be considered.
- *Septal perforation:* Excessive use of chemical cautery or repeated trauma can lead to septal perforation.

PREVENTION

- *Humidification:* Use a humidifier in the child's room to keep the nasal mucosa moist, especially in dry climates.
- *Nasal care:* Encourage the use of saline nasal sprays to maintain nasal moisture and hygiene.
- *Avoidance of trauma:* Educate children and caregivers to avoid nose picking, excessive nose blowing, and inserting foreign objects into the nose.

CONCLUSION

The management of epistaxis in children involves prompt assessment, appropriate intervention to control bleeding, and preventive measures to avoid recurrence. Proper technique, aftercare, and education are crucial for successful outcomes.

FURTHER READING

1. Béquignon E, Teissier N, Gauthier A, Brugel L, De Kermadec H, Coste A, Prulière-Escabasse V. Emergency department care of childhood epistaxis. Emerg Med J. 2017;34(8):543-8.
2. Higgins TS, Hwang PH, Kingdom TT, Orlandi RR, Stammberger H, Han JK. Systematic review of topical vasoconstrictors in endoscopic sinus surgery. Laryngoscope. 2011;121(2):422-32.
3. Shieh A, Cranford JA, Weyand AC, Bohm LA, Tomlinson SE. Risk factors and management outcomes in pediatric epistaxis at an emergency department. J Emerg Med. 2024;66(2):97-108.
4. Svider P, Arianpour K, Mutchnick S. Management of epistaxis in children and adolescents: avoiding a chaotic approach. Pediatr Clin North Am. 2018;65:607-21.
5. Tunkel DE, Anne S, Payne SC, Ishman SL, Rosenfeld RM, Abramson PJ, et al. Clinical Practice Guideline: Nosebleed (Epistaxis). Otolaryngol Head Neck Surg. 2020;162(1_suppl):S1-S38.

CHAPTER 3

Procedure for Management of Nasal Injury in Children

INTRODUCTION

Nasal injuries are common in children and can result from falls, sports activities, or other trauma. These injuries range from minor bruises and lacerations to nasal fractures. Nasal fractures are the most frequent type of facial fracture. The nose's prominence and anterior position on the face make it particularly vulnerable to injury. This chapter provides a comprehensive guide to the diagnosis and management of nasal fractures in both adult and pediatric populations. Proper assessment and management are essential to prevent complications and ensure optimal healing.

ETIOLOGY AND EPIDEMIOLOGY

Nasal fractures typically result from direct blows to the nose, falls, or motor vehicle accidents. In adults, fights and sports injuries are the leading causes, followed by falls and vehicle crashes. Alcohol consumption is often a contributing factor in many cases.

ANATOMY AND PATHOPHYSIOLOGY (FIG. 1)

The nose is supported by cartilage anteriorly and inferiorly and by bone posteriorly and superiorly. Despite the largely cartilaginous structure, the nasal bones are usually involved in fractures. The mechanism of injury influences the fracture pattern. A direct frontal blow can cause fractured bones to telescope posteriorly, while a laterally directed injury can cause depression on the impact side and outward displacement on the opposite side.

CLINICAL PRESENTATION AND DIAGNOSTIC APPROACH

Patients with nasal fractures typically present with concern about a broken nose. They may

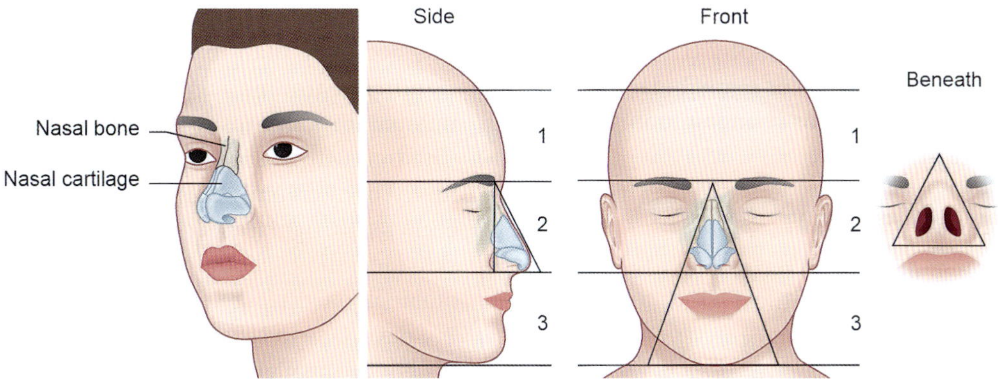

Fig. 1: Nasal structure.

have minimal continued hemorrhage, tender ecchymotic swelling over the nasal bones or anterior maxillary spine, and possibly a visible or palpable nasal deformity.

- *History:* When evaluating a potential nasal fracture, it is crucial to obtain a comprehensive history. This should include: The mechanism of injury, any previous nasal surgeries or injuries, and patient's baseline nasal function and appearance.
- *Physical examination:* Begin with a general assessment, screening for associated injuries such as cervical spine injuries, other facial fractures, or eye injuries. Look for uncommon findings that may indicate more severe trauma, such as cerebrospinal fluid leak, subcutaneous emphysema, mental status changes, malocclusion, or limited extraocular movement. Perform an external nasal examination, looking for deformity, edema, and ecchymosis of the nose and periorbital structures. Palpate for crepitus, indentation, or irregularity of the nasal bone. Conduct an internal nasal examination using good lighting, suction, and vasoconstriction with topical anesthesia. Remove any clots and assess for septal hematoma or deviation.
- *Imaging studies:* Routine radiographs are generally not recommended due to their limited utility in nasal fractures. Computed tomography (CT) scans are indicated if facial or mandibular fractures are suspected or if uncommon findings are present.

MANAGEMENT

The management of nasal fractures depends on the type and severity of the injury:

- *Nondisplaced fractures (for suspected or possible nondisplaced fractures with no nasal deformity):* Prescribe analgesics, recommend cold packs and head elevation, advise avoiding contact sports for 6 weeks, schedule follow-up in 3–5 days if marked swelling prevents thorough assessment.
- *Displaced fractures (for suspected displaced fractures or visible nasal deformity):* Refer for otolaryngologic or plastic surgery consultation, discuss immediate or delayed reduction (often more accurate between 5 and 10 days postinjury when swelling subsides).
- *Septal hematoma:* Septal hematomas require immediate attention. Immediate drainage is necessary to prevent septal necrosis and saddle-nose deformity. Otolaryngologic consultation is advisable due to potential for serious complications.
- *Associated injuries:* Isolated anterior nasal spine fractures generally do not require activity restriction. For lacerations over nasal fractures, consider closure with antibiotic prophylaxis.

SPECIAL CONSIDERATIONS IN PEDIATRIC PATIENTS

- Nasal fractures in children present unique challenges. They are less common in young children due to the pliable cartilaginous structure of their noses. Radiographic examination has even less accuracy than in adults. However, significant trauma can lead to growth retardation of the nose and midface.
- Children with posttraumatic nasal asymmetry, bony crepitus, epistaxis, periorbital ecchymosis, significant edema, or overlying skin lacerations should be referred to an otolaryngologist for re-examination within 2–4 days. Due to faster bone healing rates in children, realignment should ideally be performed within 4 days of injury.

COMPLICATIONS AND FOLLOW-UP

Proper follow-up is crucial in the management of nasal fractures. Patients should be monitored for infection, persistent deformity, and nasal airway obstruction. Schedule follow-up examinations to assess healing and functional outcomes. In pediatric cases, consider long-term follow-up to monitor for growth abnormalities. When dealing with nasal fractures, it is important to consider the possibility of physical abuse, especially in children and women. Document findings thoroughly, including photographs when possible, and follow local protocols for reporting suspected abuse cases.

CONCLUSION

Effective management of nasal fractures requires careful clinical assessment, appropriate use of imaging studies, and timely intervention when necessary. While many cases can be managed conservatively, proper referral and follow-up are crucial to ensure optimal functional and aesthetic outcomes. By understanding the nuances of nasal fracture management, healthcare providers can significantly improve patient outcomes and quality of life.

FURTHER READING

1. Borner U, Anschuetz L, Kaiser N, Rieke A, Dubach P, Caversaccio M. Blunt nasal trauma in children: a frequent diagnostic challenge. Eur Arch Otorhinolaryngol. 2019;276(1):85-91.
2. Cakabay T, Ustun Bezgin S. Pediatric nasal traumas: contribution of epidemiological features to detect the distinction between nasal fractures and nasal soft tissue injuries. J Craniofac Surg. 2018l;29(5):1334-37.
3. Higuera S, Lee EI, Cole P, Hollier LH Jr, Stal S. Nasal trauma and the deviated nose. Plast Reconstr Surg. 2007;120(7 Suppl 2): 64S-75S.
4. Navaratnam R, Davis T. The Role of ultrasound in the diagnosis of pediatric nasal fractures. J Craniofac Surg 2019; 30(7):2099 2101.
5. Wright RJ, Murakami CS, Ambro BT. Pediatric nasal injuries and management. Facial Plast Surg. 2011t;27(5):483-9.

CHAPTER 4

Procedure for Management of Foreign Body in Ear in Children

INTRODUCTION

Foreign bodies in the ear are a common pediatric problem, often resulting from the child inserting objects into their ear canal out of curiosity. Prompt and appropriate management is crucial to prevent complications such as infection, damage to the ear canal or tympanic membrane, and hearing loss.

INDICATIONS

- Observation or suspicion of a foreign body in the ear canal
- Symptoms such as ear pain, hearing loss, discharge, bleeding, or a sense of fullness in the ear

CONTRAINDICATIONS

- Foreign body, causing significant trauma or embedded in the ear canal
- Suspected perforation of the tympanic membrane
- Presence of a button battery in the ear canal (requires immediate specialized care)
- Patient uncooperativeness, requiring sedation or general anesthesia

EQUIPMENT AND SUPPLIES

- Sterile gloves
- Otoscope with bright light source
- Suction device (if available)
- Irrigation syringe with saline solution (if appropriate for the type of foreign body)
- Alligator forceps or bayonet forceps
- Right-angle hook or cerumen loop
- Topical anesthetic (e.g., lidocaine spray)
- Magnifying glass or loupe (optional)
- Personal protective equipment (PPE)

PREPARATION

- *Explain the procedure:*
  - Inform the child (if age-appropriate) and caregivers about the situation, the procedure, its purpose, and what to expect.
  - Obtain informed consent from the caregivers.
- *Positioning:*
  - Position the child sitting upright or slightly reclined with the head tilted toward the unaffected side to allow easy access to the affected ear.
  - Use an assistant to help hold the child still during the procedure if necessary.

PROCEDURE STEPS

1. *Initial assessment:*
   a. Conduct a thorough history and physical examination to determine the type and location of the foreign body.
   b. Use an otoscope to inspect the ear canal and visualize the foreign body.
2. *Preparation:* Apply a topical anesthetic to minimize discomfort during the procedure.

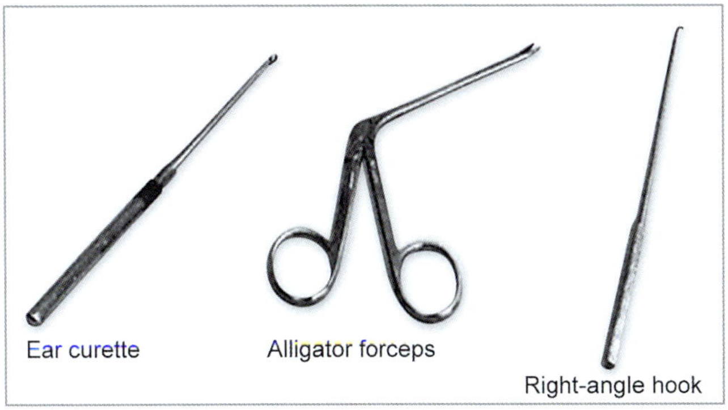

Fig. 1: The right-angle hook is best suited for removing hard objects from the ear, whereas alligator forceps work best on soft objects.

3. *Removal techniques:*
   a. *Manual removal with instruments* **(Fig. 1)**:
      i. *Preparation:* Ensure adequate visualization of the foreign body using an otoscope and a bright light source.
      ii. *Procedure:*
         - Using appropriate tools (alligator forceps, bayonet forceps, right-angle hook, or cerumen loop), carefully grasp or hook the foreign body.
         - Gently extract the foreign body, ensuring not to push it further into the ear canal.
         - If the foreign body is fragile or likely to break, consider using suction to remove it intact.
   b. *Irrigation method* ***(Fig. 2)****:*
      i. *Indications:* Suitable for small, nonabsorbent objects and objects not likely to swell or expand when wet
      ii. *Procedure:*
         - Fill an irrigation syringe with saline solution at body temperature.
         - Tilt the child's head to allow the ear canal to be irrigated effectively.

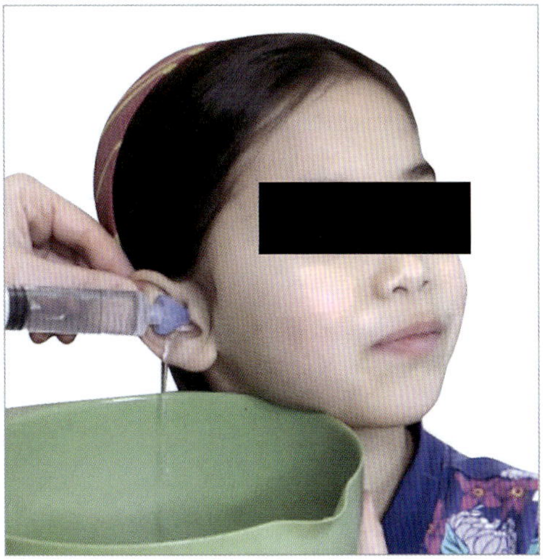

Fig. 2: Foreign body removal by syringing.

         - Gently irrigate the ear canal to flush out the foreign body. Avoid excessive force to prevent tympanic membrane perforation.
         - Use a catch basin or towel to collect the saline and foreign body.
   c. *Suction method:*
      i. *Indications:* Suitable for small, loose foreign bodies
      ii. *Procedure:*
         - Use a soft suction catheter connected to a suction device.

- Gently insert the suction catheter into the ear canal near the foreign body and apply suction to remove the object.

4. *Postprocedure care:*
   a. *Inspection:* Re-examine the ear canal to ensure complete removal of the foreign body.
   b. *Observation:* Monitor the child for any signs of distress, pain, or complications.
   c. *Wound care:* If there is minor bleeding or irritation, apply antibiotic ointment to the ear canal.

AFTERCARE

- *Monitoring:*
  - Observe the child for signs of ear pain, discharge, or infection postremoval.
  - Provide instructions to caregivers on monitoring for any delayed complications.
- *Follow-up:*
  - Schedule a follow-up appointment with a healthcare provider to ensure complete resolution and healing of the ear canal.
  - Further evaluation may be necessary, if there are recurrent episodes of foreign body insertion.
- *Education:*
  - Educate caregivers and children about the risks of inserting objects into the ear.
  - Encourage supervision and safe play practices to prevent future incidents.

COMPLICATIONS

- *Infection:* Secondary infection due to retained foreign body or trauma during removal
- *Tympanic membrane perforation:* Risk of perforation, if excessive force is used during removal
- *Ear canal damage:* Trauma to the ear canal can occur during removal.
- *Residual hearing loss:* Possible, if there is significant trauma or infection

PREVENTION

- *Supervision:* Close supervision of young children during playtime.
- *Education:* Teach children about the dangers of inserting objects into their ears.
- *Safe toys:* Provide age-appropriate toys that do not have small detachable parts.

CONCLUSION

The management of ear foreign bodies in children involves prompt and careful removal to prevent complications. Proper technique, adequate aftercare, and education are crucial for successful outcomes and preventing recurrence.

FURTHER READING

1. Marin JR, Trainor JL. Foreign body removal from the external auditory canal in a pediatric emergency department. Pediatr Emerg Care. 2006;22(9):630-4.
2. McLaughlin R, Ullah R, Heylings D. Comparative prospective study of foreign body removal from external auditory canals of cadavers with right angle hook or cyanoacrylate glue. Emerg Med J. 2002;19(1):43-5.
3. Schulze SL, Kerschner J, Beste D. Pediatric external auditory canal foreign bodies: a review of 698 cases. Otolaryngol Head Neck Surg. 2002;127:73-8.
4. Steele D. Foreign body removal from the external auditory canal. In: Textbook of Pediatric Emergency Procedures, 2nd edition, King C, Henretig FM (Eds), Lippincott, Williams & Willkins, Philadelphia 2008. p.589.
5. Thompson SK, Wein RO, Dutcher PO. External auditory canal foreign body removal: management practices and outcomes. Laryngoscope 2003;113(11):1912-5.

CHAPTER 5

Procedure for Management of Cerumen Impaction in Children

INTRODUCTION

Cerumen impaction is a common condition in children where earwax accumulates and becomes hardened, blocking the ear canal. This can cause discomfort, hearing loss, and even infection if left untreated. Proper management involves safe and effective removal of the impacted cerumen to relieve symptoms and restore normal ear function.

INDICATIONS

- Symptoms of ear discomfort, fullness, or pain
- Hearing loss or muffled hearing
- Visible earwax blocking the ear canal
- Need to visualize the ear canal and tympanic membrane (e.g., before hearing tests or ear infection evaluation)

CONTRAINDICATIONS

- Signs of ear infection (e.g., fever and ear discharge), requiring antibiotic therapy
- History of ear surgery or perforated tympanic membrane
- Presence of foreign body in the ear canal
- Severe pain or bleeding, indicating a more serious condition, requiring specialist care

EQUIPMENT AND SUPPLIES

- Sterile gloves
- Otoscope with bright light source
- Cerumenolytic agents (e.g., hydrogen peroxide, carbamide peroxide, saline, or olive oil)
- Bulb syringe or irrigation kit
- Warm water
- Sterile gauze pads
- Cotton-tipped applicators
- Ear curette or loop (optional)
- Towel or waterproof drape
- Personal protective equipment (PPE)

PREPARATION

- *Explain the procedure:*
    - Inform the child (if age-appropriate) and caregivers about the condition, the removal procedure, its purpose, and what to expect.
    - Obtain informed consent from the caregivers.
- *Positioning:*
    - Position the child comfortably, ideally seated with their head tilted to the side to allow easy access to the affected ear.
    - Use an assistant, if necessary, to help hold the child still during the procedure.

PROCEDURE STEPS

1. *Initial assessment:*
    a. Conduct a thorough history and physical examination to assess the extent of the cerumen impaction.
    b. Use an otoscope to visualize the ear canal and confirm the presence of impacted cerumen.
2. *Cerumenolytic agents:*
    a. *Application:*
        i. Instill a few drops of a cerumenolytic agent (e.g., hydrogen peroxide,

carbamide peroxide, saline, or olive oil) into the affected ear.

ii. Instruct the child to keep the affected ear facing up and remain in this position for 5–10 minutes to allow the agent to soften the earwax.

iii. Cerumenolytic agents can be used alone or in combination with irrigation for more effective removal.

3. *Irrigation method* ***(Fig. 1)****:*
   a. *Preparation:*
      i. Fill a bulb syringe or irrigation kit with warm water (body temperature) to avoid dizziness or discomfort.
      ii. Place a towel or waterproof drape around the child's shoulder to catch any water or debris.
   b. *Procedure:*
      i. Gently pull the pinna (outer ear) backward and upward to straighten the ear canal in older children or straight back in younger children.
      ii. Carefully irrigate the ear canal by directing the water along the upper wall of the ear canal, avoiding direct pressure on the tympanic membrane.
      iii. Allow the water and loosened cerumen to drain out of the ear, using sterile gauze pads to catch the fluid.
      iv. Repeat the irrigation process as needed until the cerumen is flushed out and the ear canal is clear.
4. *Manual removal (if necessary):*
   a. *Preparation* ***(Fig. 2)****:* If irrigation is insufficient or contraindicated, use an ear curette or loop for manual removal.
   b. *Procedure:*
      i. Gently insert the curette or loop into the ear canal, carefully scooping out the softened cerumen.
      ii. Avoid inserting the instrument too deeply to prevent injury to the ear canal or tympanic membrane.
      iii. Use an otoscope to visualize the ear canal and guide the removal process.
5. *Postprocedure care:*
   a. *Inspection:* Re-examine the ear canal with an otoscope to ensure complete removal of the cerumen and check for any signs of injury.
   b. *Drying:* Gently dry the ear canal with a cotton-tipped applicator or allow the ear to air dry.

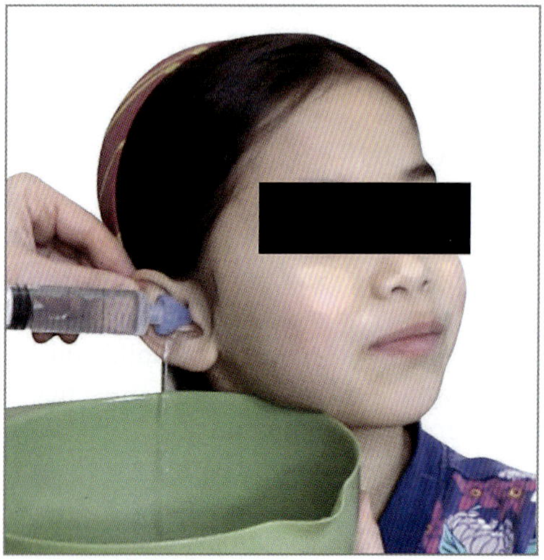

Fig. 1: Cerumen removal by syringing.

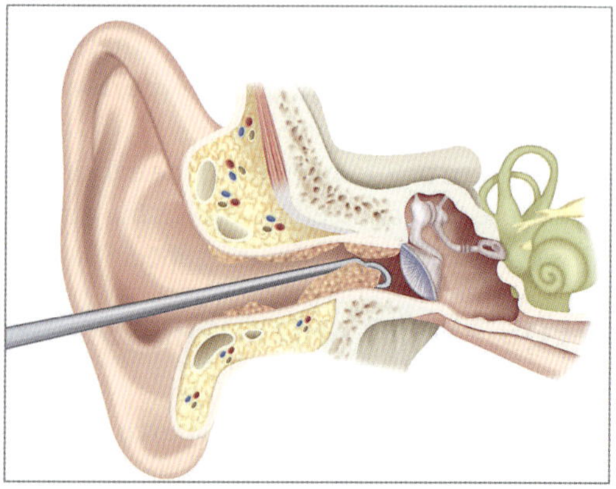

Fig. 2: Manual cerumen removal.

c. *Reassurance:* Reassure the child and caregivers that the procedure is complete and provide instructions for preventing future cerumen impaction.

AFTERCARE

- *Monitoring:*
  - Observe the child for any signs of discomfort, pain, or complications following the procedure.
  - Provide instructions to caregivers on monitoring the ear for signs of infection or recurrence of symptoms.
- *Preventive care:*
  - Advise caregivers to avoid using cotton swabs or other objects in the ear canal to prevent further impaction.
  - Recommend regular ear hygiene practices, such as using ear drops periodically to keep the cerumen soft and easier to remove naturally.
- *Follow-up:*
  - Schedule a follow-up appointment if there are concerns about persistent symptoms or if the child has a history of recurrent cerumen impaction.
  - Further evaluation by an otolaryngologist may be necessary for children with chronic or complicated cases.

COMPLICATIONS

- *Infection:* Risk of secondary infection if the ear canal is not properly cared for after removal
- *Ear canal injury:* Potential for injury to the ear canal or tympanic membrane if the procedure is not performed correctly
- *Pain:* Persistent pain may require further evaluation and management.
- *Vertigo:* Improper irrigation techniques, such as using cold water, can cause dizziness or vertigo.

PREVENTION

- *Safe ear care:* Educate caregivers and children about safe ear care practices, including avoiding the use of cotton swabs or other objects in the ear.
- *Regular ear hygiene:* Recommend the use of ear drops or cerumenolytic agents periodically to prevent cerumen buildup.

CONCLUSION

The management of cerumen impaction in children involves safe and effective removal of the impacted earwax to relieve symptoms and restore normal ear function. Proper technique, aftercare, and caregiver education are crucial for successful outcomes and preventing complications.

FURTHER READING

1. Aaron K, Cooper TE, Warner L, Burton MJ. Ear drops for the removal of ear wax. Cochrane Cochrane Database Syst Rev. 2018;7(7):CD012171.
2. Clegg AJ, Loveman E, Gospodarevskaya E, Harris P, Bird A, Bryant J, et al. The safety and effectiveness of different methods of earwax removal: a systematic review and economic evaluation. Health Technol Assess. 2010;14(28):1-192
3. Hand C, Harvey I. The effectiveness of topical preparations for the treatment of earwax: a systematic review. Br J Gen Pract. 2004;54:(508)862-7.
4. Memel D, Langley C, Watkins C, Laue B, Birchall M, Bachmann M. Effectiveness of ear syringing in general practice: a randomized controlled trial and patients' experiences. Br J Gen Pract. 2002;52(484):906-1
5. Oron Y, Zwecker-Lazar I, Levy D, Kreitler S, Roth Y. Cerumen removal: comparison of cerumenolytic agents and effect on cognition among the elderly. Arch Gerontol Geriatr. 2011;52(2):228-32.

CHAPTER 6

Procedure for Management of Ocular Foreign Body in Children

INTRODUCTION

An ocular foreign body is a common pediatric emergency that involves the presence of a foreign object in the eye. Prompt and careful removal is essential to prevent complications such as infection, corneal abrasion, or vision impairment. This chapter outlines the procedure for managing an ocular foreign body in children.

INDICATIONS

- Observation or suspicion of a foreign body in the eye
- Symptoms such as eye pain, redness, tearing, photophobia, or a sensation of something in the eye
- Visible foreign body on the ocular surface or under the eyelids

CONTRAINDICATIONS

- Suspected penetration or perforation of the globe
- Foreign body embedded in the cornea or deeper structures of the eye
- Chemical burns requiring immediate specialized care
- Significant trauma to the eye or orbit requiring ophthalmologic consultation

EQUIPMENT AND SUPPLIES

- Sterile gloves
- Sterile saline solution or eye wash
- Cotton-tipped applicators
- Irrigation syringe with sterile saline (if necessary)
- Magnifying glass or loupe
- Bright light source or slit lamp (if available)
- Sterile gauze pads
- Fluorescein strips and blue light (for corneal abrasion assessment)
- Topical anesthetic eye drops (e.g., proparacaine)
- Small forceps (e.g., jeweler's forceps) or foreign body removal spud
- Antibiotic eye drops or ointment
- Analgesics (if necessary)
- Eye patch (optional)
- Personal protective equipment (PPE)

PREPARATION

- *Explain the procedure:*
  - Inform the child (if age-appropriate) and caregivers about the situation, the procedure, its purpose, and what to expect.
  - Obtain informed consent from the caregivers.
- *Positioning:* Position the child comfortably, ideally seated or lying down with the head supported. Use an assistant if necessary to help hold the child still during the procedure.

PROCEDURE STEPS

1. *Initial assessment:*
   a. Conduct a thorough history and physical examination to determine

the type and location of the foreign body.

b. Inspect the eye using a bright light source or slit lamp to visualize the foreign body.

2. *Preparation:* Instill topical anesthetic eye drops to minimize discomfort during the procedure.
3. *Removal techniques:*
   a. *Irrigation method* ***(Fig. 1)****:*
      i. *Indications:* Suitable for small, loose foreign bodies on the conjunctiva or cornea
      ii. *Procedure:*
         - Fill an irrigation syringe/bottle with sterile saline solution.
         - Gently irrigate the eye, directing the saline from the inner canthus (near the nose) to the outer canthus to flush out the foreign body.
         - Use a catch basin or towel to collect the saline and foreign body.

   b. *Cotton-tipped applicator method* ***(Figs. 2A to E)****:*
      i. *Preparation:* Ensure adequate visualization of the foreign body using a magnifying glass or loupe.

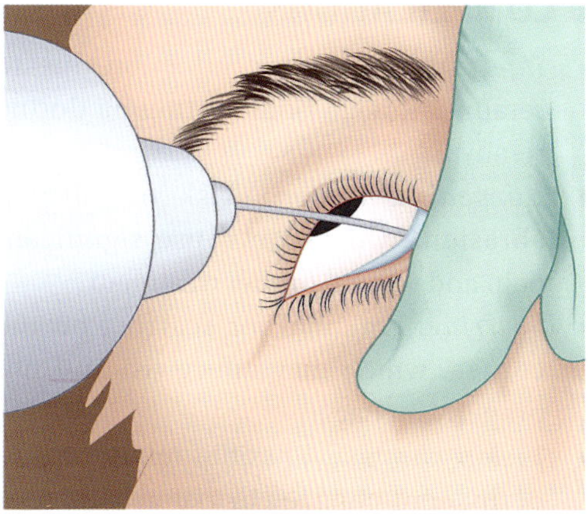

Fig. 1: Eye irrigation with squeeze bottle.

      ii. *Procedure:*
         - Moisten the tip of a sterile cotton-tipped applicator with saline.
         - Gently touch the foreign body with the moistened applicator and lift it away from the ocular surface.
         - Avoid applying excessive pressure to prevent corneal abrasion.

   c. *Forceps or spud method:*
      i. *Preparation:* If the foreign body is embedded or difficult to remove with irrigation or a cotton-tipped applicator, use small forceps or a foreign body removal spud.
      ii. *Procedure:*
         - Using jeweler's forceps or a spud, carefully grasp or dislodge the foreign body.
         - Ensure steady hands and a cooperative patient to avoid further injury.

4. *Postprocedure care:*
   a. *Inspection:* Re-examine the eye to ensure complete removal of the foreign body.
   b. *Fluorescein staining:* Instill a fluorescein strip into the eye and examine with a blue light to check for corneal abrasions.
   c. *Observation:* Monitor the child for any signs of discomfort, persistent foreign body sensation, or complications.

AFTERCARE

- *Monitoring:*
  - Observe the child for signs of eye pain, discharge, or vision changes postremoval.
  - Provide instructions to caregivers on monitoring for any delayed complications.

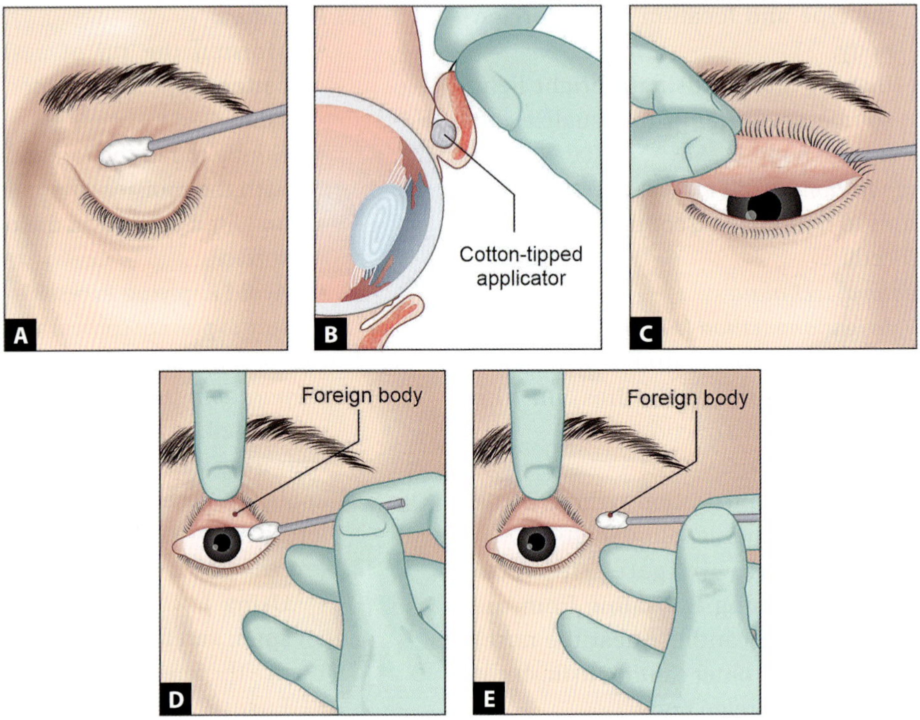

Figs. 2A to E: Conjunctival foreign body removal. (A) A cotton-tipped applicator is placed above the upper lid; (B) Lid eversion with the patient looking downward; (C) Push down on the applicator to reveal a foreign body hidden under the tarsal plate; (D and E) The moistened applicator touches the foreign body, lifting it away.

- *Medication:*
  - Prescribe antibiotic eye drops or ointment to prevent infection.
  - Administer appropriate analgesics for pain relief if necessary.
- *Follow-up:*
  - Schedule a follow-up appointment with an ophthalmologist to ensure complete resolution and healing of the ocular surface.
  - Further evaluation may be necessary if there are recurrent episodes of foreign body sensation or eye discomfort.
- *Education:*
  - Educate caregivers and children about the risks of inserting or exposing the eyes to foreign objects.
  - Encourage protective eyewear during activities that pose a risk of eye injury.

COMPLICATIONS

- *Infection:* Secondary infection due to retained foreign body or trauma during removal
- *Corneal abrasion:* Risk of corneal abrasion, which can cause significant pain and require further treatment
- *Scarring:* Potential for scarring on the cornea, which may affect vision if not properly managed
- *Vision changes:* Possible temporary or permanent changes in vision if there is significant trauma or infection.

PREVENTION

- *Protective eyewear:* Encourage the use of protective eyewear during activities that pose a risk of eye injury.
- *Education:* Teach children about the dangers of inserting objects into their eyes and the importance of eye safety.
- *Supervision:* Ensure close supervision of young children during playtime, especially when handling small objects.

CONCLUSION

The management of ocular foreign bodies in children involves prompt and careful removal to prevent complications. Proper technique, adequate aftercare, and education are crucial for successful outcomes and preventing recurrence.

FURTHER READING

1. Ambikkumar A, Arthurs B, El-Hadad C. Corneal foreign bodies. CMAJ. 2022 21;194(11):E419.
2. Jones G. Foreign bodies in the eye. Accid Emerg Nurs. 1998;6(2):66-9.
3. Marsden J. Care of patients with minor eye trauma. Emerg Nurse. 1998;6(7):10-3.
4. Marsden J. Ophthalmic trauma in the emergency department. Accid Emerg Nurs. 2002;10(3):136-42
5. Owens JK, Scibilia J, Hezoucky N. Corneal foreign bodies—first aid, treatment, and outcomes. Skills review for an occupational health setting. AAOHN J. 2001;49(5):226-30.

CHAPTER 7

Procedure for Eye Drop Administration in Children

INTRODUCTION

Administering eye drops to children can be challenging due to their natural aversion to the procedure. Proper technique and a calm approach are essential to ensure effective delivery of medication and minimize discomfort or distress.

INDICATIONS

- Prescription of eye drops for conditions such as conjunctivitis, allergies, infections, or other ocular conditions
- Prophylactic or therapeutic use of eye drops postsurgery or injury

CONTRAINDICATIONS

- Known hypersensitivity or allergy to the prescribed eye drop medication
- Presence of eye trauma requiring specialist intervention

EQUIPMENT AND SUPPLIES

- Sterile gloves (optional, for personal protection)
- Eye drop medication
- Clean tissue or cotton pad
- Personal protective equipment (PPE) if required

PREPARATION

- *Explain the procedure:*
  - Inform the child (if age-appropriate) and caregivers about the need for eye drops, their purpose, and what to expect during administration.
  - Obtain informed consent from the caregivers.
- *Positioning:*
  - Position the child comfortably, ideally lying down or reclining with their head supported.
  - Ensure the child's head is slightly tilted back and the eyes are looking up.

PROCEDURE STEPS

1. *Initial assessment:*
   a. Wash your hands thoroughly with soap and water.
   b. Ensure the eye drop bottle is at room temperature to minimize discomfort.
2. *Preparation of the medication:*
   a. Check the eye drop bottle for the correct medication and expiration date.
   b. Shake the bottle gently if the medication requires it (check the label for instructions).
3. *Instilling the eye drops:*
   a. For older children (cooperative) **(Fig. 1)**:
      i. *Procedure:*
         - Ask the child to lie down or tilt their head back while looking up.
         - Gently pull down the lower eyelid with one hand to create a small pocket.
         - Hold the eye drop bottle with the other hand, resting the

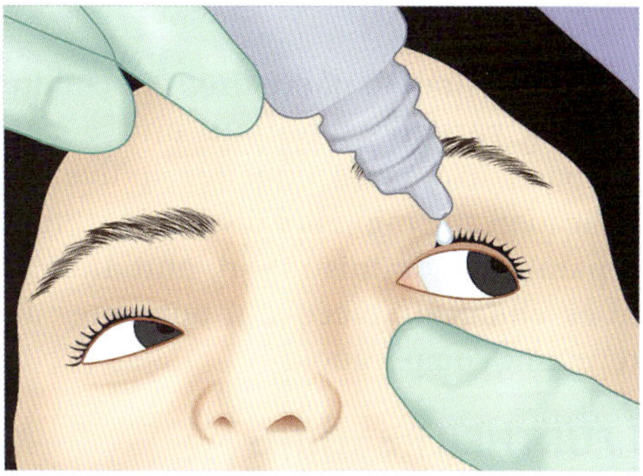

Fig. 1: Eye drop administration in a cooperative child.

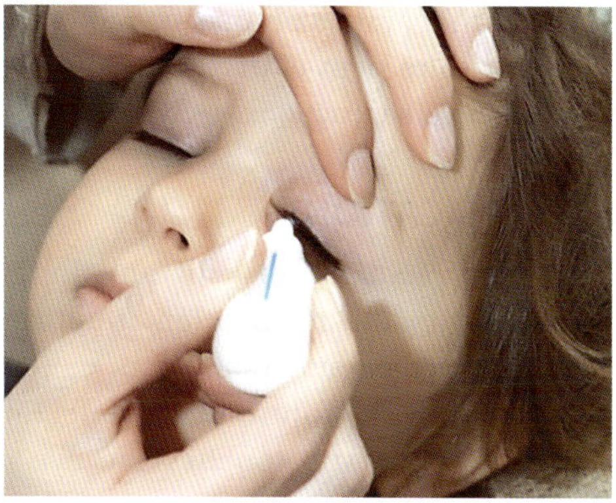

Fig. 2: Eye drop administration in an uncooperative child.

hand on the child's forehead for stability.
- Squeeze the prescribed number of drops into the pocket formed by the lower eyelid, being careful not to touch the eye or eyelashes with the dropper tip.
- Release the lower eyelid and ask the child to close their eyes gently for a minute or two to allow the medication to spread evenly.
- Use a clean tissue or cotton pad to wipe away any excess liquid around the eye.

b. For younger children or infants (uncooperative) **(Fig. 2)**:

i. *Procedure:*
- Have the child lie down with their head stabilized, possibly with the help of a caregiver.
- Hold the child's head gently but firmly with one hand.
- With the other hand, pull down the lower eyelid to create a small pocket.
- Quickly and accurately squeeze the prescribed number of drops into the pocket.
- If the child is unable to keep their eyes open, place the drops at the inner corner of the closed eyelids. When the child opens their eyes, the drops will flow into the eye.
- Allow the child to close their eyes gently, then wipe away any excess liquid with a clean tissue or cotton pad.

POSTADMINISTRATION CARE

- *Monitoring:*
  - Observe the child for any immediate adverse reactions, such as redness, swelling, or discomfort.
  - Provide instructions to caregivers on monitoring for signs of an allergic reaction or worsening symptoms.
- *Cleaning:*
  - Clean the tip of the eye drop bottle with a clean tissue after use to prevent contamination.
  - Replace the cap on the bottle tightly and store it as directed, usually in a cool, dry place.
- *Follow-up:*
  - Schedule follow-up appointments as necessary to monitor the child's response to treatment.

- Further evaluation may be required if there are signs of persistent infection or adverse reactions.

COMPLICATIONS

- *Allergic reaction:* Risk of an allergic reaction to the medication, requiring prompt medical attention
- *Infection:* Risk of introducing infection if the dropper tip touches the eye or surrounding areas
- *Discomfort:* Temporary stinging or burning sensation after administration

PREVENTION

- *Hygiene:* Ensure proper hand hygiene before and after administration.
- *Avoid contamination:* Prevent the dropper tip from touching any surface, including the eye, to avoid contamination.
- *Correct storage:* Store eye drops according to manufacturer's instructions to maintain efficacy and safety.

CONCLUSION

The administration of eye drops in children requires careful technique and a calm approach to ensure effective delivery of medication and minimize discomfort. Proper preparation, administration, and aftercare are essential for successful outcomes and preventing complications.

FURTHER READING

1. Eye drops: How to give eye drops to a child: https://www.aboutkidshealth.ca/eye-drops-how-to-give-eye-drops-to-a-child
2. How to give your child eye drops: https://www.gosh.nhs.uk/conditions-and-treatments/medicines-information/how-give-your-child-eye-drops/
3. How to Put in Eye Drops: https://www.aao.org/eye-health/treatments/how-to-put-in-eye-drops
4. Scared of Eye Drops? Tips for Anxious Kids and Adults: https://www.aao.org/eye-health/tips-prevention/tips-eyedrop-anxiety-scared-kids-adults
5. Tips to Make Eye Drops Easier for Kids and Parents: https://health.choc.org/tips-make-eye-drops-easier-kids-parents/

CHAPTER 8

Procedure for Management of Paraphimosis in Children

INTRODUCTION

Paraphimosis is a urological emergency where the foreskin, once retracted behind the glans penis, cannot be returned to its normal position **(Fig. 1)**. This condition can lead to constriction, pain, and compromised blood flow to the glans penis, requiring immediate intervention to prevent serious complications such as ischemia or necrosis.

INDICATIONS

- Retracted foreskin that cannot be returned to its original position
- Swelling, pain, and discoloration of the glans penis
- Signs of compromised blood flow such as ischemia or necrosis.

CONTRAINDICATIONS

- Severe infection or ulceration, requiring surgical intervention
- Suspected traumatic injury to the penis, needing specialist care.

EQUIPMENT AND SUPPLIES

- Sterile gloves
- Antiseptic solution (e.g., povidone-iodine or chlorhexidine)
- Lubricant (e.g., water-soluble jelly)
- Sterile gauze pads
- Local anesthetic (e.g., lidocaine gel)
- Syringe and needle (for local anesthesia)
- Osmotic agents (e.g., granulated sugar or 50% dextrose solution)
- Cold compress or ice pack
- Hemostatic agents (if necessary)

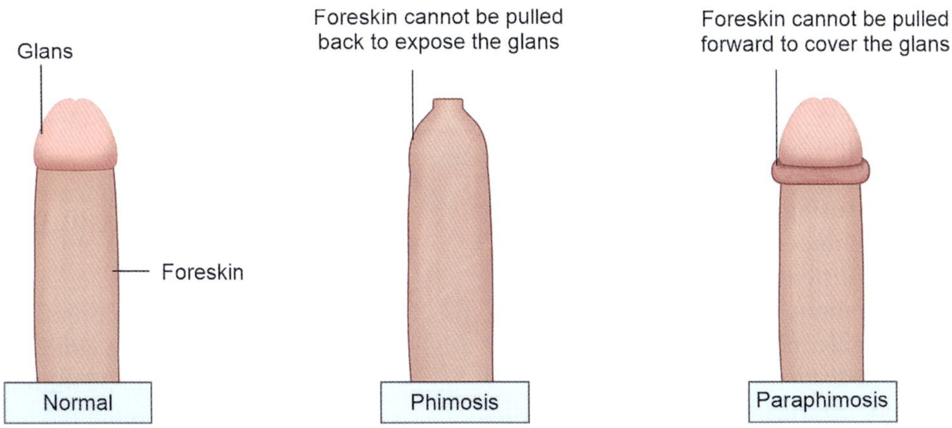

Fig. 1: Phimosis and paraphimosis.

- Small hemostat (if necessary)
- Personal protective equipment (PPE).

PREPARATION

- *Explain the procedure:*
    - Inform the child (if age-appropriate) and caregivers about the condition, the procedure, its purpose, and what to expect.
    - Obtain informed consent from the caregivers.
- *Positioning:* Position the child in a comfortable, supine position with the genital area exposed and supported.
- *Pain management:* Administer an appropriate analgesic or sedative if necessary to alleviate pain and anxiety.

PROCEDURE STEPS

1. *Initial assessment:*
    a. Conduct a thorough history and physical examination to confirm the diagnosis of paraphimosis.
    b. Inspect the penis for signs of ischemia, necrosis, or severe swelling.
2. *Cleansing:* Clean the genital area with an antiseptic solution to reduce the risk of infection.
3. *Reduction techniques:*
    a. *Manual reduction* **(Fig. 2)**:
        i. *Preparation:* Apply a topical anesthetic (e.g., lidocaine gel) to the affected area and allow it to take effect.
        ii. *Compression:* Gently compress the glans penis with your fingers or using sterile gauze for several minutes to reduce swelling.
        iii. *Lubrication:* Apply a generous amount of lubricant to the glans penis and foreskin.
        iv. *Reduction:*
            - Using both thumbs, place them on the glans penis while your fingers wrap around the shaft of the penis.
            - Apply gentle, steady pressure to push the glans back into the foreskin while simultaneously pulling the foreskin forward over the glans.

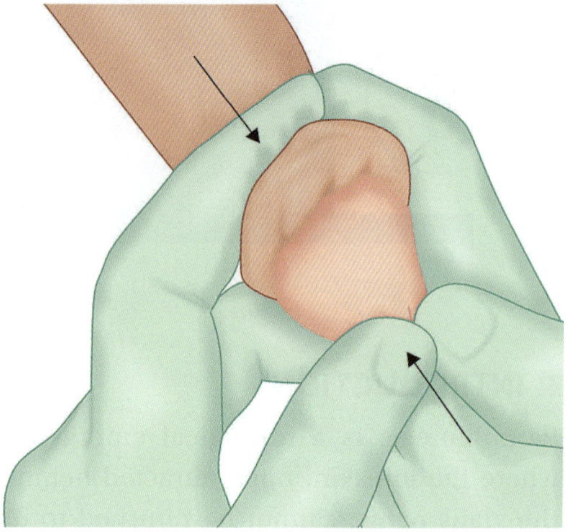

Fig. 2: Manual reduction of paraphimosis by counter pressure between thumbs and fingers.

    b. *Osmotic agents:*
        i. *Indications:* Useful for reducing swelling before manual reduction
        ii. *Procedure:*
            - Apply granulated sugar or a gauze pad soaked in 50% dextrose solution to the glans penis.
            - Leave in place for 30 minutes to 1 hour to help reduce edema through osmotic action.
            - Follow with manual reduction as described above.
    c. *Cold compress:*
        i. *Indications:* It helps to reduce swelling.
        ii. *Procedure:*
            - Apply a cold compress or ice pack wrapped in a cloth to the glans penis for 10–15 minutes.
            - Follow with manual reduction as described above.

4. *Postreduction care:*
   a. *Inspection:* Re-examine the penis to ensure the foreskin has returned to its normal position and assess for any residual swelling or signs of ischemia.
   b. *Observation:* Monitor the child for any signs of discomfort, pain, or recurrence of paraphimosis.

AFTERCARE

- *Monitoring:*
  - Observe the child for signs of pain, swelling, or recurrence of paraphimosis postreduction.
  - Provide instructions to caregivers on monitoring for any delayed complications.
- *Wound care:*
  - Advise on proper genital hygiene to prevent infections.
  - If there are minor abrasions or irritation, recommend the application of a mild antiseptic ointment.
- *Activity modification:* Advise the child to avoid activities that may result in trauma to the genital area until fully healed.
- *Follow-up:* Schedule a follow-up appointment with a healthcare provider to ensure complete resolution and evaluate for any underlying conditions such as phimosis.
- *Education:*
  - Educate caregivers on the importance of gentle handling of the foreskin.
  - Explain the potential need for circumcision or other surgical interventions if recurrent episodes occur or if phimosis is present.

COMPLICATIONS

- *Recurrence:* Risk of recurrent paraphimosis, requiring further medical or surgical intervention.
- *Infection:* Secondary infection due to minor abrasions or trauma during reduction.
- *Ischemia/necrosis:* Prolonged paraphimosis can lead to compromised blood flow and tissue necrosis, necessitating urgent surgical management.
- *Pain and discomfort:* Residual pain or discomfort may occur postreduction, requiring analgesia.

PREVENTION

- *Proper foreskin care:* Educate caregivers and older children on the proper retraction and replacement of the foreskin during hygiene practices.
- *Avoid forceful retraction:* Advise against forceful retraction of the foreskin in young children.
- *Regular monitoring:* Monitor for signs of phimosis and seek medical advice if difficulties in retracting the foreskin are noticed.

CONCLUSION

The management of paraphimosis in children involves prompt and careful reduction to prevent serious complications. Proper technique, postoperative care, and caregiver education are crucial for successful outcomes and preventing recurrence.

FURTHER READING

1. Chambers P. Paraphimosis reduction. In: Textbook of Pediatric Emergency Procedures, 2nd ed, King C, Henretig FM (Eds), Lippincott, Williams & Wilkins, Philadelphia 2008. p.904.
2. Choe JM. Paraphimosis: current treatment options. Am Fam Physician 2000;62 (12):2623-6, 2628.
3. McCollough M, Sharieff GQ. Abdominal surgical emergencies in infants and young children. Emerg Med Clin North Am. 2003;21(4):909-35.
4. Reynard JM, Barua JM. Reduction of paraphimosis the simple way—the Dundee technique. BJU Int. 1999;83(7):859-60.
5. Vunda A, Lacroix LE, Schneider F, Manzano S, Gervaix A. Videos in clinical medicine. Reduction of paraphimosis in boys. N Engl J Med. 2013;368(13):e16.

CHAPTER 9

Procedure for Zipper Injury in Children

INTRODUCTION

Zipper injuries are a common pediatric emergency, particularly involving the genital area. These injuries can cause significant pain, distress, and potential complications if not managed appropriately. Prompt and effective management is crucial to relieve pain and prevent further injury.

EPIDEMIOLOGY

Zipper injuries predominantly affect boys, commonly involving the foreskin or shaft of the penis. Girls may also sustain injuries, typically involving the labia. The majority of these incidents occur in children under the age of 10.

CLINICAL PRESENTATION

Symptoms

- *Pain:* Acute pain at the site of injury
- *Swelling and bruising:* Localized swelling and possible bruising of the affected area.
- *Bleeding:* Minor to moderate bleeding may occur.
- *Entrapment:* The skin or genital tissue is caught within the zipper mechanism.

History and Examination

- Obtain a detailed history of the incident, including the type of clothing involved and the duration of entrapment.
- Perform a gentle and thorough examination to assess the extent of injury and identify the precise location of the entrapment.

DIAGNOSIS

Clinical Diagnosis

Based on history and physical examination, visual inspection reveals the entrapment and associated tissue injury.

MANAGEMENT

General Principles

- *Pain relief:* Administer analgesics to alleviate pain and distress.
- *Calm environment:* Keep the child calm and still to prevent further injury.

Specific Management

- *Preparation:*
  - *Explain the procedure:* Explain the procedure to the child (if age-appropriate) and caregivers, emphasizing the steps to minimize anxiety.
  - *Positioning:* Position the child comfortably, ensuring easy access to the injury site.
- *Analgesia and anesthesia:*
  - Administer age-appropriate analgesia (e.g., oral ibuprofen or acetaminophen).

- Topical anesthetic cream (e.g., lidocaine) can be applied to the area to provide localized pain relief.
- In some cases, sedation may be necessary, particularly if the child is highly distressed or uncooperative.

▪ *Removal techniques:*
- *Cutting the zipper* **(Figs. 1 and 2)**:
  - *Tools needed:* Small wire cutters or heavy-duty scissors
  - *Procedure:*
    - Carefully cut through the median bar of the zipper or the zipper's teeth adjacent to the entrapped skin.
    - Gently separate the zipper halves to release the trapped tissue.
- *Mineral oil or lubricant method:*
  - *Tools needed:* Mineral oil, petroleum jelly, or a similar lubricant.
  - *Procedure:*
    - Apply a generous amount of lubricant to the zipper and entrapped tissue.
    - Allow the lubricant to penetrate for a few minutes.
    - Gently attempt to slide the zipper mechanism backward to free the trapped tissue.
- *Screwdriver method (for metal zippers):*
  - *Tools needed:* Small flat-head screwdriver
  - *Procedure:*
    - Insert the tip of the screwdriver into the space between the zipper slider and the trapped tissue.
    - Carefully twist the screwdriver to widen the gap, allowing the tissue to be freed.

▪ *Postremoval care:*
- *Assessment:* Re-examine the area for any residual injury, bleeding, or signs of infection.

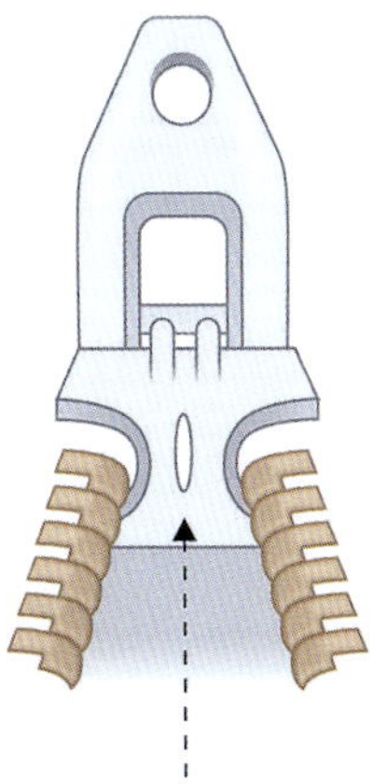

Fig. 1: Penile zipper injury management. If the penile skin is caught in the mobile zipper head, apply local anesthesia such as prilocaine or lignocaine. Use the wire cutter to cut through the median bar of the zipper fastener. The front and back plates of the fastener will then fall apart allowing the zipper to be separated.

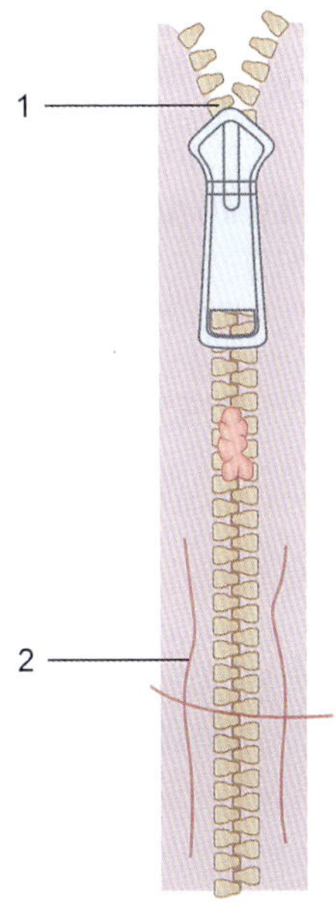

Fig. 2: Penile zipper injury management. If the penile skin is caught between the interlocking teeth of the zipper, cut the zipper inferior to the entrapment (at point 2) site to enable two interlocking rows of the teeth to be gently pulled apart releasing the skin.

    - *Wound care:* Cleanse the area with a mild antiseptic solution and apply a sterile dressing if needed.
    - *Pain management:* Continue pain relief as required.
- *Complications:*
    - Monitor for potential complications such as infection, tissue necrosis, or significant bleeding.
    - Advise caregivers on signs of infection to watch for, such as increased redness, swelling, or discharge.

PREVENTION

- *Education:* Educate parents and caregivers about the risks of zipper injuries and encourage supervision during dressing.
- *Safety measures:* Recommend clothing with protective fabric behind zippers or alternatives such as Velcro or elastic waistbands for younger children.

CONCLUSION

Management of zipper injuries in children involves prompt pain relief, careful extraction of entrapped tissue, and appropriate aftercare to prevent complications. Educating caregivers on preventive measures can reduce the incidence of these distressing injuries.

FURTHER READING

1. Fein JA, Zderic SA. Management of zipper injuries. In: Textbook of Pediatric Emergency Procedures, 2nd ed, King C, Henretig FM (Eds), Lippincott, Williams & Wilkins, Philadelphia, PA, USA 2008. p.908.
2. Kanegaye JT, Schonfeld N. Penile zipper entrapment: a simple and less threatening approach using mineral oil. Pediatr Emerg Care. 1993;9(2):90-1.
3. Maurice MJ, Cherullo EE. A novel, nonoperative treatment for delayed penile zipper injury. Am J Emerg Med. 2013;31(2):419-20.
4. Oquist M, Buck L, Michel K, Ouellette L, Emery M, Bush C. Comparative analysis of five methods of emergency zipper release by experienced versus novice clinicians. Am J Emerg Med. 2017;35(5):783-4.
5. Raveenthiran V. Releasing of zipper-entrapped foreskin: a novel nonsurgical technique. Pediatr Emerg Care. 2007;23:(7) 463-4.

CHAPTER 10

Procedure for Detorsion of Testes in Children

INTRODUCTION

Testicular torsion is a surgical emergency where the spermatic cord twists, cutting off the blood supply to the testicle **(Figs. 1A and B)**. Prompt diagnosis and intervention are crucial to salvage the testicle and prevent long-term complications such as testicular atrophy or infertility. Manual detorsion is a temporizing measure that can relieve pain and restore blood flow until definitive surgical management can be performed.

INDICATIONS

- Acute onset of scrotal pain and swelling, typically in a child or adolescent
- High suspicion of testicular torsion based on clinical presentation and physical examination
- Immediate intervention is required while awaiting surgical exploration.

CONTRAINDICATIONS

- Delay in definitive surgical management
- Suspected or confirmed nonviable testicle
- Signs of infection or abscess in the scrotal area.

EQUIPMENT AND SUPPLIES

- Sterile gloves
- Analgesics (e.g., intravenous or oral pain medication)

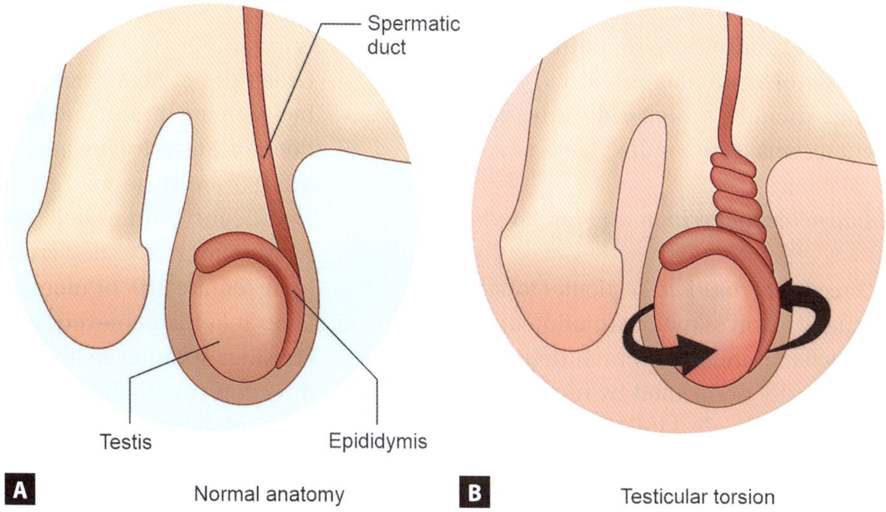

Figs. 1A and B: Torsion of testes.

- Sedation (if necessary, based on the child's anxiety and pain level)
- Doppler ultrasound (if available) to confirm diagnosis and assess blood flow
- Surgical consultation and preparation for possible emergency surgery.

PREPARATION

- *Explain the procedure:*
  - Inform the child (if age-appropriate) and caregivers about the condition, the need for immediate intervention, and the procedure itself.
  - Obtain informed consent from the caregivers.
- *Positioning:* Position the child supine with the scrotum exposed and supported.
- *Pain management:*
  - Administer appropriate analgesics to alleviate pain.
  - Sedation may be considered in highly anxious or uncooperative children to facilitate the procedure.

PROCEDURE STEPS

1. *Initial assessment:* Conduct a thorough physical examination to confirm the diagnosis of testicular torsion. Typical findings include a high-riding testicle, absent cremasteric reflex, and severe scrotal pain.
2. *Manual detorsion technique* ***(Figs. 2A and B):***
   a. *Direction of rotation:* Testicular torsion usually involves medial rotation of the testicle. Therefore, manual detorsion is typically performed by rotating the affected testicle laterally (outward, away from the midline). This is commonly described as the "open book" technique.

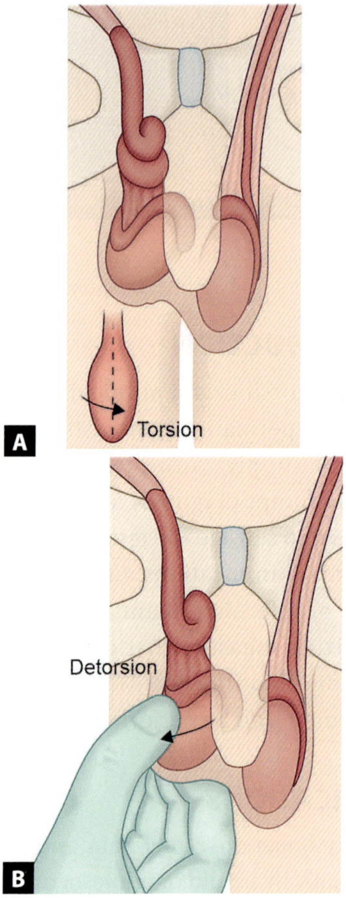

Figs. 2A and B: Manual detorsion of testes.

   b. *Procedure:*
      i. Grasp the affected testicle gently between the thumb and forefinger.
      ii. Rotate the testicle outward (laterally) in a 180° arc. If the child experiences significant pain relief, continue rotating until the testicle is untwisted (may require 360° or more).
      iii. If no relief is achieved after 180°, consider rotating in the opposite direction (medially), as some torsions may involve atypical rotation.
   c. *Observation:* After attempting detorsion, assess the child for pain relief and monitor the testicle for changes in

position and blood flow. Use Doppler ultrasound, if available, to confirm the restoration of blood flow.

3. *Confirmation and further management:*
   a. *Successful detorsion:* If manual detorsion is successful and blood flow is restored, the pain should significantly decrease. Immediate surgical consultation is still necessary to perform orchiopexy (fixation of the testicle) to prevent recurrence.
   b. *Unsuccessful detorsion or recurrence:* If manual detorsion is unsuccessful or if there is any doubt about the adequacy of detorsion, immediate surgical exploration and detorsion are required.

POSTPROCEDURE CARE

- *Monitoring:*
  - Continuously monitor the child for signs of pain relief and restore blood flow to the testicle.
  - Prepare for emergency surgical exploration regardless of the success of manual detorsion.
- *Definitive surgical management:* Surgical exploration and orchiopexy of both testicles are necessary to prevent recurrence and to address any potential complications from the torsion.
- *Pain management:*
  - Continue administering pain relief as needed.
  - Provide supportive care and reassurance to the child and caregivers.
- *Education and follow-up:*
  - Educate caregivers about the signs and symptoms of testicular torsion and the importance of seeking immediate medical attention if symptoms recur.
  - Schedule follow-up appointments to monitor recovery and assess testicular function.

COMPLICATIONS

- *Recurrence:* High risk of recurrent torsion without surgical fixation
- *Testicular atrophy:* Prolonged torsion can lead to irreversible damage and atrophy of the testicle.
- *Infertility:* Potential long-term complication if both testicles are affected or if there is significant damage.

PREVENTION

- *Education:* Educate caregivers and adolescents about the importance of early recognition and prompt treatment of testicular pain.
- *Prophylactic orchiopexy:* Consider prophylactic fixation in patients with a history of torsion or anatomical predisposition.

CONCLUSION

Manual detorsion of the testes is an emergency procedure that can provide immediate relief and restore blood flow in cases of testicular torsion. However, definitive surgical management is crucial to prevent recurrence and ensure the long-term viability of the testicle.

FURTHER READING

1. Dias Filho AC, Oliveira Rodrigues R, Riccetto CL, Oliveira PG. Improving Organ Salvage in Testicular Torsion: Comparative Study of Patients Undergoing vs Not Undergoing Preoperative Manual Detorsion. J Urol. 2017;197(3 Pt 1):811-17
2. Lukosiute-Urboniene A, Nekrosius D, Dekeryte I, Kilda A, Malcius D. Clinical risk

factors for testicular torsion and a warning against falsely reassuring ultrasound scans: a 10-year single-centre experience.Emerg Med J. 2023;40(2):134-9. 2022 Dec 16.
3. Nelson CP, Williams JF, Bloom DA. The cremasteric reflex: a useful but imperfect sign in testicular torsion. J Pediatr Surg. 2003;38(8):1248-9.
4. Scheier E. Manual detorsion in pediatric testicular torsion: A narrative review of the literature. Urologia. 2024;91(3):628-31.
5. Weiss DA, Jacobstein CR. Genitourinary emergencies. In: Fleisher and Ludwig's Textbook of Pediatric Emergency Medicine, 7th ed, Shaw KN, Bachur RG (Eds), Wolters Kluwer, Philadelphia 2016. p.1353.

CHAPTER 11

Manual Reduction of Obstructed Inguinal Hernia

INTRODUCTION

An inguinal hernia occurs when a portion of the intestine protrudes through an opening in the abdominal muscles. While many inguinal hernias are reducible, some may become obstructed, meaning that the protruding intestine becomes trapped and cannot easily be pushed back into the abdomen. This condition is particularly concerning as it can lead to strangulation of the intestine, cutting off its blood supply and resulting in tissue death. The manual reduction of an obstructed inguinal hernia is a delicate procedure that requires specific techniques and considerations to ensure patient safety and successful resolution of the obstruction.

ANATOMY OF INGUINAL HERNIA

To understand the manual reduction process, it is essential to have a clear grasp of the anatomy involved. The inguinal canal is a passage in the anterior abdominal wall, which in men conveys the spermatic cord and in women the round ligament of the uterus. An inguinal hernia occurs when abdominal contents, such as the intestines, protrude through this canal. Obstruction occurs when these contents cannot return to the abdominal cavity due to swelling or constriction at the hernia neck.

INDICATIONS FOR MANUAL REDUCTION

Manual reduction is indicated in cases where the hernia is obstructed but not strangulated, as indicated by the absence of signs such as severe pain, fever, or changes in skin color over the hernia site. Manual reduction should be considered a temporary measure to relieve symptoms before definitive surgical repair can be performed.

CONTRAINDICATIONS

Manual reduction is contraindicated if there is suspicion of strangulation or if the patient shows signs of peritonitis, including severe abdominal pain, tenderness, and systemic signs of infection such as fever and tachycardia. In such cases, immediate surgical intervention is required.

TECHNIQUE OF MANUAL REDUCTION (FIGS. 1A TO C)

- *Preparation:*
    - Ensure the patient is in a comfortable supine position.
    - Provide adequate analgesia or sedation as necessary to relieve discomfort and reduce muscle tension.
    - Apply warm compresses to the hernia site to help relax the abdominal muscles.

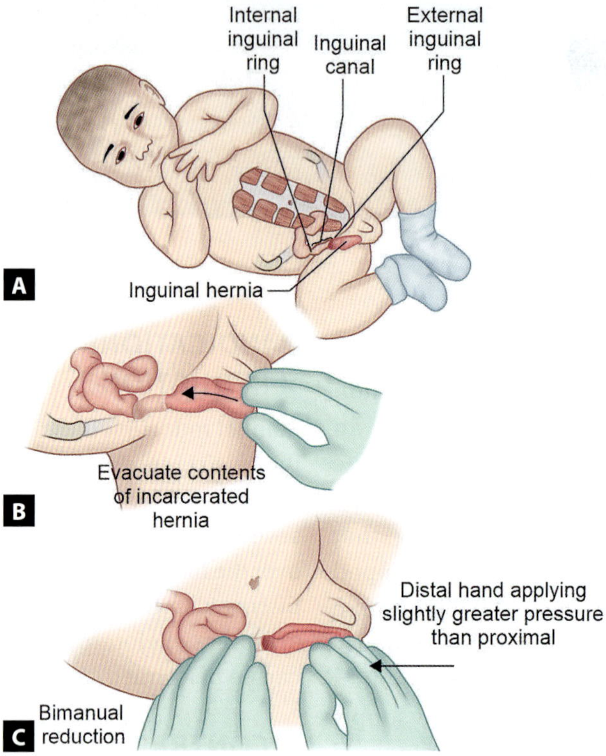

Figs. 1A to C: Manual reduction of inguinal hernia.

- *Reduction process:*
  - *Gentle pressure:* Begin by applying gentle, steady pressure over the hernia with the palm of the hand. The pressure should be directed upward and inward toward the inguinal canal.
  - *Taxis maneuver:* Using the other hand, manipulate the proximal part of the hernia sac to guide the intestine back into the abdominal cavity. The movements should be smooth and avoid any jerky or forceful actions.
  - *Slow and steady:* Maintain steady pressure for several minutes. If the reduction is not successful within a few minutes, re-evaluate the situation. Prolonged or forceful attempts can cause additional injury.
  - *Successful reduction:* Successful reduction is usually indicated by a softening of the hernia mass and a palpable movement of the herniated contents back into the abdomen. The patient may also report immediate relief from pain and discomfort.

POSTREDUCTION CARE

After successful reduction, monitor the patient closely for signs of recurrence or complications. Advise the patient to avoid activities that increase intra-abdominal pressure, such as heavy lifting or straining. Schedule a follow-up appointment for surgical repair, as the hernia is likely to recur without definitive treatment.

COMPLICATIONS

Complications of manual reduction include:

- *Failure of reduction:* Inability to reduce the hernia indicates possible strangulation or irreducibility due to adhesions.
- *Bowel injury:* Forceful reduction can cause bowel injury or perforation.
- *Recurrence:* Even with successful reduction, there is a high risk of recurrence, necessitating surgical intervention.

CONCLUSION

Manual reduction of an obstructed inguinal hernia is a critical skill in acute care settings. While it can provide temporary relief and prevent strangulation, it is essential to follow appropriate techniques and recognize contraindications to avoid complications. Ultimately, surgical repair remains the definitive treatment to prevent recurrence and ensure patient safety.

FURTHER READING

1. Abdulhai SA, Glenn IC, Ponsky TA. Incarcerated Pediatric Hernias. Surg Clin North Am. 2017;97(1):129-45.
2. Gahukamble DB, Khamage AS. Early versus delayed repair of reduced incarcerated inguinal hernias in the pediatric population. J Pediatr Surg. 1996;31(9):1218-20.
3. Lau ST, Lee YH, Caty MG. Current management of hernias and hydroceles. Semin Pediatr Surg. 2007;16 (1):50-7.
4. Moss RL, Hatch EI Jr. Inguinal hernia repair in early infancy. Am J Surg 1991;161(5):596-9.
5. Stringer MD, Higgins M, Capps SN, Holmes SJ. Irreducible inguinal hernia. Br J Surg 1991;78(4):504-5.
6. Stylianos S, Jacir NN, Harris BH. Incarceration of inguinal hernia in infants prior to elective repair. J Pediatr Surg. 1993;28(4):582-3.

CHAPTER 12

Procedure for Rectal Prolapse Reduction in Children

INTRODUCTION

Rectal prolapse reduction is a procedure to manually reposition the prolapsed rectal tissue back into its normal anatomical position. This procedure is often necessary to alleviate discomfort and prevent complications such as edema, ulceration, and strangulation of the prolapsed tissue **(Fig. 1)**.

INDICATIONS

- Acute rectal prolapse with visible protrusion of rectal tissue
- Prolapse, causing significant discomfort or pain
- Prolapse that does not spontaneously reduce

CONTRAINDICATIONS

- Signs of strangulation or ischemia of the prolapsed tissue (e.g., darkened or necrotic tissue)
- Suspected bowel perforation
- Severe infection or sepsis associated with the prolapse

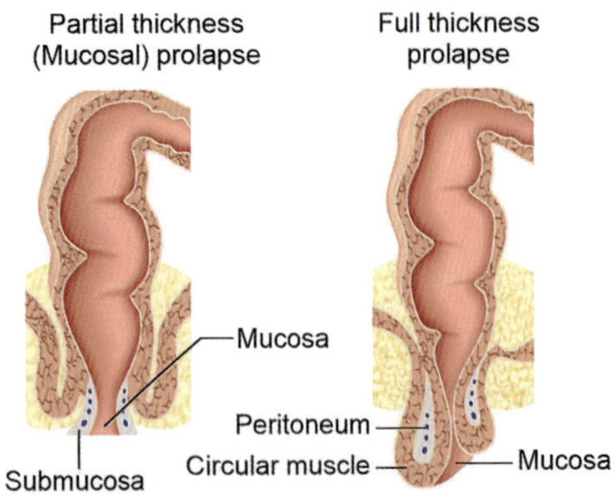

Fig. 1: Prolapse reduction—partial and complete.

EQUIPMENT AND SUPPLIES

- Sterile gloves
- Lubricant (e.g., water-soluble jelly)
- Gauze pads
- Warm saline solution or warm water
- Anesthetic gel or topical anesthetic (if necessary)
- Sedation (if required for uncooperative or distressed children)

PREPARATION

- *Explain the procedure:*
  - Inform the child (if age-appropriate) and caregivers about the procedure, its purpose, and what to expect.
  - Obtain informed consent from the caregivers.
- *Positioning:* Position the child in a comfortable and supportive manner, typically in the left lateral decubitus (side-lying) position or the knee-chest position. The position should allow easy access to the anal area.
- *Hygiene:* Ensure the anal and perineal areas are clean. Cleanse the area with warm saline or water if necessary.

PROCEDURE STEPS (FIG. 2)

1. *Initial assessment:* Assess the prolapsed tissue for signs of edema, ischemia, or

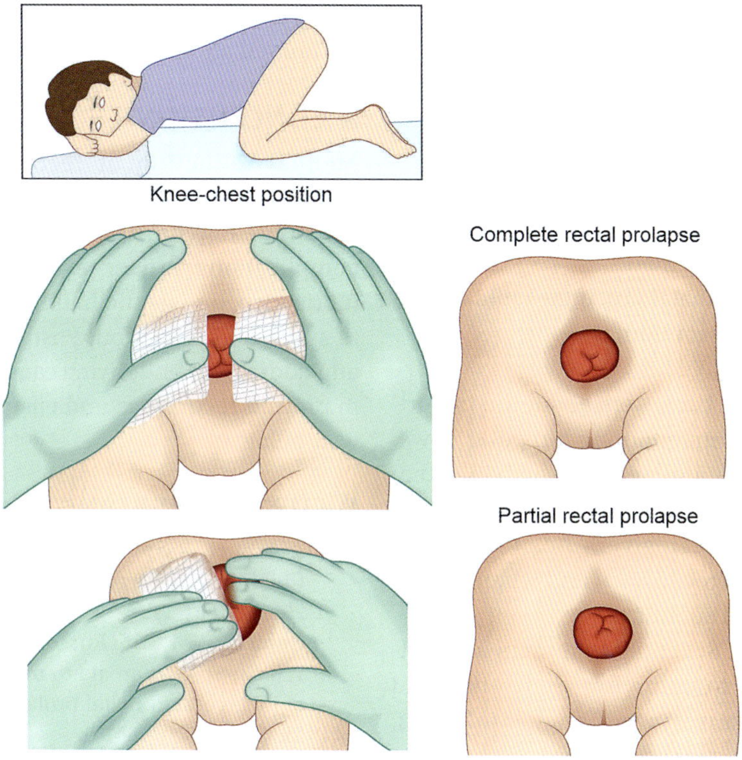

Fig. 2: Manual rectal prolapse reduction.

necrosis. If the tissue appears compromised, seek surgical consultation immediately.

2. *Lubrication:* Apply a generous amount of lubricant to the prolapsed rectal tissue and the surrounding anal area to reduce friction and facilitate reduction.
3. *Manual reduction:*
    a. Using sterile gloves, gently grasp the prolapsed rectum with a gauze pad to improve grip.
    b. Gradually and gently apply continuous pressure to the prolapsed tissue, pushing it inward toward the anus.
    c. Use the fingertips to guide the prolapsed tissue back through the anal sphincter. Apply gentle, steady pressure rather than forceful pushing to avoid injury.
4. *Warm compress (if needed):* If the tissue is edematous and difficult to reduce, apply warm saline-soaked gauze to the prolapsed area for a few minutes to reduce swelling before attempting reduction again.
5. *Postreduction care:*
    a. Once the prolapse is successfully reduced, encourage the child to lie quietly for a few minutes to ensure the tissue remains in place.
    b. Observe for any immediate recurrence or complications.

AFTERCARE

- *Observation:*
    - Monitor the child for any signs of pain, discomfort, or reprolapse.
    - Assess for complications such as bleeding or signs of infection.

- *Diet and hydration:* Encourage a high-fiber diet and adequate fluid intake to prevent constipation and reduce the risk of recurrence.
- *Medications:*
  - Consider prescribing stool softeners or laxatives to prevent straining during bowel movements.
  - Provide analgesics, if the child experiences discomfort.
- *Education:*
  - Educate caregivers about the importance of maintaining a regular bowel regimen and avoiding activities that increase intra-abdominal pressure.
  - Instruct caregivers on recognizing signs of recurrence and when to seek medical attention.
- *Follow-up:* Schedule follow-up appointments to monitor for recurrence and manage any underlying conditions, contributing to the prolapse.

COMPLICATIONS

- *Recurrence:* Common, especially if underlying factors are not addressed.
- *Ulceration and infection:* Prolonged prolapse can lead to mucosal damage and secondary infection.
- *Strangulation:* Rare but serious; it requires immediate surgical intervention.

CONCLUSION

Manual reduction of rectal prolapse in children is a straightforward but essential procedure to relieve discomfort and prevent complications. Proper technique, adequate lubrication, and gentle handling are the keys to successful reduction. Postprocedure care and addressing underlying causes are crucial to prevent recurrence and ensure the child's well-being.

FURTHER READING

1. Azzam N, Rashid OM. Rectal Prolapse in Children: A Clinical Review. Pediatr Surg Int. 2019;35(1):1-11.
2. Coburn WM 3rd, Russell MA, Hofstetter WL. Sucrose as an aid to manual reduction of incarcerated rectal prolapse. Ann Emerg Med. 1997;30(3):347-9.
3. Morrison ZD, LaPlant M, Hess D, Segura B, Saltzman D. A systematic review of management options in pediatric rectal prolapse. J Pediatr Surg. 2019;54(9):1782-87.
4. Siafakas C, Vottler TP, Andersen JM. Rectal prolapse in pediatrics. Clin Pediatr (Phila). 1999;38(2):63-72.
5. Singh SJ, Croaker GD. Rectal Prolapse in Children. J Pediatr Surg. 2018;53(1):121-6.

CHAPTER 13

Management of Constipated Stool Impaction in Children

INTRODUCTION

Stool impaction is a condition where hardened stool becomes lodged in the rectum, making it difficult to pass **(Fig. 1)**. It can cause significant discomfort and lead to more severe complications if not treated promptly. This chapter outlines the steps for managing stool impaction in children.

INDICATIONS

- Chronic constipation with abdominal pain and distension
- Inability to pass stool for several days
- Palpable mass in the abdomen or rectum
- Symptoms such as nausea, vomiting, or poor appetite

CONTRAINDICATIONS

- Severe abdominal pain, indicating possible acute abdomen or surgical emergency
- Rectal bleeding or signs of bowel perforation
- Known or suspected bowel obstruction

EQUIPMENT AND SUPPLIES

- Sterile gloves
- Lubricant (e.g., water-soluble gel)
- Digital rectal examination (DRE) kit

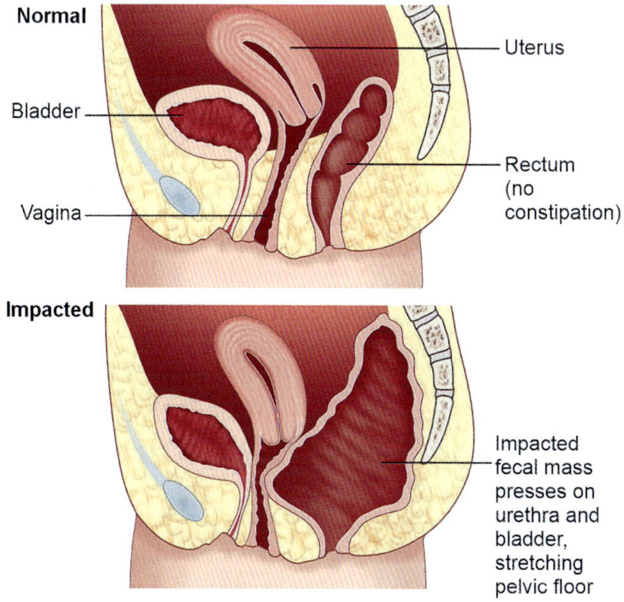

Fig. 1: Fecal impaction.

- Enema kit (e.g., phosphate, saline, or mineral oil enema)
- Oral laxatives or stool softeners [e.g., polyethylene glycol (PEG) and lactulose]
- Personal protective equipment (PPE)

PREPARATION

- *Explain the procedure:*
    - Inform the child (if age-appropriate) and caregivers about the need for the procedure, its purpose, and what to expect.
    - Obtain informed consent from the caregivers.
- *Positioning:* Position the child in a comfortable and appropriate position, such as lying on their left side with knees drawn up (Sims' position) or on their back with knees bent and feet flat.

PROCEDURE STEPS

Step 1: Digital Rectal Examination (Fig. 2)

- *Initial assessment:*
    - Conduct a thorough history and physical examination to confirm the indication for the procedure.
    - Palpate the abdomen to assess for masses and tenderness.
- *Digital rectal examination:*
    - *Preparation:*
        - Wash hands thoroughly and put on sterile gloves.
        - Apply a generous amount of lubricant to the index finger.
    - *Procedure:*
        - Gently insert the lubricated finger into the rectum.

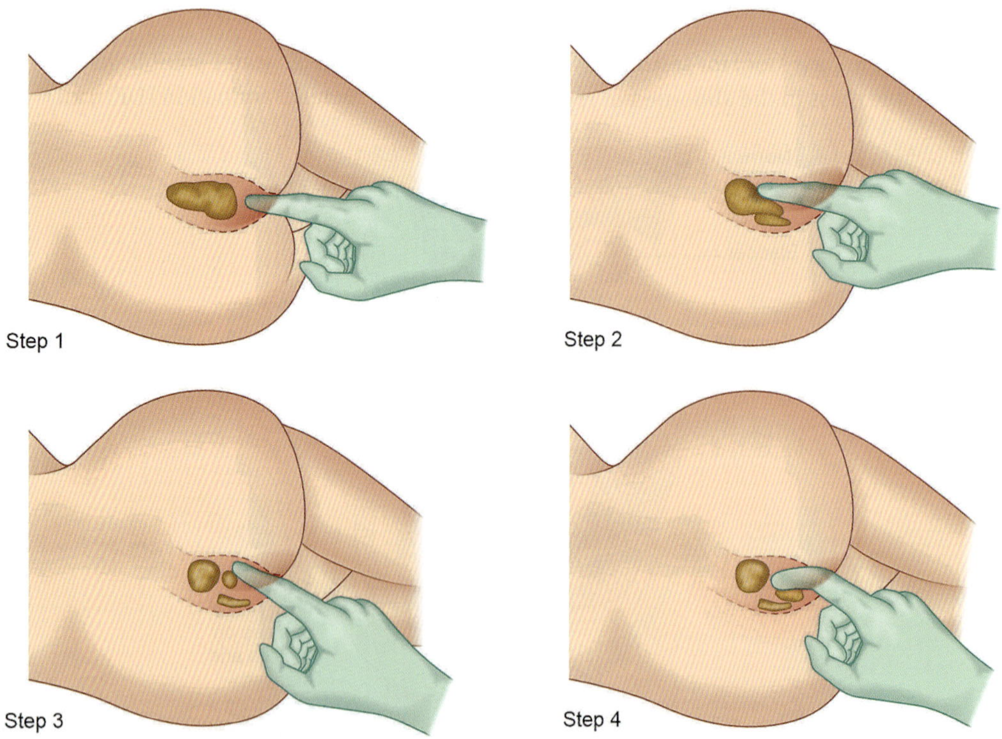

Fig. 2: Manual (digital) release of fecal impaction.

- Assess the presence, size, and consistency of the impacted stool.
- If the stool is reachable and soft, attempt gentle removal using a scooping motion. Remove small amounts at a time to minimize discomfort.
- Be cautious and gentle to avoid causing trauma to the rectal mucosa.

Step 2: Enema Administration

- *Preparation:*
  - Select the appropriate type and volume of enema solution based on the child's age and weight.
  - Warm the enema solution to body temperature to reduce discomfort.
- *Enema procedure:*
  - *Preparation:*
    - Position the child appropriately, typically lying on their left side with knees drawn up.
    - Lubricate the enema nozzle.
  - *Administration:*
    - Gently insert the enema nozzle into the rectum, aiming toward the navel.
    - Slowly administer the enema solution, encouraging the child to retain the solution for as long as possible (usually 5–10 minutes).
  - *Completion:* After the enema is administered, encourage the child to remain in position for a few minutes before using the toilet.

Step 3: Oral Laxatives or Stool Softeners

- *Selection and dosage:*
  - Choose an appropriate oral laxative or stool softener based on the child's age, weight, and severity of constipation.
  - Common options include PEG, lactulose, or milk of magnesia.
- *Administration:*
  - Administer the oral medication as prescribed, ensuring adequate hydration to aid its effectiveness.
  - Monitor the child for bowel movements and adjust the dosage as necessary based on the response.

AFTERCARE

- *Monitoring:*
  - Observe the child for any signs of discomfort, abdominal pain, or adverse reactions following the procedure.
  - Monitor bowel movements and ensure the child passes stool regularly.
- *Hydration and diet:*
  - Encourage adequate fluid intake to help soften stools.
  - Advise a diet rich in fiber, including fruits, vegetables, and whole grains, to promote regular bowel movements.
- *Education:*
  - Educate caregivers on the importance of regular bowel habits and how to recognize early signs of constipation.
  - Provide guidance on appropriate use of laxatives and stool softeners if needed.
- *Follow-up:*
  - Schedule a follow-up appointment to assess the child's progress and adjust the treatment plan as necessary.
  - Refer to a pediatric gastroenterologist if there are persistent symptoms or complications.

COMPLICATIONS

- *Rectal trauma:* Potential injury to the rectal mucosa during manual disimpaction

- *Dehydration:* Risk of dehydration with excessive use of enemas or laxatives
- *Electrolyte imbalance:* Imbalances may occur with certain types of enemas or prolonged use of laxatives.

PREVENTION

- *Regular bowel habits:* Encourage regular toilet routines, especially after meals, to establish healthy bowel habits.
- *Dietary measures:* Ensure a balanced diet with sufficient fiber and fluids to maintain soft, regular stools.
- *Physical activity:* Promote regular physical activity to help stimulate bowel function.

CONCLUSION

The management of stool impaction in children involves a combination of manual disimpaction, enemas, and oral laxatives or stool softeners. Proper technique, aftercare, and caregiver education are crucial for effective treatment and preventing recurrence.

FURTHER READING

1. Alper A, Pashankar DS. Polyethylene glycol: a game-changer laxative for children. J Pediatr Gastroenterol Nutr. 2013;57(2):134-40.
2. Bekkali NL, van den Berg MM, Dijkgraaf MG, van Wijk MP, Bongers ME, Liem O, et al. Rectal fecal impaction treatment in childhood constipation: enemas versus high doses oral PEG. Pediatrics. 2009;124(6):e1108-15.
3. Borowitz SM, Cox DJ, Kovatchev B, Ritterband LM, Sheen J, SutphenJ, et al. Treatment of childhood constipation by primary care physicians: efficacy and predictors of outcome. Pediatrics. 2005;115(4):873-7.
4. Brooks RC, Copen RM, Cox DJ, Morris J, Borowitz S, Sutphen J. Review of the treatment literature for encopresis, functional constipation, and stool-toileting refusal. Ann Behav Med. 2000;22(3):260-7.
5. Gleghorn EE, Heyman MB, Rudolph CD. No-enema therapy for idiopathic constipation and encopresis. Clin Pediatr (Phila). 1991;30(12):669-72.
6. Tabbers MM, DiLorenzo C, Berger MY, Faure C, Langendam MW, Nurko S, et al. Evaluation and treatment of functional constipation in infants and children: evidence-based recommendations from ESPGHAN and NASPGHAN.J Pediatr Gastroenterol Nutr. 2014;58(2):258-74.
7. Youssef NN, Peters JM, Henderson W, Shultz-Peters S, Lockhart DK, Di Lorenzo C . Dose response of PEG 3350 for the treatment of childhood fecal impaction. J Pediatr. 2002;141(3):410-4.

CHAPTER 14

Procedure for Umbilical Granuloma in Children

INTRODUCTION

An umbilical granuloma is a common condition in infants where a small growth of tissue forms at the base of the umbilicus after the umbilical cord has fallen off. It appears as a moist, red, or pink nodule and can cause minor irritation or discharge. Umbilical granulomas typically respond well to simple treatment methods, often performed in an outpatient setting.

INDICATIONS

- Presence of a moist, pink, or red nodule at the base of the umbilicus
- Persistent discharge from the umbilical area after the cord has fallen off
- No signs of infection, significant bleeding, or other abnormalities.

CONTRAINDICATIONS

- Signs of infection (e.g., redness, warmth, pus, and fever).
- Presence of an umbilical polyp, which is a different condition
- Significant bleeding or ulceration
- Suspected underlying anatomical abnormalities.

EQUIPMENT AND SUPPLIES

- Sterile gloves
- Alcohol swabs or antiseptic solution
- Silver nitrate sticks (75% silver nitrate and 25% potassium nitrate)
- Saline solution (for neutralizing any excess silver nitrate)
- Cotton-tipped applicators
- Gauze pads
- Adhesive bandage or dressing
- Analgesics (if necessary, though usually not required).

PREPARATION

- *Explain the procedure:*
  - Inform the caregivers about the condition, the procedure, its purpose, and what to expect.
  - Obtain informed consent from the caregivers.
- *Positioning:* Lay the infant on a clean, flat surface, such as an examination table, with the umbilical area exposed.

PROCEDURE STEPS (FIG. 1A AND B)

1. *Initial assessment:*
   a. Examine the umbilical area to confirm the diagnosis of an umbilical granuloma.
   b. Ensure there are no signs of infection, significant bleeding, or other abnormalities.
2. *Cleansing:* Clean the umbilical area with an alcohol swab or antiseptic solution to reduce the risk of infection.
3. *Application of silver nitrate:*
   a. Preparation: Put on sterile gloves and prepare a silver nitrate stick.

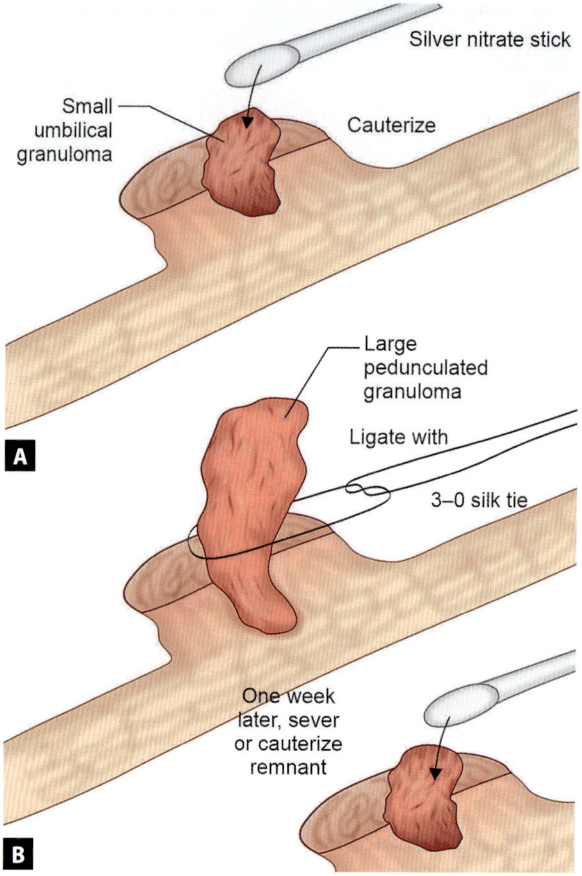

Figs. 1A and B: Umbilical granuloma ligation.

b. Application:
   i. Gently dry the area around the granuloma using a gauze pad.
   ii. Carefully apply the silver nitrate stick directly to the granuloma for a few seconds, ensuring that only the granuloma tissue is treated. Avoid contact with surrounding healthy skin to prevent chemical burns.
   iii. The treated tissue will turn a grayish color, indicating successful application.

4. *Neutralization:* If any silver nitrate comes into contact with the surrounding skin, neutralize it with saline solution using a cotton-tipped applicator to prevent irritation or burns.
5. *Postapplication care:*
   a. Wipe away any excess silver nitrate with a damp gauze pad.
   b. Observe the area for a few minutes to ensure there are no adverse reactions.

AFTERCARE

- *Monitoring:*
  - Instruct caregivers to monitor the umbilical area for signs of infection, increased redness, or persistent discharge.
  - A follow-up appointment should be scheduled to assess the response to

treatment and determine if additional applications are necessary.

- *Wound care:*
  - Advise caregivers to keep the area clean and dry. Normal bathing can continue, but the area should be gently patted dry afterward.
  - A small adhesive bandage or dressing can be applied to protect the area if there is minor discharge.
  - *Pain management:* Usually, the procedure is well-tolerated with minimal discomfort. If necessary, recommend age-appropriate analgesics (e.g., acetaminophen) for pain relief.

COMPLICATIONS

- *Chemical burns:* Accidental application of silver nitrate to surrounding skin can cause burns and irritation.
- *Infection:* Though rare, secondary infection can occur. Caregivers should watch for signs such as increased redness, warmth, swelling, or pus.
- *Recurrent granuloma:* Some granulomas may require repeated treatments with silver nitrate or alternative therapies.

ALTERNATIVE TREATMENTS

- *Salt application:* Applying common table salt to the granuloma can be an effective home remedy. Caregivers can place a small pinch of salt on the granuloma, cover it with a bandage for 30 minutes, then rinse it off. This can be repeated daily until the granuloma shrinks.
- *Ligation:* In cases where silver nitrate is not effective, a surgical tie can be placed around the base of the granuloma to cut off its blood supply, leading to its eventual fall off.
- *Cryotherapy:* Freezing the granuloma with liquid nitrogen is another option, typically performed by a healthcare provider.

CONCLUSION

The management of umbilical granuloma in infants is straightforward and typically involves the application of silver nitrate to promote the healing of the umbilical area. Ensuring proper technique and aftercare can prevent complications and promote rapid resolution of the granuloma.

FURTHER READING

1. Aydin M, Orman A, Deveci U, Taskin E. Topical clobetasol propionate may not be safe for treating umbilical granuloma in infants. Acta Paediatr. 2015;104(2):e49.
2. Bagadia J, Jaiswal S, Bhalala KB, Poojary S. Pinch of salt: A modified technique to treat umbilical granuloma. Pediatr Dermatol. 2019l;36(4):561-3.
3. Brødsgaard A, Nielsen T, Mølgaard U, Pryds O, Pedersen P. Treating infants for umbilical granuloma with topical clobetasol propionate cream. Acta Paediatr. 2015;104(2):e49-50.
4. Pomeranz A. Anomalies, abnormalities, and care of the umbilicus. Pediatr Clin North Am. 2004;51(3):819-27, xii.
5. Sheth SS, Malpani A. The management of umbilical granulomas with cryocautery. Am J Dis Child. 1990;144(2):146-7.

CHAPTER 15

Procedure for Ring Removal in Children

INTRODUCTION

Removing a ring that is stuck on a child's finger is a common emergency that can cause significant pain, swelling, and potential injury to the finger if not managed appropriately. Prompt and careful removal is crucial to prevent further complications such as compromised blood flow, nerve damage, or tissue necrosis.

INDICATIONS

- Ring stuck on a swollen finger
- Pain or discomfort due to the ring
- Circulatory compromise (e.g., discoloration, coldness, or loss of sensation in the finger)
- Traumatic injury, causing finger swelling with a ring in place.

CONTRAINDICATIONS

- Severe finger injury with associated fractures or extensive soft tissue damage
- Suspected infection around the ring area.

EQUIPMENT AND SUPPLIES

- Lubricant (e.g., soap, petroleum jelly, or hand cream)
- String or ribbon (preferably nonstretchable)
- Elastic band or dental floss
- Needle holder or hemostat
- Ring cutter (manual or electric)
- Ice pack
- Elevation device (e.g., pillows or rolled towels)
- Anesthetic cream or topical anesthetic (if necessary)
- Sterile dressing materials (for postremoval care).

PREPARATION

- *Explain the procedure:*
  - Inform the child (if age-appropriate) and caregivers about the procedure, its purpose, and what to expect.
  - Obtain informed consent from the caregivers.
- *Positioning:* Position the child comfortably with the affected hand elevated to reduce swelling.

PROCEDURE STEPS

1. *Initial measures:*
   a. *Cold therapy:* Apply an ice pack to the affected finger for 5–10 minutes to reduce swelling.
   b. *Elevation:* Keep the hand elevated above heart level to decrease edema.
2. *Lubrication method:*
   a. Apply a generous amount of lubricant around the ring and finger.
   b. Gently twist and slide the ring off the finger, using back-and-forth movements to ease it over the knuckle.
3. *String or ribbon method **(Fig. 1)**:*
   a. *String preparation:* Use a string, ribbon, or dental floss approximately 24 inches long.

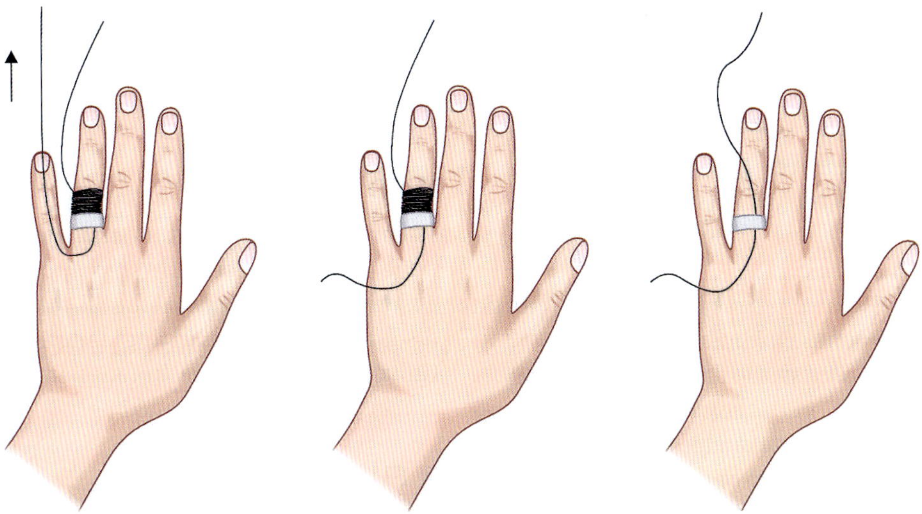

Fig. 1: Ring removal string method. *Step 1*: Pull one end of the material under the ring toward your palm, long enough for you to grab onto, and have mort of the lengths pointing toward the fingertip. *Step 2*: Tightly wrap the remaining material around your finger, starting from the ring and all the way over the knuckle. This will squeeze your finger so that the ring can fit over it. *Step 3:* Grab the end that is sticking out at bottom of the ring and slowly unravel it, the ring should move up finger as you do this.

b. *String wrapping*:
   i. Pass one end of the string under the ring using a needle holder or hemostat.
   ii. Wrap the remaining length of the string tightly around the finger, starting from the distal end (fingertip) and working proximally toward the ring. Each wrap should be snug, reducing swelling and compressing the tissue.

c. *Ring removal*: Grasp the other end of the string that is under the ring and begin unwinding it toward the fingertip. As the string unwinds, it will help slide the ring over the knuckle and off the finger.

4. *Elastic band method:*
   a. *Elastic preparation:* Use an elastic band or dental floss.
   b. *Elastic wrapping:* Similar to the string method, wrap the elastic band tightly around the finger starting from the fingertip and moving toward the ring.
   c. *Ring removal:* Slowly unwind the elastic band while pulling the ring toward the fingertip, using the same principle as the string method.

5. *Ring cutter method:*
   a. *Indications:* Use a ring cutter if other methods fail or if there is evidence of severe swelling or circulatory compromise.
   b. *Procedure:*
      i. Position the cutter's blade under the ring and carefully cut through the ring.
      ii. Avoid cutting directly over the knuckle or any area with significant swelling to prevent injury.
      iii. Once the ring is cut, gently spread the cut ends apart using pliers or a hemostat and slide the ring off the finger.

POSTREMOVAL CARE

- *Assessment:*
  - Reassess the finger for any signs of injury, swelling, or compromised circulation.
  - Look for any cuts or abrasions caused by the ring or the removal process.
- *Wound care:*
  - Cleanse any abrasions or minor wounds with mild antiseptic.
  - Apply a sterile dressing if necessary.
  - *Pain management:* Provide age-appropriate analgesics to manage any residual pain or discomfort.
  - *Monitoring:* Monitor the finger for signs of circulation return and watch for any delayed swelling or injury.

COMPLICATIONS

- *Skin abrasions:* Minor cuts or abrasions may occur during the removal process.
- *Swelling and bruising:* Transient swelling or bruising is possible postremoval.
- *Circulatory compromise:* Rare but serious complication requiring immediate medical attention.

PREVENTION

- *Proper ring size:* Ensure children wear properly sized rings that can be easily removed.
- *Avoid wearing rings during physical activity:* Advise against wearing rings during activities that could cause finger swelling or injury.
- *Education:* Educate caregivers on the risks of rings and the importance of regular checks to ensure they can be easily removed.

CONCLUSION

The management of a stuck ring on a child's finger involves a step-by-step approach to ensure safe and effective removal, minimizing discomfort and preventing complications. Utilizing appropriate techniques and tools is crucial for a successful outcome.

FURTHER READING

1. Chiu TF, Chu SJ, Chen SG, Chen SL, Chen TM. Use of a Penrose drain to remove an entrapped ring from a finger under emergent conditions. Am J Emerg Med. 2007;25(6):722-3.
2. Emesih J, Staple L. A Novel Cutting Device for Ring Removal: Case Study. Journal of Emergency Medical Services. Sept, 14, 2023. https://www.jems.com/equipment-gear/a-novel-cutting-device-for-ring-removal-case-study/
3. Kalkan A, Kose O, Tas M, Meric G. Review of techniques for the removal of trapped rings on fingers with a proposed new algorithm. Am J Emerg Med. 2013;31(11):1605-11.
4. Mittage, Ruddy RM. Illustrated techniques of pediatric emergency procedures. In: Textbook of Pediatric Emergency Medicine, 7th ed, Fleisher GR, Ludwig S, Henretig FM (Eds), Wolters Kluwer, Philadelphia 2016. p.47e.
5. Walter J, DeBoer M, Koops J, Hamel LL, Rupp PE, Westgard BC. Quick cuts: A comparative study of two tools for ring tourniquet removal. Am J Emerg Med. 2021:46:238-24.

CHAPTER 16

Procedure for Subungual Hematoma in Children

INTRODUCTION

A subungual hematoma is a collection of blood beneath a fingernail or toenail, usually resulting from a crush injury **(Fig. 1)**. This condition can cause significant pain and discomfort due to increased pressure under the nail. Prompt and appropriate management is necessary to relieve pain and prevent complications such as nail deformity or infection.

INDICATIONS

- Visible collection of blood under the nail (subungual hematoma)
- Significant pain or throbbing associated with the hematoma
- Hematoma involving >50% of the nail surface
- Traumatic injury to the finger or toe causing the hematoma

CONTRAINDICATIONS

- Suspected fracture of the distal phalanx (requires imaging and possible referral)

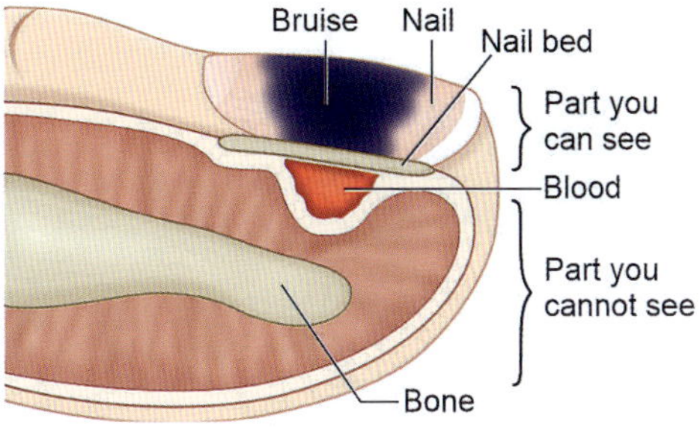

Fig. 1: Subungual hematoma.

- Signs of infection (e.g., redness, warmth, and pus)
- Compromised nail bed or surrounding tissue integrity
- Underlying nail or skin disease (e.g., psoriasis and eczema)

EQUIPMENT AND SUPPLIES

- Sterile gloves
- Antiseptic solution (e.g., povidone-iodine or alcohol swabs)
- An 18-gauge needle or large paper clip (for trephination)
- Lighter or sterile heat source (if using a paper clip)
- Electrocautery device (optional)
- Sterile gauze pads
- Bandage or adhesive strip
- Analgesics (e.g., acetaminophen or ibuprofen)
- Antibiotic ointment (if necessary)

PREPARATION

- *Explain the procedure:*
  - Inform the child (if age-appropriate) and caregivers about the procedure, its purpose, and what to expect.
  - Obtain informed consent from the caregivers.
- *Positioning:* Position the child comfortably, ensuring easy access to the affected finger or toe.
- *Pain management:* Administer appropriate analgesics (e.g., oral acetaminophen

or ibuprofen) to alleviate pain before the procedure.

PROCEDURE STEPS

1. *Initial assessment:* Examine the affected digit for signs of fracture, infection, or extensive soft tissue damage. If a fracture is suspected, obtain an X-ray before proceeding with the trephination.
2. *Cleansing:* Clean the affected digit thoroughly with an antiseptic solution to minimize the risk of infection.
3. *Trephination techniques:*
   a. *Needle method:*
      i. *Tool preparation:* Use a sterile 18-gauge needle.
      ii. *Procedure:*
         - Gently place the needle over the hematoma and apply downward pressure while twisting back and forth.
         - Continue until the needle punctures the nail and releases the blood. Be careful not to press too hard to avoid damaging the nail bed.
         - Allow the blood to drain completely, using sterile gauze to absorb it.

   b. *Heated paper clip method* ***(Figs. 2A to D)****:*
      i. *Tool preparation:* Straighten a paper clip and sterilize it by heating

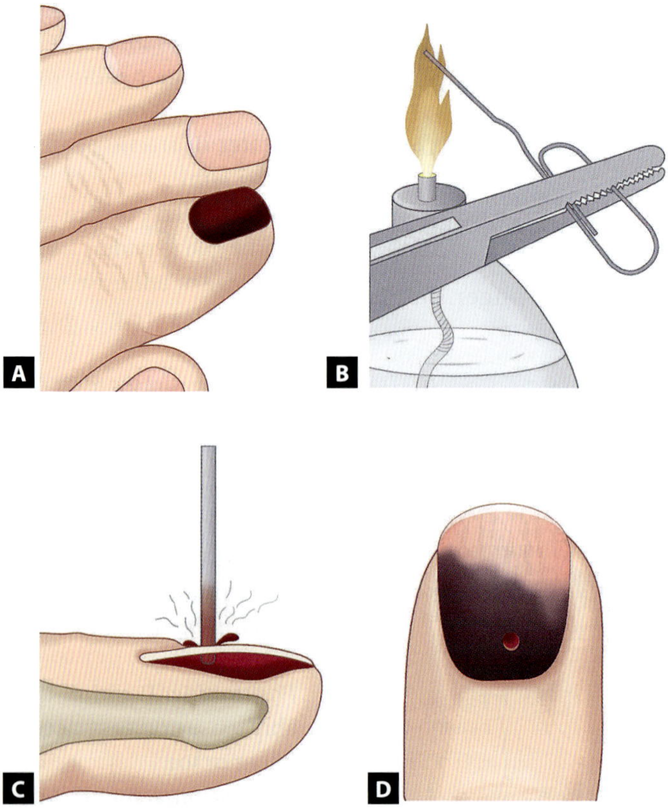

Figs. 2A to D: Subungual hematoma drainage.

the tip until it is red hot using a lighter or flame.

ii. *Procedure:*
   - Once the paper clip is sufficiently hot, gently touch the heated tip to the nail over the hematoma.
   - Allow the heat to burn a small hole through the nail, releasing the blood.
   - Remove the paper clip immediately after the hole is created to prevent further tissue damage.
   - Allow the blood to drain completely, using sterile gauze to absorb it.

c. *Electrocautery method:*
   i. *Tool preparation:* Use an electrocautery device if available.
   ii. *Procedure:*
      - Carefully apply the tip of the electrocautery device to the nail over the hematoma.
      - Activate the device to create a small hole in the nail, allowing the blood to drain.
      - Use sterile gauze to absorb the draining blood.

4. *Postprocedure care:*
   a. *Cleansing:* Clean the area again with an antiseptic solution.
   b. *Dressing:* Apply a sterile bandage or adhesive strip to protect the area and keep it clean.
   c. *Monitoring:* Observe for signs of infection, such as increased redness, warmth, swelling, or discharge.

AFTERCARE

- *Pain management:* Continue administering oral analgesics as needed for pain relief.
- *Activity modification:* Advise the child to avoid activities that may traumatize the affected nail further.
- *Follow-up:*
  - Schedule a follow-up appointment to monitor healing and ensure no complications arise.
  - Instruct caregivers to watch for signs of infection and seek medical attention if any concerns develop.
- *Nail care:* The nail may eventually fall off as the underlying nail bed heals and a new nail grows. Educate caregivers on proper nail care and what to expect during the healing process.

COMPLICATIONS

- *Infection:* Risk of infection at the site of trephination.
- *Nail deformity:* Potential for nail deformity or discoloration as the nail grows out.
- *Persistent pain:* Pain may persist if the hematoma is not completely drained or if there is an underlying fracture.

PREVENTION

- *Protective gear:* Encourage the use of protective gear during activities that pose a risk of finger or toe injuries.
- *Safety education:* Educate children and caregivers on safety measures to prevent crush injuries.

CONCLUSION

The management of subungual hematoma in children involves prompt assessment, effective pain relief, and careful trephination to relieve pressure and prevent complications. Proper aftercare and monitoring are crucial for optimal recovery.

FURTHER READING

1. Ashbell TS, Kleinert HE, Putcha SM, Kutz JE. The deformed finger nail, a frequent result of failure to repair nail bed injuries. J Trauma. 1967;7(2):177-90.

2. Helms A, Brodell RT. Surgical pearl: prompt treatment of subungual hematoma by decompression. J Am Acad Dermatol. 2000; 42(3):508-9.
3. Kaya TI, Tursen U, Baz K, Ikizoglu G. Extra-fine insulin syringe needle: an excellent instrument for the evacuation of subungual hematoma. Dermatol Surg. 2003;29(11):1141-3.
4. Patel L. Management of simple nail bed lacerations and subungual hematomas in the emergency department. Pediatr Emerg Care. 2014t;30(10):742-5.
5. Roser SE, Gellman H. Comparison of nail bed repair versus nail trephination for subungual hematomas in children. J Hand Surg Am. 1999;24(6):1166-70.

CHAPTER 17

Procedure for Management of Paronychia in Children

INTRODUCTION

Paronychia is an infection of the periungual tissues, typically caused by bacteria or fungi, leading to redness, swelling, and pain around the nail. Prompt and appropriate management is crucial to prevent the spread of infection and alleviate symptoms.

INDICATIONS

- Redness, swelling, and pain around the nail
- Presence of pus or abscess formation
- Symptoms persisting despite initial conservative treatment.

CONTRAINDICATIONS

- Severe systemic symptoms indicating a more extensive infection, requiring hospital admission
- Signs of deep space infection of the hand, requiring specialist intervention.

EQUIPMENT AND SUPPLIES

- Sterile gloves
- Antiseptic solution (e.g., povidone-iodine or chlorhexidine)
- Sterile gauze pads
- Cotton-tipped applicators
- Local anesthetic (e.g., lidocaine)
- Syringe and needle for local anesthesia
- Scalpel or sterile needle
- Hemostats (if needed)
- Sterile saline solution
- Antibiotic ointment
- Adhesive bandage or sterile dressing
- Pain management (oral analgesics)
- Personal protective equipment (PPE).

PREPARATION

- *Explain the procedure:*
    - Inform the child (if age-appropriate) and caregivers about the condition, the procedure, its purpose, and what to expect.
    - Obtain informed consent from the caregivers.
- *Positioning:* Position the child comfortably, ideally seated or lying down with the affected digit easily accessible.
- *Pain management:*
    - Administer appropriate analgesics before the procedure.
    - Consider local anesthesia to minimize pain during the procedure.

PROCEDURE STEPS

1. *Initial assessment:*
    a. Conduct a thorough history and physical examination to assess the extent of the infection.
    b. Inspect the affected area for signs of abscess formation, such as fluctuance or visible pus.
2. *Cleansing:* Clean the area around the infected nail with an antiseptic solution to reduce the risk of infection.

3. *Anesthesia:*
   a. Administer local anesthesia by injecting lidocaine around the base of the affected finger or toe.
   b. Ensure adequate anesthesia before proceeding with the drainage.
4. *Incision and drainage* ***(Fig. 1)****:*
   a. *Needle drainage (for mild cases)*:
      i. *Procedure:*
         - Use a sterile needle to puncture the area of maximal fluctuance or pus collection.
         - Gently press around the area to express the pus.
         - Use a cotton-tipped applicator to help remove any remaining pus.
   b. *Scalpel drainage (for more severe cases)*:
      i. *Procedure:*
         - Make a small incision at the edge of the nail fold where the abscess is located using a sterile scalpel.
         - Allow the pus to drain out naturally, gently expressing any remaining pus if necessary.
         - If the abscess is deep, use hemostats to gently open the incision and ensure complete drainage.
5. *Irrigation and dressing:*
   a. Irrigate the wound with sterile saline solution to flush out any remaining debris or pus.
   b. Apply a thin layer of antibiotic ointment to the area.
   c. Cover the wound with a nonadherent dressing to protect it and promote healing.
   d. Secure the dressing with an adhesive bandage or gauze wrap.

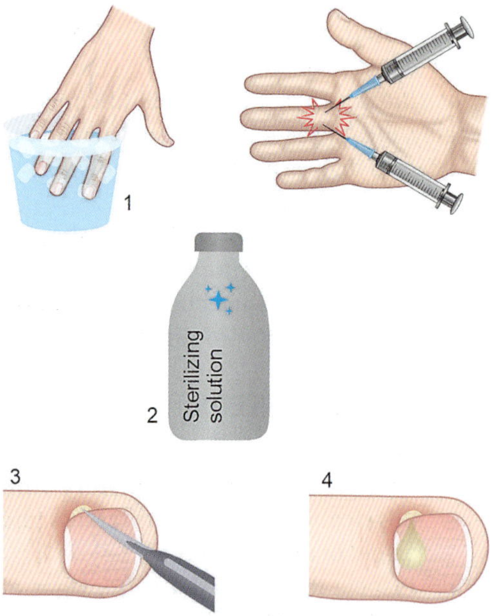

Fig. 1: Procedure for draining a finger paronychia. (1) Numb the finger with ice water or a digital nerve block; (2) Clean the cuticle with sterilizing solution; (3) Stab under the skin parallel to the nail with the #11 blade; (4) Pus will escape from the incision.

POSTPROCEDURE CARE

- *Monitoring:*
  - Observe the child for signs of infection, such as increased redness, swelling, warmth, or discharge.
  - Provide instructions to caregivers on monitoring the wound for signs of infection and ensuring proper wound care.
- *Pain management:*
  - Prescribe appropriate oral analgesics for pain relief.
  - Advise caregivers to elevate the affected limb and apply cold compresses to reduce swelling and pain.
- *Wound care:*
  - Instruct caregivers on proper wound care, including changing the dressing daily and keeping the area clean and dry.

    - Recommend the use of a protective covering or shoe for toe injuries to prevent further trauma.
- *Antibiotic therapy:* Consider prescribing oral antibiotics if there are signs of a spreading infection or if the child has a weakened immune system.
- *Follow-up:*
    - Schedule a follow-up appointment to monitor healing and assess for any complications.
    - Further evaluation may be necessary if there are concerns about persistent infection or delayed healing.

COMPLICATIONS

- *Infection spread:* Risk of the infection spreading to deeper tissues or other parts of the body.
- *Nail deformity:* Improper healing may result in nail deformities or abnormal regrowth.
- *Chronic paronychia:* Recurrent episodes of infection requiring further evaluation and management.
- *Pain:* Persistent pain may require further evaluation and management.

PREVENTION

- *Proper nail care:* Encourage proper nail care, including regular trimming and avoiding biting or picking at nails.
- *Hygiene:* Emphasize the importance of good hand and foot hygiene to prevent infections.
- *Protection:* Advise wearing protective gloves when handling chemicals or performing activities that may injure the nails.

CONCLUSION

The management of paronychia in children involves prompt and careful treatment to ensure proper healing, prevent infection, and minimize pain. Proper technique, aftercare, and caregiver education are crucial for successful outcomes.

FURTHER READING

1. Ogunlusi JD, Oginni LM, Ogunlusi OO. DAREJD simple technique of draining acute paronychia. Tech Hand Up Extrem Surg. 2005;9(2):120-1.
2. Pierrart J, Delgrande D, Mamane W, Tordjman D, Masmejean EH. Acute felon and paronychia: Antibiotics not necessary after surgical treatment. Prospective study of 46 patients. Hand Surg Rehabil. 2016;35(1):40-3.
3. Shaw J, Body R. Best evidence topic report. Incision and drainage preferable to oral antibiotics in acute paronychial nail infection? Emerg Med J. 2005;22(11):813-4.
4. Tosti R, Ilyas AM. Empiric antibiotics for acute infections of the hand. J Hand Surg Am. 2010;35(1):125-8.
5. Wollina U. Acute paronychia: comparative treatment with topical antibiotic alone or in combination with corticosteroid. J Eur Acad Dermatol Venereol. 2001;15(1):82-4

CHAPTER 18

Management of Ingrowing Toenail in Children

INTRODUCTION

An ingrowing toenail (onychocryptosis) occurs when the edge of a toenail grows into the surrounding skin, causing pain, inflammation, and sometimes infection. It most commonly affects the big toe and can result from improper nail trimming, tight footwear, or injury. Prompt and effective treatment is crucial to alleviate symptoms and prevent complications.

INDICATIONS FOR TREATMENT

- Pain or discomfort in the affected toe
- Signs of infection (redness, swelling, and pus)
- Difficulty walking or participating in activities due to toe pain
- Recurrent ingrowing toenails.

CONTRAINDICATIONS

- Severe infection requiring systemic antibiotics or surgical intervention
- Allergy to local anesthetics (for surgical treatments)
- Peripheral vascular disease or diabetes (increased risk of complications).

EQUIPMENT AND SUPPLIES

- Sterile gloves
- Antiseptic solution (e.g., povidone-iodine or chlorhexidine)
- Sterile gauze pads and dressings
- Nail scissors or clippers
- Nail elevator or cotton swabs
- Antibiotic ointment
- Cotton or dental floss for packing
- Bandages or adhesive strips
- Personal protective equipment (PPE).

PREPARATION

- *Explain the procedure:*
    - Inform the child (if age-appropriate) and caregivers about the nature of the condition, the treatment options, and what to expect during the procedure.
    - Obtain informed consent from the caregivers.
- *Positioning:* Position the child comfortably, ideally seated or lying down with the affected foot elevated and accessible.

PROCEDURE STEPS

Conservative Treatment

- *Initial assessment:*
    - Conduct a thorough history and physical examination to assess the extent of the ingrowing toenail and any signs of infection.
    - Inspect the nail fold for redness, swelling, and discharge.
- *Soaking:* Soak the affected foot in warm, soapy water for 15–20 minutes, 3–4 times daily to soften the nail and reduce inflammation.
- *Nail trimming* ***(Figs. 1 and 2)****:*

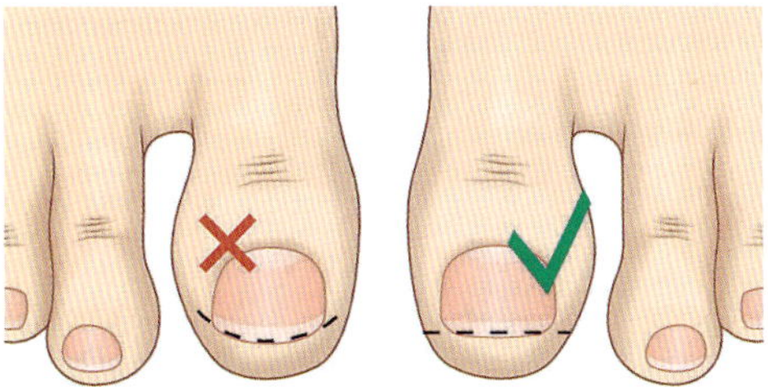

Fig. 1: Ingrowing toenail trimming.

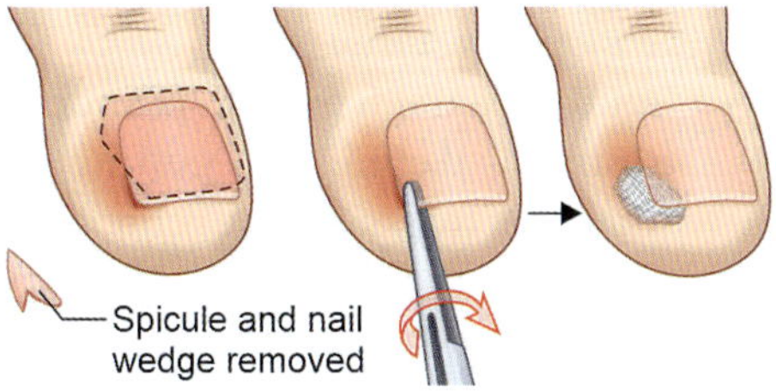

Fig. 2: Ingrowing toenail spicule and nail wedge removal.

- *Preparation:*
  - Wash hands thoroughly and put on sterile gloves.
  - Clean the affected toe with an antiseptic solution.
- *Procedure:*
  - Trim the toenail straight across using sterile nail scissors or clippers. Avoid rounding the edges, as this can exacerbate the problem. Cutting the nails straight across the top encourages the nails to grow back down the sides, into the skin, rather than outward at the top.
  - Gently lift the edge of the ingrowing nail using a nail elevator or a cotton swab.
  - Place a small piece of cotton or dental floss under the nail edge to help lift it away from the skin.

- *Antibiotic application:*
  - Apply a thin layer of antibiotic ointment to the affected area to prevent infection.
  - Cover the toe with a sterile gauze pad and secure it with a bandage or adhesive strip.
- *Pain Management:* Provide appropriate oral analgesics for pain relief if needed.
  - *Follow-up:*
    - Instruct caregivers on proper foot care and monitoring for signs of infection.
    - Schedule a follow-up appointment to assess healing and adjust treatment if necessary.

Surgical Treatment (for Severe or Recurrent Cases)

- *Initial assessment:*
  - Conduct a thorough history and physical examination to determine the need for surgical intervention.
  - Confirm the presence of significant pain, recurrent ingrowing toenail, or severe infection.
- *Preparation:*
  - Explain the surgical procedure to the child and caregivers, including potential risks and benefits.
  - Obtain informed consent from the caregivers.
- *Anesthesia:* Administer local anesthesia (e.g., lidocaine) to the affected toe to numb the area.
- *Partial nail avulsion* **(Fig. 3)***:*
  - *Preparation:*
    - Clean the affected toe with an antiseptic solution.
    - Elevate the edge of the ingrowing nail using a nail elevator.
  - *Procedure:*
    - Using sterile scissors or nail clippers, carefully trim away the affected portion of the nail.
    - Remove any granulation tissue or debris from the nail fold.

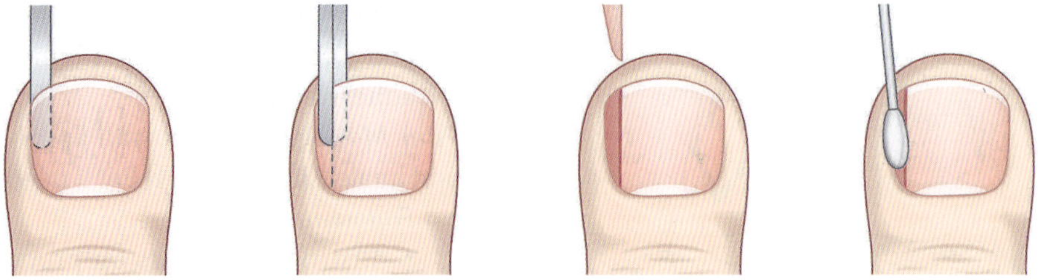

Fig. 3: Partial nail avulsion.

- Apply phenol or another chemical to the nail matrix to prevent regrowth of the affected nail edge if necessary.

- *Postprocedure care:*
  - Apply antibiotic ointment to the treated area.
  - Cover the toe with a sterile gauze pad and secure it with a bandage or adhesive strip.
  - Provide instructions on wound care, including keeping the area clean and dry.
- *Follow-up*:
  - Schedule follow-up appointments to monitor healing and assess for any complications.
  - Instruct caregivers on proper foot care and signs of infection to watch for.

AFTERCARE

- *Monitoring:*
  - Continuously monitor the child for signs of infection or complications.
  - Observe for pain, swelling, redness, or discharge from the treated area.
- *Hygiene and care:*
  - Instruct caregivers to keep the treated area clean and dry.
  - Encourage wearing loose, comfortable footwear to avoid pressure on the affected toe.
- *Pain management:* Provide appropriate oral analgesics for pain relief if needed.
- *Prevention of recurrence:*
  - Educate caregivers on proper nail trimming techniques (cutting nails straight across, avoiding rounding the edges).
  - Recommend appropriate footwear that provides adequate space for the toes.

COMPLICATIONS

- *Infection:* Potential for bacterial infection if the nail is not properly cared for
- *Recurrence:* Risk of the ingrowing toenail recurring, especially if proper nail care is not followed
- *Pain:* Persistent pain may require further evaluation and management.

PREVENTION

- *Proper nail care:* Trim toenails straight across and avoid cutting them too short.
- *Footwear:* Wear shoes that fit well and provide adequate room for the toes.
- *Foot hygiene:* Maintain good foot hygiene to prevent infections and other complications.

CONCLUSION

The management of ingrowing toenails in children involves a combination of conservative and, in some cases, surgical treatments to alleviate pain, prevent infection, and avoid recurrence. Proper technique, aftercare, and caregiver education are crucial for successful outcomes and preventing complications.

FURTHER READING

1. Gutiérrez-Mendoza D, De Anda Juárez M,Ávalos VF, Martínez GR, Domínguez-Cherit J. "Cotton nail cast": a simple solution for mild and painful lateral and distal nail embedding. Dermatol Surg. 2015;41(3):411-4.
2. Haneke E. Controversies in the treatment of ingrown nails. Dermatol Res Pract. 2012; 2012:783924.
3. Lencastre A, Iorizzo M, Caucanas M, Cunha N, Trakatelli MG, Zaraa I, et al. Topical steroids for the treatment of retronychia. J Eur Acad Dermatol Venereol. 2019;33(9): e320-e322.
4. Nishioka K, Katayama I, Kobayashi Y, Takijiri C, Nishioka K. Taping for embedded toenails. Br J Dermatol. 1985;113(2):246-7.
5. Woo SH, Kim IH. Surgical pearl: nail edge separation with dental floss for ingrown toenails. J Am Acad Dermatol. 2004;50(6): 939-40.

CHAPTER 19

Procedure for Management of Fingernail and Toenail Avulsion in Children

INTRODUCTION

Nail avulsion, where a fingernail or toenail is partially or completely detached from the nail bed, is a common injury in children. This can result from trauma such as crushing injuries, stubbing, or catching the nail on an object. Proper management is crucial to ensure healing, prevent infection, and minimize pain.

INDICATIONS

- Partial or complete avulsion of the fingernail or toenail
- Symptoms such as pain, bleeding, and exposure of the nail bed
- Visible trauma to the nail and surrounding tissue.

CONTRAINDICATIONS

- Suspected fracture of the distal phalanx, requiring imaging and orthopedic consultation
- Severe tissue damage or extensive lacerations, requiring surgical intervention
- Signs of infection, requiring antibiotic therapy.

EQUIPMENT AND SUPPLIES

- Sterile gloves
- Antiseptic solution (e.g., povidone-iodine or chlorhexidine)
- Sterile gauze pads
- Cotton-tipped applicators
- Local anesthetic (e.g., lidocaine)
- Syringe and needle for local anesthesia
- Small forceps
- Scissors or nail nippers
- Splint (if necessary)
- Nonadherent dressing
- Antibiotic ointment
- Adhesive bandage or dressing
- Pain management (oral analgesics)
- Personal protective equipment (PPE).

PREPARATION

- *Explain the procedure:*
  - Inform the child (if age-appropriate) and caregivers about the condition, the procedure, its purpose, and what to expect.
  - Obtain informed consent from the caregivers.
- *Positioning:* Position the child comfortably, ideally seated or lying down with the affected digit easily accessible.
- *Pain management:*
  - Administer appropriate analgesics before the procedure.
  - Consider local anesthesia to minimize pain during the procedure.

PROCEDURE STEPS

- *Initial assessment:*
  - Conduct a thorough history and physical examination to assess the extent of the injury.

- Inspect the nail bed, surrounding tissue, and check for any signs of underlying fracture or severe damage.

- *Cleansing:* Clean the affected area thoroughly with an antiseptic solution to reduce the risk of infection.
- *Anesthesia:*
  - Administer local anesthesia by injecting lidocaine around the base of the affected finger or toe.
  - Ensure adequate anesthesia before proceeding with the nail avulsion.
- *Removal of avulsed nail:*
  - *Partial avulsion:*
    - If part of the nail is still attached, use small forceps to gently lift and trim the loose portion using scissors or nail nippers.
    - Be careful not to damage the underlying nail bed.
  - *Complete avulsion:*
    - If the entire nail is detached, gently remove it using forceps.
    - Clean the nail bed and remove any debris or foreign material.
- *Inspection and debridement*:
  - Inspect the nail bed for any lacerations, hematomas, or foreign bodies.
  - Debride any necrotic or damaged tissue to promote healing.
- *Dressing the wound:*
  - Apply a thin layer of antibiotic ointment to the nail bed.
  - Cover the area with a nonadherent dressing to protect the wound and promote healing.
  - Secure the dressing with an adhesive bandage or gauze wrap.
- *Splinting (if necessary):* If there is significant soft tissue injury or if the digit requires immobilization, apply a splint to protect the area and prevent further injury.

POSTPROCEDURE CARE

- *Monitoring:*
  - Observe the child for signs of infection, excessive pain, or complications.
  - Provide instructions to caregivers on monitoring the wound for signs of infection, such as increased redness, swelling, warmth, or discharge.
- *Pain management:*
  - Prescribe appropriate oral analgesics for pain relief.
  - Advise caregivers to elevate the affected limb and apply cold compresses to reduce swelling and pain.
- *Wound care:*
  - Instruct caregivers on proper wound care, including changing the dressing daily and keeping the area clean and dry.
  - Recommend the use of a protective covering or shoe for toe injuries to prevent further trauma.
- *Follow-up:*
  - Schedule a follow-up appointment to monitor healing and assess for any complications.
  - Further evaluation may be necessary if there are concerns about infection, delayed healing, or regrowth of the nail.
- *Activity modification:*
  - Advise the child to avoid activities that may cause further injury to the affected digit until it has healed.
  - Encourage gentle use of the affected digit to promote circulation and healing.

COMPLICATIONS

- *Infection:* Risk of secondary infection if the wound is not properly cared for.
- *Nail deformity:* Improper healing may result in nail deformities or abnormal regrowth.

- *Delayed healing:* Factors such as underlying health conditions or improper wound care can delay healing.
- *Pain:* Persistent pain may require further evaluation and management.

PREVENTION

- *Safety measures:* Encourage the use of protective gear during sports and physical activities.
- *Supervision:* Supervise young children to prevent injuries from falls or accidents.
- *Education:* Educate caregivers and children on the importance of nail care and injury prevention.

CONCLUSION

The management of fingernail and toenail avulsion in children involves prompt and careful treatment to ensure proper healing, prevent infection, and minimize pain. Proper technique, aftercare, and caregiver education are crucial for successful outcomes.

FURTHER READING

1. Al-Anazi AF. Fingertip injuries in paediatric patients—experiences at an emergency centre in Saudi Arabia. J Pak Med Assoc. 2013; 63:675.
2. Antevy PM, Saladino RA. Management of finger injuries. In: King C, Henretig FM (Eds). Textbook of Pediatric Emergency Procedures, 2nd edition, Lippincott, Williams & Wilkins, Philadelphia 2008. pp 939.
3. Fukumasa H, Kobayashi M, Okahata Y, Nishiyama K. Epidemiology of Pediatric Hand Injury at a Pediatric Department in Japan. Pediatr Emerg Care. 2022;38:582.
4. Jester N, Han S, Singh M, Rao AA, Sokhal B, Ma Y, et al. Outcomes of Composite Grafts for Pediatric Fingertip Amputations: A Systematic Review. Indian J Plast Surg. 2023; 56:310.
5. Yorlets RR, Busa K, Eberlin KR, Raisolsadat MA, Bae DS, Waters PM, et al. Fingertip Injuries in Children: Epidemiology, Financial Burden, and Implications for Prevention. Hand (NY). 2017;12:342.

CHAPTER 20

Procedure for Fishhook Removal in Children

INTRODUCTION

Fishhook injuries are common in children, especially in those who participate in fishing activities. Removing a fishhook requires careful technique to prevent further tissue damage and minimize pain. This chapter outlines the procedure for safely removing a fishhook from a child's skin.

INDICATIONS

- Fishhook embedded in the skin
- Visible portion of the fishhook protruding from the skin
- Pain, discomfort, or risk of infection from the embedded fishhook

CONTRAINDICATIONS

- Fishhook embedded in or near sensitive areas, such as the eye, face, or genitals (requires specialist care)
- Deeply embedded fishhook near major blood vessels, nerves, or joints
- Signs of infection, requiring antibiotic treatment and possible surgical intervention

EQUIPMENT AND SUPPLIES

- Sterile gloves
- Antiseptic solution (e.g., povidone-iodine or chlorhexidine)
- Sterile gauze pads
- Local anesthetic (e.g., lidocaine)
- Syringe and needle for local anesthesia
- Needle driver or hemostat
- Wire cutters or heavy-duty scissors
- Sterile saline solution
- Antibiotic ointment
- Adhesive bandage or sterile dressing
- Pain management (oral analgesics)
- Personal protective equipment (PPE)

PREPARATION

- *Explain the procedure:*
  - Inform the child (if age-appropriate) and caregivers about the injury, the removal procedure, its purpose, and what to expect.
  - Obtain informed consent from the caregivers.
- *Positioning:* Position the child comfortably, ideally seated or lying down with the affected area easily accessible.
- *Pain management:*
  - Administer appropriate analgesics before the procedure.
  - Consider local anesthesia to minimize pain.

PROCEDURE STEPS

1. *Initial assessment:*
   a. Conduct a thorough history and physical examination to assess the extent of the injury.
   b. Determine the type and location of the fishhook, noting whether it is barbed or barbless.

2. *Cleansing:* Clean the area around the embedded fishhook with an antiseptic solution to reduce the risk of infection.
3. *Anesthesia:*
   a. Administer local anesthesia by injecting lidocaine around the base of the embedded fishhook.
   b. Ensure adequate anesthesia before proceeding with the removal.
4. *Removal techniques:*
   a. *Back-out method (for barbless hooks):*
      i. *Procedure:*
         - Gently grasp the exposed part of the hook with a needle driver or hemostat.
         - Apply steady, backward pressure to slide the hook out along the path of entry.
         - If resistance is encountered, do not force the hook, switch to another method.
   b. *String-yank method (for barbed hooks)* ***(Fig. 1)****:*
      i. *Preparation:*
         - Tie a length of string around the midpoint of the bend of the hook.
         - Have an assistant stabilize the affected body part and apply gentle downward pressure on the hook shank.
      ii. *Procedure:*
         - While maintaining pressure on the shank to flatten the barb, give a quick, firm yank on the string to pull the hook out in the direction of entry.
         - This method requires careful coordination and should be done quickly to minimize pain.
   c. *Needle-cover method (for deeply embedded barbed hooks)* ***(Fig. 2)****:*
      i. *Procedure:*
         - Insert an 18 g needle along the entry path of the hook until the needle covers the barb.

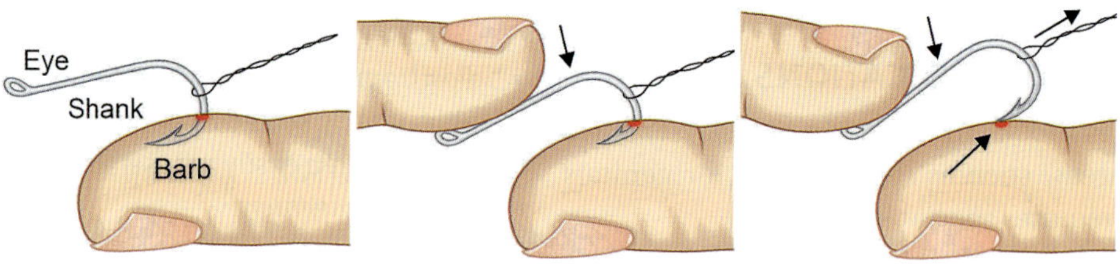

Fig. 1: Fishhook removal—string yank technique.

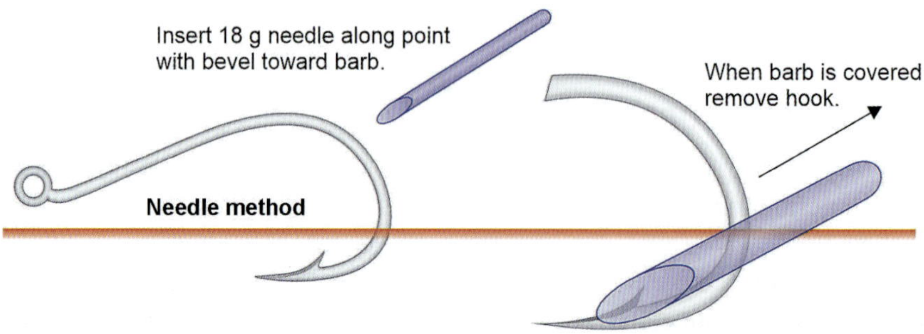

Fig. 2: Fishhook removal—needle-cover method.

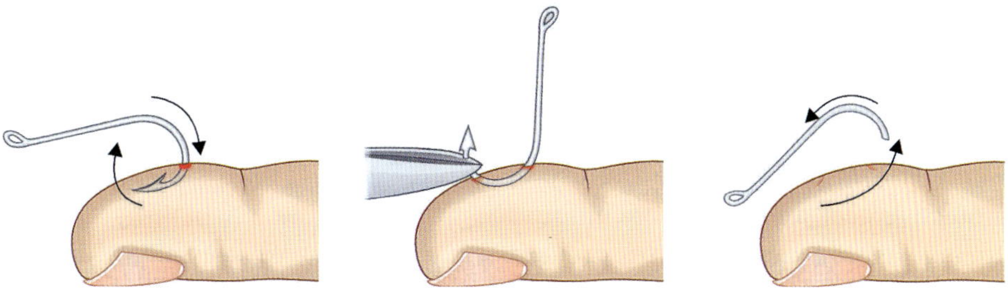

Fig. 3: Fishhook removal—advance and cut technique.

   - Advance the hook until the barb is inside the needle.
   - Withdraw the needle and hook together.
   - This method may require precision and patience.

d. *Advance-and-cut method (for barbed hooks with significant embedding)* ***(Fig. 3):***
   i. *Procedure:*
      - Push the hook forward to advance the barb through the skin until it emerges.
      - Use wire cutters or heavy-duty scissors to cut off the barb.
      - Withdraw the remaining hook shaft backward through the original entry wound.

5. *Postremoval care:*
   a. *Inspection:* Examine the wound to ensure no part of the hook remains.
   b. *Cleaning:* Irrigate the wound with sterile saline solution to flush out any debris.
   c. *Dressing:* Apply a thin layer of antibiotic ointment to the wound and cover it with a sterile dressing or adhesive bandage.

AFTERCARE

- *Monitoring:*
  - Observe the child for signs of infection, such as increased redness, swelling, warmth, or discharge.
  - Provide instructions to caregivers on monitoring the wound for signs of infection and ensuring proper wound care.
- *Pain management:*
  - Prescribe appropriate oral analgesics for pain relief.
  - Advise caregivers to elevate the affected limb and apply cold compresses to reduce swelling and pain.
- *Wound care:*
  - Instruct caregivers on proper wound care, including changing the dressing daily and keeping the area clean and dry.
  - Recommend follow-up with a healthcare provider if there are any concerns about the wound.
- *Activity modification:*
  - Advise the child to avoid activities that may cause further injury to the affected area until it has healed.
  - Encourage gentle use of the affected limb to promote circulation and healing.

COMPLICATIONS

- *Infection:* Risk of secondary infection if the wound is not properly cared for.
- *Tissue damage:* Improper removal techniques can cause additional tissue damage.
- *Retained hook fragments:* Incomplete removal can lead to retained fragments, requiring further intervention.

- *Pain:* Persistent pain may require further evaluation and management.

PREVENTION

- *Safety measures:* Encourage the use of protective gear and proper techniques during fishing activities to prevent injuries.
- *Supervision:* Supervise young children during fishing activities to prevent accidents.
- *Education:* Educate caregivers and children on the importance of fishing safety and injury prevention.

CONCLUSION

The management of fishhook injuries in children involves prompt and careful removal to prevent further tissue damage and minimize pain. Proper technique, aftercare, and caregiver education are crucial for successful outcomes and preventing complications.

FURTHER READING

1. Diekema DS. Fishhook removal. In: King C, Henretig FM (Eds). Textbook of Pediatric Emergency Procedures, 2nd edition, Lippincott, Williams and Wilkins, Baltimore, 2008. p. 1102.
2. Mittiga MR, Ruddy RM. Removal of fish hooks. In: Shaw KN, Bachur RG (Eds). Fleisher and Ludwig's Textbook of Pediatric Emergency Medicine, 7th edition, Lippincott Williams and Wilkins, Philadelophia, 2016. p. 48e.
3. Prats M, O'Connell M, Wellock A, Kman NE. Fishhook removal: case reports and a review of the literature. J Emerg Med. 2013;44:e375.
4. Su E. Removal of a barbed fishhook. In: Diekema RA, Fiser DH, Selbst SM (Eds). Illustrated Textbook of Pediatric Emergency and Critical Care Procedures. Mosby, St. Louis 1997. p. 727.
5. Watari T, Sekine I, Tokuda Y. Fish hook injury: an easy removal using the string yank technique. BMJ Case Rep. 2017; 2017.

CHAPTER 21

Procedure for Management of Hair Tourniquets in Children

INTRODUCTION

A hair tourniquet occurs when a strand of hair or thread wraps tightly around an appendage such as a toe, finger, or penis, leading to pain, swelling, and potential tissue damage due to constriction of blood flow. This condition requires prompt recognition and intervention to prevent serious complications.

INDICATIONS

- Visible strand of hair or thread tightly wrapped around an appendage (toe, finger, and penis)
- Signs of constriction including swelling, redness, and pain in the affected area
- Child's irritability or crying without an apparent cause

CONTRAINDICATIONS

- Severe tissue damage or necrosis indicating the need for surgical intervention
- Signs of infection (e.g., purulence, excessive warmth, and fever)

EQUIPMENT AND SUPPLIES

- Sterile gloves
- Magnifying glass or loupe
- Bright light source
- Fine-tipped forceps or tweezers
- Small, blunt-tipped scissors or surgical blade
- Antiseptic solution (e.g., povidone-iodine or alcohol swabs)
- Lubricant (e.g., water-soluble jelly)
- Hair removal cream (optional)
- Sterile gauze pads
- Bandage or adhesive strip
- Analgesics (if necessary)
- Sedation (if necessary for an uncooperative or distressed child)

PREPARATION

- *Explain the procedure:*
  - Inform the caregivers about the condition, the need for immediate intervention, and the procedure itself.
  - Obtain informed consent from the caregivers.
- *Positioning:*
  - Position the child comfortably and securely, ensuring easy access to the affected appendage.
  - Consider employing an assistant to help hold the child still during the procedure.

PROCEDURE STEPS

1. *Initial assessment:*
   a. Examine the affected area carefully to identify the hair or thread causing the constriction.
   b. Assess the degree of swelling, redness, and any signs of compromised circulation.
2. *Cleansing:* Clean the affected area with an antiseptic solution to reduce the risk of infection.

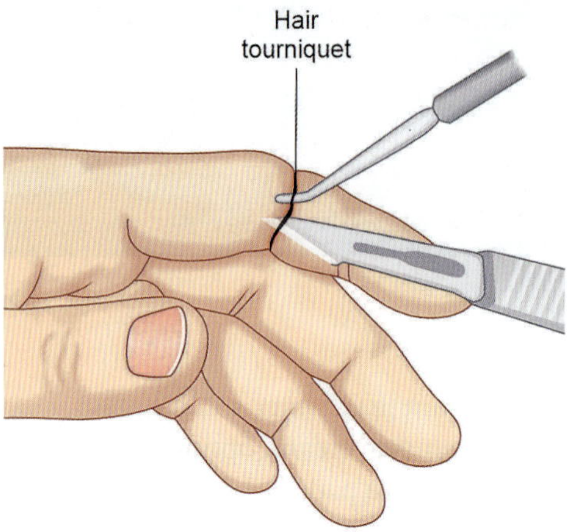

Fig. 1: Manual hair torniquet removal.

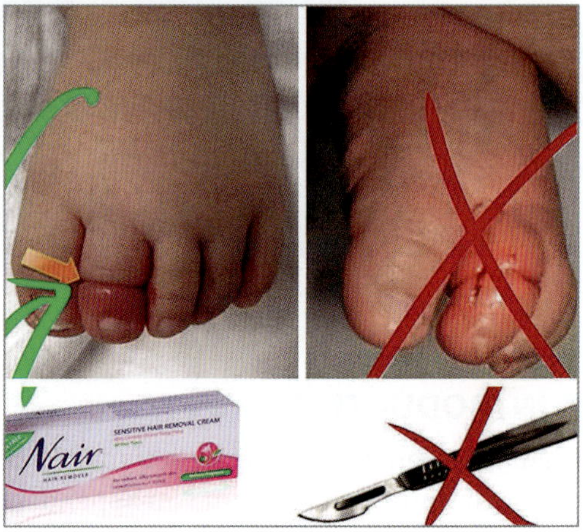

Fig. 2: Cream hair torniquet removal.

3. *Removal techniques:*
   a. *Manual removal* ***(Fig. 1)****:*
      i. *Visualization:* Use a magnifying glass or loupe and a bright light source to clearly visualize the hair or thread.
      ii. *Lubrication:* Apply a water-soluble jelly to the affected area to ease the removal process.
      iii. *Dissection:*
         - Using fine-tipped forceps or tweezers, gently grasp the hair or thread.
         - Carefully cut the hair or thread using small, blunt-tipped scissors or a surgical blade. Take care not to damage the underlying skin.
         - Gradually unwind and remove the hair or thread.
   b. Hair removal cream (for hair tourniquets) **(Fig. 2)**:
      i. *Application:* Apply a small amount of hair removal cream to the affected area, following the product's instructions. This method can help dissolve the hair if it is difficult to visualize or grasp.
      ii. *Waiting time:* Allow the cream to sit for the recommended time, usually a few minutes.
      iii. *Removal:* Wipe away the cream along with the dissolved hair using a damp, sterile gauze pad.
4. *Postremoval care:*
   a. *Cleansing:* Cleanse the area again with an antiseptic solution.
   b. *Inspection:* Inspect the site to ensure complete removal of the hair or thread and to assess any residual damage.
   c. *Dressing:* Apply a sterile bandage or adhesive strip to protect the area and keep it clean.

AFTERCARE

- *Monitoring:*
  - Instruct caregivers to monitor the affected area for signs of infection or persistent swelling.
  - Schedule a follow-up appointment to assess healing and ensure no further complications.
- *Wound care:*
  - Advise caregivers to keep the area clean and dry.

  - Recommend gentle cleaning and application of an antiseptic ointment if necessary.
- *Pain management:*
  - Provide age-appropriate analgesics for pain relief if the child experiences discomfort postprocedure.
- *Education:*
  - Educate caregivers on the importance of regular inspection of digits and other appendages for hair or thread, especially in infants and young children.
  - Highlight preventive measures such as regularly checking for and removing loose hairs from the child's environment.

COMPLICATIONS

- *Infection:* Though rare, secondary infection can occur if the hair or thread has caused a break in the skin.
- *Tissue damage:* Prolonged constriction can lead to tissue necrosis, requiring more extensive medical or surgical intervention.
- *Recurrence:* Emphasize the importance of vigilance to prevent recurrence.

PREVENTION

- *Regular inspection:* Caregivers should regularly inspect their child's fingers, toes, and other appendages for any signs of hair or thread entanglement.
- *Hair management:* Parents with long hair should ensure loose hairs are removed from the child's clothing, bedding, and environment.
- *Appropriate clothing:* Avoid using clothing with loose threads that could wrap around a child's appendages.

CONCLUSION

The management of hair tourniquets in children involves prompt and careful removal of the constricting hair or thread to prevent complications. Proper technique, adequate aftercare, and caregiver education are crucial for effective treatment and prevention of recurrence.

FURTHER READING

1. Adjei NN, Lynn AY, Grimshaw A, Brault MA, Dugan K, Vash-Margita A. Systematic Literature Review of Pediatric Male and Female Genital Hair Thread Tourniquet Syndrome. Pediatr Emerg Care. 2022;38:e799
2. Bean JF, Hebal F, Hunter CJ. A single center retrospective review of hair tourniquet syndrome and a proposed treatment algorithm. J Pediatr Surg. 2015;50:1583.
3. Martonovich N, Khatib M, Assaf M. Hair tourniquet syndrome: A retrospective study. Pediatr Dermatol. 2023;40:125.
4. Pahwa HS, Kumar A, Srivastava R, Kumar S, Goel A, Ahmad A. Partial penile amputation due to penile tourniquet syndrome in a child troubled with primary nocturnal enuresis—a rare emergency. Urology. 2013;81:653.
5. Pantuck AJ, Kraus SL, Barone JG. Hair strangulation injury of the penis. Pediatr Emerg Care. 1997;13:423

CHAPTER 22

Superficial Splinter Removal in Children

INTRODUCTION

Superficial splinters are common injuries in children, typically resulting from contact with wood, glass, metal, or other foreign materials. Prompt and careful removal is important to prevent infection and alleviate pain.

INDICATIONS

- Visible splinter in the skin
- Pain, redness, or swelling around the site of the splinter
- Discomfort or difficulty using the affected area

CONTRAINDICATIONS

- Deeply embedded splinter, requiring surgical intervention
- Signs of infection (e.g., increased redness, warmth, and pus), requiring antibiotic therapy
- Location near sensitive areas such as the eye, requiring specialist care

EQUIPMENT AND SUPPLIES

- Sterile gloves
- Antiseptic solution (e.g., povidone-iodine or chlorhexidine)
- Sterile gauze pads
- Cotton-tipped applicators
- Tweezers or fine-tipped forceps
- Needle (for stubborn splinters)
- Magnifying glass or loupe (optional)
- Sterile saline solution
- Antibiotic ointment
- Adhesive bandage or sterile dressing
- Pain management (oral analgesics)
- Personal protective equipment (PPE)

PREPARATION

- *Explain the procedure:*
    - Inform the child (if age-appropriate) and caregivers about the splinter, the removal procedure, its purpose, and what to expect.
- Obtain informed consent from the caregivers.
- *Positioning:* Position the child comfortably, ideally seated or lying down with the affected area easily accessible.
- *Pain management:* Administer appropriate analgesics before the procedure if the child is in significant pain.

PROCEDURE STEPS

1. *Initial assessment:*
    - Conduct a thorough history and physical examination to assess the location and extent of the splinter.
    - Inspect the affected area for signs of infection or deeper embedding.
2. *Cleansing:* Clean the area around the splinter with an antiseptic solution to reduce the risk of infection.
3. *Splinter removal:*
    a. *For visible and easily accessible splinters* ***(Fig. 1)****:*

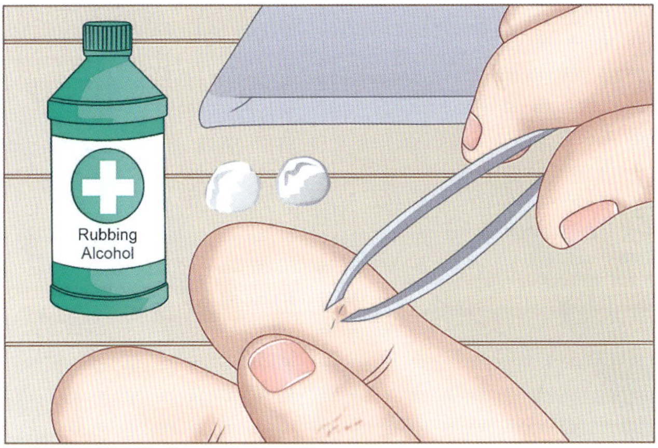

Fig. 1: Superficial splinter removal with tweezers.

i. *Procedure:*
   - Use tweezers or fine-tipped forceps to grasp the exposed end of the splinter.
   - Gently pull the splinter out along the path it entered to avoid breaking it.
   - If the splinter is difficult to grasp, use a magnifying glass or loupe to enhance visibility.

b. *For partially embedded splinters*:
   i. *Procedure:*
   - If part of the splinter is embedded beneath the skin, use a sterile needle to gently lift the skin over the splinter.
   - Once the splinter is exposed, use tweezers or forceps to grasp and remove it.
   - Be careful to avoid breaking the splinter, as this can make removal more difficult.

c. *For deeply embedded splinters* ***(Figs. 2A to D)***

4. *Postremoval care:*
   a. *Inspection:* Examine the wound to ensure no part of the splinter remains.
   b. *Cleaning:* Irrigate the wound with sterile saline solution to flush out any debris.
   c. *Dressing:* Apply a thin layer of antibiotic ointment to the area.
   d. *Bandaging:* Cover the wound with a nonadherent dressing or adhesive bandage to protect it and promote healing.

AFTERCARE

- *Monitoring:*
  - Observe the child for signs of infection, such as increased redness, swelling, warmth, or discharge.
  - Provide instructions to caregivers on monitoring the wound and ensuring proper wound care.
- *Pain management:*
  - Prescribe appropriate oral analgesics for pain relief.
  - Advise caregivers to keep the affected area clean and dry.
- *Wound care:*
  - Instruct caregivers on proper wound care, including changing the dressing daily and keeping the area clean.
  - Recommend avoiding activities that may cause further injury to the affected area until it has healed.

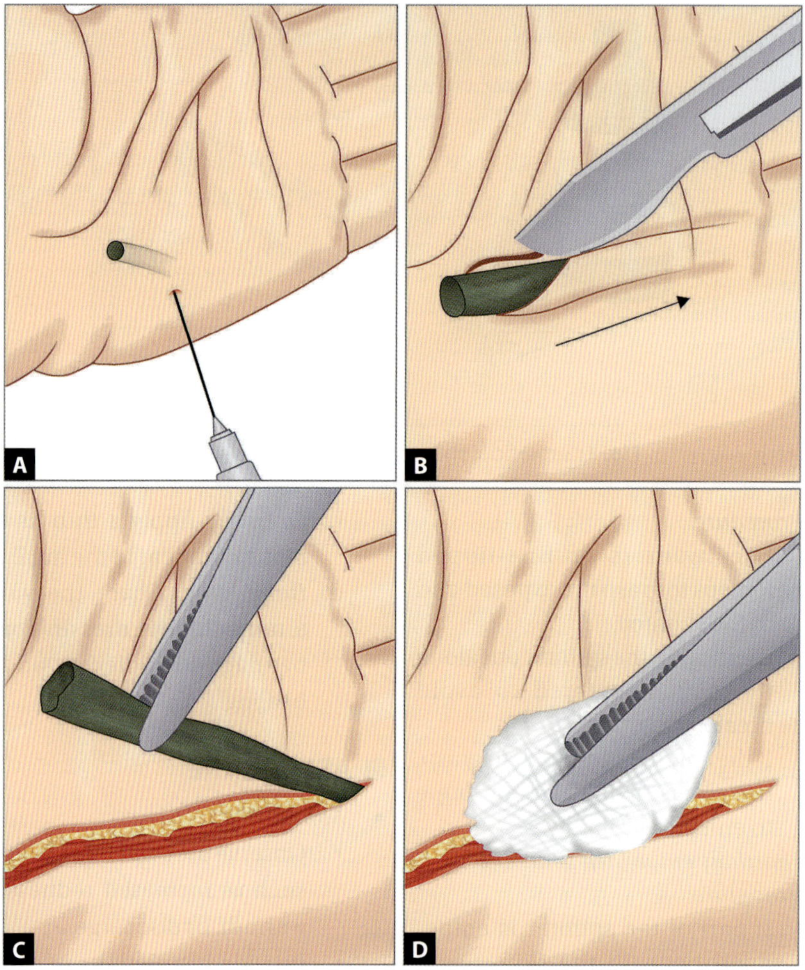

Figs. 2A to D: Deep splinter removal. (A) Inject with a local anesthetic; (B) Incise down to the sliver; (C) Lift the sliver out with forceps; (D) Clean the wound track with a wet gauze sponge.

- *Follow-up:*
  - Schedule a follow-up appointment if there are concerns about infection or if the splinter was deeply embedded.
  - Further evaluation may be necessary if there are signs of persistent infection or delayed healing.

COMPLICATIONS

- *Infection:* Risk of secondary infection if the wound is not properly cared for.
- *Incomplete removal:* Retained splinter fragments may cause ongoing pain or infection.
- *Tissue damage:* Improper removal techniques can cause additional tissue damage.
- *Pain:* Persistent pain may require further evaluation and management.

PREVENTION

- *Safety measures:* Encourage the use of protective gear, such as gloves, when handling materials that can cause splinters.

- *Education:* Teach children about the risks of playing with or handling rough or sharp objects.
- *Supervision:* Supervise young children during activities that may expose them to splinters.

CONCLUSION

The management of superficial splinters in children involves prompt and careful removal to prevent further tissue damage and minimize pain. Proper technique, aftercare, and caregiver education are crucial for successful outcomes and preventing complications.

FURTHER READING

1. Al-Anazi AF. Fingertip injuries in paediatric patients—experiences at an emergency centre in Saudi Arabia. J Pak Med Assoc. 2013; 63:675.
2. Antevy PM, Saladino RA. Management of finger injuries. In: King C, Henretig FM (Eds). Textbook of Pediatric Emergency Procedures, 2nd edition, Lippincott, Williams & Wilkins, Philadelphia 2008. p. 939.
3. Fukumasa H, Kobayashi M, Okahata Y, Nishiyama K. Epidemiology of Pediatric Hand Injury at a Pediatric Department in Japan. Pediatr Emerg Care. 2022;38:582.
4. Jester N, Han S, Singh M, Rao AA, Sokhal B, Ma Y, et al. Outcomes of Composite Grafts for Pediatric Fingertip Amputations: A Systematic Review. Indian J Plast Surg. 2023; 56:310.
5. Yorlets RR, Busa K, Eberlin KR, Raisolsadat MA, Bae DS, Waters PM, et al. Fingertip Injuries in Children: Epidemiology, Financial Burden, and Implications for Prevention. Hand (NY). 2017;12:342.

CHAPTER 23

Management of Warts and Calluses in Children

INTRODUCTION

Warts and calluses are common skin conditions in children. Warts are caused by the human papillomavirus (HPV) and can appear on any part of the body, while calluses are thickened areas of skin that develop due to repeated friction or pressure, commonly on the hands and feet. This chapter outlines the identification, treatment, and prevention of warts and calluses in children **(Figs. 1A and B)**.

WARTS

Etiology and Types

- *Common warts (verruca vulgaris):* Rough, raised lesions that commonly appear on the hands and fingers
- *Plantar warts:* Hard, grainy growths that appear on the soles of the feet
- *Flat warts:* Small, smooth, flat lesions that typically appear on the face, arms, or legs
- *Filiform warts:* Finger-like projections that often appear on the face or neck

Indications for Treatment

- Pain or discomfort
- Functional impairment or interference with activities
- Cosmetic concerns or social stigma
- Rapid spread or multiple warts
- Immunocompromised status

Contraindications for Certain Treatments

- Allergies to treatment components (e.g., salicylic acid)
- Peripheral vascular disease or diabetes (for aggressive treatments)
- Pregnancy (some treatments are contraindicated)

Equipment and Supplies

- Sterile gloves
- Alcohol swabs
- Salicylic acid preparations (liquid, gel, and pads)
- Cryotherapy device (liquid nitrogen)
- Duct tape
- Emery board or pumice stone
- Personal protective equipment (PPE)

Treatment Options

- *Topical treatments:*
    - *Salicylic acid:* Apply daily to the wart after soaking the area in warm water and gently filing down the wart with an emery board or pumice stone.
    - *Duct tape occlusion therapy:* Apply a piece of duct tape over the wart for 6 days, then remove, soak, and debride the area. Repeat as needed.
- *Cryotherapy:*
    - *Procedure:*
        - Clean the area with an alcohol swab.
        - Apply liquid nitrogen to the wart using a cryotherapy device or cotton-tipped applicator.
        - Repeat every 2–3 weeks until the wart resolves.

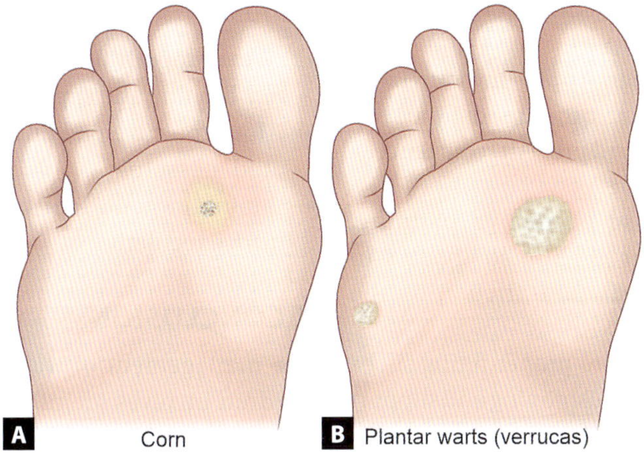

Figs. 1A and B: Corns and warts. There are a few ways we as podiatrists can differentiate between a corn and a wart. (A) *Corn:* These are hardened layers of skin and hurts more when you applied direct pressure on it; (B) *Warts:* These have small, tiny dots within the lesion (blood vessels). Warts hurt more when you squeeze the sides like a pimple. Warts bleed a lot easier.

- *Other treatments:*
    - *Cantharidin:* It is applied by a healthcare provider, causing a blister to form under the wart, leading to its removal.
    - *Imiquimod cream:* It enhances the immune response to the wart, used primarily for genital warts but sometimes for recalcitrant warts elsewhere.

Aftercare and Monitoring

- Monitor for signs of infection or adverse reactions.
- Instruct caregivers on proper home care and when to seek further medical advice.
- Follow up to assess treatment effectiveness and repeat treatments as necessary.

CALLUSES

Etiology and Types

- *Causes:* Repeated friction, pressure, or irritation, typically on the hands and feet
- *Types:* Hard calluses on the soles or palms, and soft calluses between the toes

Indications for Treatment

- Pain or discomfort
- Functional impairment
- Cosmetic concerns

Contraindications for Certain Treatments

- Peripheral vascular disease or diabetes (increased risk of complications)
- Presence of infection or ulceration

Equipment and Supplies

- Sterile gloves
- Alcohol swabs
- Pumice stone or emery board
- Moisturizing creams or lotions
- Protective padding or orthotic devices
- PPE

Treatment Options

- *Self-care measures:*
    - *Soaking and filing:* Soak the affected area in warm, soapy water for 10–15 minutes, then gently file down the

callus with a pumice stone or emery board.
    - *Moisturizing:* Apply moisturizing cream or lotion to the area daily to keep the skin soft and prevent recurrence.
- *Protective measures:*
    - *Padding:* Use protective padding, moleskin, or cushioned insoles to reduce pressure and friction on the affected area.
    - *Footwear:* Ensure proper-fitting shoes with adequate cushioning and support to prevent callus formation.
- *Professional treatments*:
    - *Debridement:* A healthcare provider may carefully trim away excess thickened skin with a scalpel.
    - *Orthotic devices:* Custom orthotics may be recommended to redistribute pressure and prevent recurrence.

Aftercare and Monitoring

- Advise caregivers on appropriate footwear and protective measures to prevent recurrence.
- Monitor for signs of infection or complications, especially in high-risk children (e.g., those with diabetes).
- Regular follow-up may be necessary for persistent or recurrent calluses.

PREVENTION

Warts

- Avoid direct contact with warts, including not picking at them.
- Keep your feet clean and dry; change socks daily.
- Use flip-flops or shoes in communal showers and locker rooms.
- Do not share personal items such as towels or razors.

Calluses

- Wear properly fitting shoes with adequate cushioning and support.
- Use protective padding to reduce friction and pressure.
- Maintain good foot hygiene and moisturize regularly.

CONCLUSION

The management of warts and calluses in children involves identifying the condition, selecting appropriate treatments, and implementing preventive measures. Proper technique, aftercare, and caregiver education are crucial for successful outcomes and preventing recurrence.

FURTHER READING

1. Bae JM, Kang H, Kim HO, Park YM. Differential diagnosis of plantar wart from corn, callus and healed wart with the aid of dermoscopy. Br J Dermatol. 2009;160:220.
2. Freeman DB. Corns and calluses resulting from mechanical hyperkeratosis. Am Fam Physician. 2002;65:2277.
3. Gijón-Noguerón G, García-Paya I, Morales-Asencio JM, Jiménez-Cebrián A, Ortega-Ávila AB, Cervera-Marín JA. Short-term effect of scalpel debridement of plantar callosities versus treatment with salicylic acid patches: The EMEDESCA randomized controlled trial. J Dermatol. 2017;44:706.
4. Stephenson J, Farndon L, Concannon M. Analysis of a trial assessing the long-term effectiveness of salicylic acid plasters compared with scalpel debridement in facilitating corn resolution in patients with multiple corns. J Dermatol. 2016;43:662.
5. Sterling JC, Gibbs S, Haque Hussain SS, Mohd Mustapa MF, Handfield-Jones SE. British Association of Dermatologists' guidelines for the management of cutaneous warts 2014. Br J Dermatol. 2014;171:696.

CHAPTER 24

Management of Simple Lacerations in Children

INTRODUCTION

Simple lacerations are common injuries in children, often resulting from falls, cuts, or minor accidents. These injuries typically involve the skin and sometimes the subcutaneous tissues. Proper management is essential to ensure optimal healing, minimize scarring, and prevent infection.

INDICATIONS

- Open wound with clean, straight edges
- Minor cuts involving the skin and superficial tissues
- Bleeding that can be controlled with simple measures.

CONTRAINDICATIONS

- Deep lacerations involving muscles, tendons, or nerves, requiring specialist care
- Signs of infection (e.g., pus, increased redness, and swelling), requiring antibiotic therapy
- Severe bleeding or wounds with irregular, jagged edges, needing more complex repair.

EQUIPMENT AND SUPPLIES

- Sterile gloves
- Antiseptic solution (e.g., povidone-iodine or chlorhexidine)
- Sterile gauze pads
- Cotton-tipped applicators
- Local anesthetic (e.g., lidocaine)
- Syringe and needle for local anesthesia
- Suture kit or alternative closure materials (e.g., adhesive strips and tissue adhesive)
- Stapler and staple remover (if using staples)
- Fine-tipped forceps
- Scissors
- Sterile saline solution
- Antibiotic ointment
- Adhesive bandage or sterile dressing
- Pain management (oral analgesics)
- Personal protective equipment (PPE)

PREPARATION

- *Explain the procedure:*
    - Inform the child (if age-appropriate) and caregivers about the injury, the procedure for closure, its purpose, and what to expect.
    - Obtain informed consent from the caregivers.
- *Positioning:* Position the child comfortably, ideally seated or lying down with the affected area easily accessible.
- *Pain management:* Administer appropriate analgesics before the procedure if the child is in significant pain.

PROCEDURE STEPS

1. *Initial assessment:*
    a. Conduct a thorough history and physical examination to assess the location and extent of the laceration.

   b. Inspect the affected area for signs of deeper injury, foreign bodies, or infection.
2. *Cleansing:*
   a. Clean the area around the laceration with an antiseptic solution to reduce the risk of infection.
   b. Irrigate the wound thoroughly with sterile saline solution to remove debris and contaminants.
3. *Anesthesia:*
   a. Administer local anesthesia by injecting lidocaine around the edges of the laceration.
   b. Ensure adequate anesthesia before proceeding with the closure.
4. *Wound closure:*
   a. *Suturing (for deeper or gaping wounds):*
      i. *Preparation:* Assemble the suture kit and ensure all instruments are sterile.
      ii. *Procedure:*
         - Using fine-tipped forceps, gently approximate the wound edges.
         - Insert the needle at a 90° angle to the skin and pass it through both wound edges.
         - Tie the suture using an appropriate knot technique (e.g., simple interrupted, vertical mattress).
         - Continue suturing along the length of the laceration, ensuring even tension to approximate the wound edges without causing ischemia.
         - Trim the suture ends to leave about 0.5 cm of suture material above the knot.
   b. *Adhesive strips (for superficial or small lacerations)* ***(Figs. 1A and B)****:*
      i. *Procedure:*
         - Ensure the skin is dry before applying adhesive strips.
         - Align the wound edges and apply adhesive strips perpendicular to the laceration.
         - Space the strips evenly along the length of the wound.
   c. *Tissue adhesive (for clean, straight lacerations)* ***(Figs. 2A to C)****:*
      i. *Procedure:*
         - Align the wound edges and apply tissue adhesive in a thin layer over the wound.

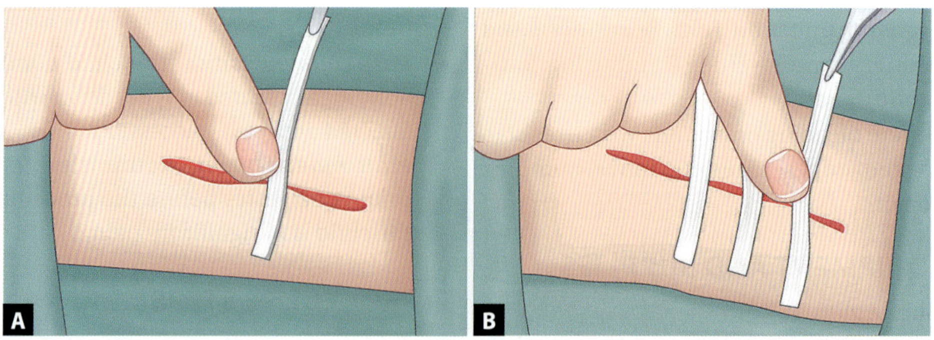

Figs. 1A and B: Adhesive tape application. (A) The tape is placed on one side of the wound at its midpoint while the clinician grasps it with forceps in the dominant hand. The opposite wound edge is then gently apposed by pushing with a finger of the nondominant hand; (B) The remaining open sections of the wound are bisected by additional tape strips until the strips are within 2–5 mm of each other.

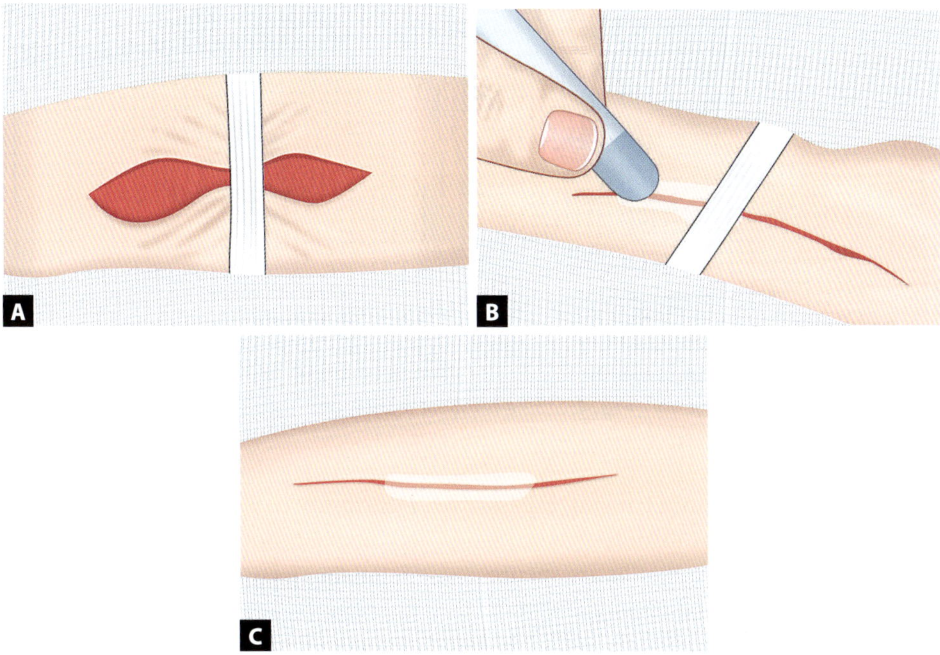

Figs. 2A to C: Tissue glue application. (A) The wound is bisected with a strip of surgical tape; (B) The wound limbs on either side of the tape are glued; (C) The strip is removed, and the central portion of the wound is glued. Some practitioners prefer to leave the tape strip and apply the adhesive over it.

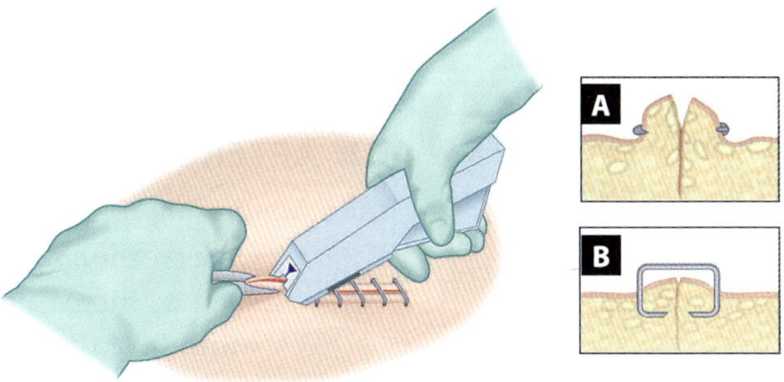

Figs. 3A and B: Wound closure by stapling.

- Hold the wound edges together for about 30 seconds until the adhesive sets.
- Avoid getting adhesive inside the wound to prevent foreign body reaction.

d. *Stapling (for long or high-tension lacerations)* ***(Figs. 3 and 4)***:

i. *Preparation:* Ensure the stapler is sterile and ready for use.

ii. *Procedure:*
- Align the wound edges using forceps or manually.
- Place the stapler over the wound and apply steady pressure to insert the staples evenly across the wound.
- Ensure staples are spaced appropriately to hold the wound edges

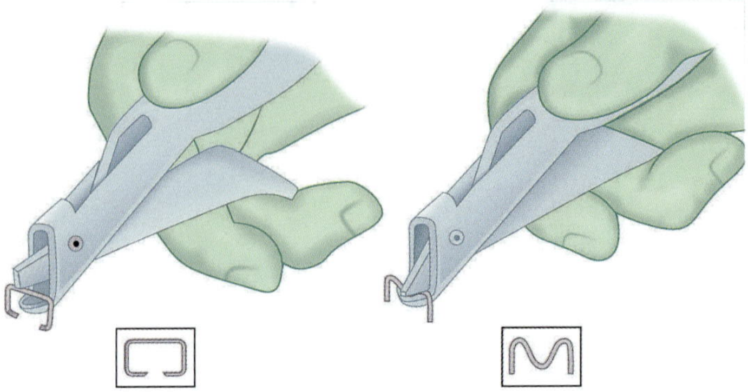

Fig. 4: Staple removal technique.

together without causing excess tension on the skin.
- Verify that the staples are secure and the wound edges are approximated well.

e. *Hair tying apposition (for scalp lacerations)* ***(Figs. 5A to D)***:
   i. *Preparation:* Identify and isolate strands of hair on either side of the scalp laceration.
   ii. *Procedure:*
   - Clean the area thoroughly with antiseptic solution.
   - Select several strands of hair (4–6 strands) on each side of the wound.
   - Twist the hair strands together to create a hair bundle on each side of the laceration.
   - Tie the hair bundles together over the wound using a surgeon's knot or similar secure knot to approximate the wound edges.
   - Ensure the wound edges are well approximated and secure. Hair tying is especially useful for small, superficial scalp lacerations and avoids the need for sutures or staples.

5. *Postclosure care:*
   a. *Inspection:* Examine the wound to ensure proper alignment and closure.
   b. *Cleaning:* Clean the surrounding skin with antiseptic to remove any residual blood or adhesive.
   c. *Dressing:* Apply a thin layer of antibiotic ointment to the wound and cover it with a sterile dressing or adhesive bandage.

AFTERCARE

- *Monitoring:*
  - Observe the child for signs of infection, such as increased redness, swelling, warmth, or discharge.
  - Provide instructions to caregivers on monitoring the wound and ensuring proper wound care.
- *Pain management:*
  - Prescribe appropriate oral analgesics for pain relief.
  - Advise caregivers to keep the affected area elevated if possible to reduce swelling.
- *Wound care:*
  - Instruct caregivers on proper wound care, including keeping the wound

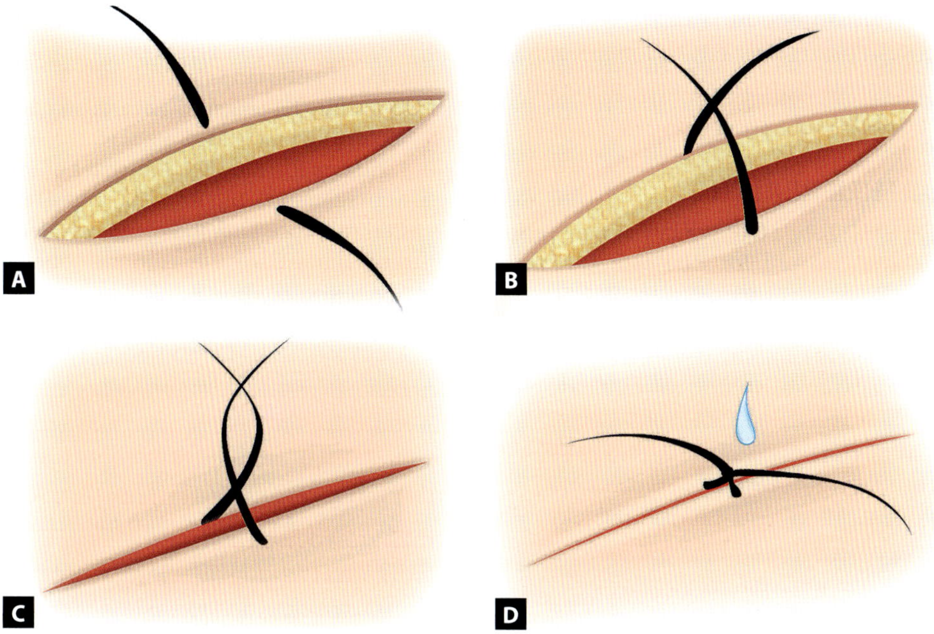

Figs. 5A to D: Hair apposition technique. (A) Choose four to five strands of hair in a bundle on either side of the scalp laceration; (B) Using artery forceps, cross the strands; (C) Make a single twist to appose wound; (D) Secure with a single drop of glue.

clean and dry, and changing the dressing as needed.
    - Recommend avoiding soaking the wound in water (e.g., baths and swimming) until it has healed.
- *Follow-up:*
    - Schedule a follow-up appointment for suture or staple removal if these methods were used (typically 5–7 days for facial wounds and 7–10 days for other areas).
    - Further evaluation may be necessary if there are signs of infection or delayed healing.

COMPLICATIONS

- *Infection:* Risk of secondary infection if the wound is not properly cared for.
- *Scarring:* Improper closure or care can lead to more prominent scarring.
- *Dehiscence:* Wound reopening due to inadequate closure or excessive tension.
- *Allergic reaction:* Possible reaction to suture material, adhesive, or staple metal.

PREVENTION

- *Safety measures:* Encourage the use of protective gear during activities that may cause injuries.
- *Education:* Teach children about the importance of safety to prevent cuts and lacerations.
- *Supervision:* Supervise young children during activities that may expose them to risks of injury.

CONCLUSION

The management of simple lacerations in children involves prompt and careful closure to ensure proper healing, minimize scarring, and prevent infection. Proper technique, aftercare, and caregiver education are crucial for successful outcomes and preventing complications.

FURTHER READING

1. Eliya MC, Banda GW. Primary closure versus delayed closure for non bite traumatic wounds within 24 hours post injury. Cochrane Database Syst Rev. 2011:(9):CD008574.
2. Hollander JE, Singer AJ, Valentine S. Comparison of wound care practices in pediatric and adult lacerations repaired in the emergency department. Pediatr Emerg Care. 1998;14(1):15-8.
3. Hollander JE, Singer AJ. Laceration management. Ann Emerg Med. 1999;34(3):356-67.
4. Lammers RL, Aldy KN. Principles of Wound Management. In: Roberts and Hedges' Clinical Procedures in Emergency Medicine and Acute Care, 7th edition, Roberts JR, Custalow CB, Thomsen TW (Eds), Elsevier, Philadelphia 2019. p.621.
5. Mankowitz SL. Laceration Management. J Emerg Med. 2017 Sep;53(3):369-82.

CHAPTER 25

Management of Simple Tongue and Lip Lacerations in Children

INTRODUCTION

Tongue and lip lacerations are common injuries in children, often resulting from falls, sports activities, or accidental bites. Proper management is crucial to ensure optimal healing, minimize scarring, and prevent infection.

PROCEDURE FOR SIMPLE TONGUE LACERATION

Indications

- Laceration of the tongue with minimal tissue loss
- Bleeding that can be controlled with simple measures
- Lacerations <2 cm in length, not involving the tongue base or deep muscle layers.

Contraindications

- Deep lacerations involving muscle or large vessels requiring specialist care
- Signs of infection (e.g., pus, increased redness, and swelling)
- Lacerations causing significant functional impairment or involving the base of the tongue.

Equipment and Supplies

- Sterile gloves
- Antiseptic solution (e.g., saline or chlorhexidine)
- Sterile gauze pads
- Cotton-tipped applicators
- Local anesthetic (e.g., lidocaine gel or injection)
- Syringe and needle for local anesthesia
- Absorbable sutures (e.g., 4-0 or 5-0 Vicryl)
- Fine-tipped forceps
- Needle holder
- Scissors
- Suction apparatus (optional)
- Oral antiseptic rinse
- Pain management (oral analgesics).

Preparation

- *Explain the procedure:*
    - Inform the child (if age-appropriate) and caregivers about the injury, the procedure for closure, its purpose, and what to expect.
    - Obtain informed consent from the caregivers.
- *Positioning:* Position the child comfortably, ideally seated or lying down with their head supported.
- *Pain management:* Administer appropriate analgesics before the procedure if the child is in significant pain.

Procedure Steps

1. *Initial assessment:*
    a. Conduct a thorough history and physical examination to assess the location and extent of the laceration.
    b. Inspect the tongue for signs of deeper injury, foreign bodies, or infection.

2. *Cleansing:* Clean the area around the laceration with an antiseptic solution to reduce the risk of infection.
3. *Anesthesia:*
   a. Administer local anesthesia using lidocaine gel or an injection around the laceration site.
   b. Ensure adequate anesthesia before proceeding with the closure.
4. *Wound closure:*
   a. Suturing (for deeper or gaping wounds):
      i. *Preparation:* Assemble the suture kit and ensure all instruments are sterile.
      ii. *Procedure:*
         - Using fine-tipped forceps, gently approximate the wound edges.
         - Insert the needle at a 90° angle to the tissue and pass it through both wound edges.
         - Tie the suture using an appropriate knot technique (e.g., simple interrupted).
         - Continue suturing along the length of the laceration, ensuring even tension to approximate the wound edges without causing ischemia.
         - Trim the suture ends to leave about 0.5 cm of suture material above the knot.
         - Absorbable sutures are preferred for tongue lacerations to avoid the need for removal.
5. *Postclosure care:*
   a. *Inspection:* Examine the wound to ensure proper alignment and closure.
   b. *Cleaning:* Clean the surrounding area with an antiseptic to remove any residual blood.
   c. *Oral care:* Advise rinsing the mouth with an oral antiseptic rinse to maintain cleanliness.

Aftercare

- *Monitoring:*
  - Observe the child for signs of infection, such as increased redness, swelling, warmth, or discharge.
  - Provide instructions to caregivers on monitoring the wound and ensuring proper oral hygiene.
- *Pain management:*
  - Prescribe appropriate oral analgesics for pain relief.
  - Recommend cold compresses or ice pops to reduce swelling and numb the area.
- *Wound care:*
  - Instruct caregivers on proper oral care, including rinsing the mouth with an antiseptic rinse after meals.
  - Recommend a soft diet to avoid trauma to the healing wound.
- *Follow-up:* Schedule a follow-up appointment to monitor healing and assess for any complications.

PROCEDURE FOR SIMPLE LIP LACERATION

Indications

- Laceration of the lip with minimal tissue loss
- Bleeding that can be controlled with simple measures
- Lacerations involving the vermilion border, requiring careful approximation.

Contraindications

- Deep lacerations involving muscle or large vessels requiring specialist care
- Signs of infection (e.g., pus, increased redness, and swelling)
- Lacerations causing significant functional impairment or involving the inner mucosal surface extensively.

Procedure Steps

1. *Initial assessment:*
   a. Conduct a thorough history and physical examination to assess the location and extent of the laceration.
   b. Inspect the lip for signs of deeper injury, foreign bodies, or infection.
2. *Cleansing:* Clean the area around the laceration with an antiseptic solution to reduce the risk of infection.
3. *Anesthesia:*
   a. Administer local anesthesia using lidocaine with epinephrine around the laceration site.
   b. Ensure adequate anesthesia before proceeding with the closure.
3. *Wound closure:*
   - Suturing (for deeper or gaping wounds):
     i. *Preparation:* Assemble the suture kit and ensure all instruments are sterile.
     ii. *Procedure:*
       - Using fine-tipped forceps, gently approximate the wound edges.
       - Insert the needle at a 90° angle to the skin and pass it through both wound edges.
       - For lacerations involving the vermilion border, align the border carefully to ensure a smooth cosmetic result.
       - Tie the suture using an appropriate knot technique (e.g., simple interrupted).
       - Continue suturing along the length of the laceration, ensuring even tension to approximate the wound edges without causing ischemia.
       - Trim the suture ends to leave about 0.5 cm of suture material above the knot.
       - Use nonabsorbable sutures for skin closure and absorbable sutures for mucosal closure.
5. *Postclosure care:*
   a. *Inspection:* Examine the wound to ensure proper alignment and closure.
   b. *Cleaning:* Clean the surrounding area with an antiseptic to remove any residual blood.
   c. *Oral care:* Advise rinsing the mouth with an oral antiseptic rinse to maintain cleanliness.

Aftercare

- *Monitoring:*
  - Observe the child for signs of infection, such as increased redness, swelling, warmth, or discharge.
  - Provide instructions to caregivers on monitoring the wound and ensuring proper oral hygiene.
- *Pain management:*
  - Prescribe appropriate oral analgesics for pain relief.
  - Recommend cold compresses to reduce swelling and numb the area.
- *Wound care:*
  - Instruct caregivers on proper oral care, including rinsing the mouth with an antiseptic rinse after meals.
  - Recommend a soft diet to avoid trauma to the healing wound.
- *Follow-up:*
  - Schedule a follow-up appointment for suture removal if nonabsorbable sutures were used (typically 5–7 days for facial wounds).
  - Further evaluation may be necessary if there are signs of infection or delayed healing.

COMPLICATIONS

- *Infection:* Risk of secondary infection if the wound is not properly cared for

- *Scarring:* Improper closure or care can lead to more prominent scarring.
- *Dehiscence:* Wound reopening due to inadequate closure or excessive tension
- *Functional impairment:* Possible impact on speech or eating if the wound does not heal properly

PREVENTION

- *Safety measures:* Encourage the use of protective gear during activities that may cause injuries.
- *Education:* Teach children about the importance of safety to prevent cuts and lacerations.
- *Supervision:* Supervise young children during activities that may expose them to risks of injury.

CONCLUSION

The management of simple tongue and lip lacerations in children involves prompt and careful closure to ensure proper healing, minimize scarring, and prevent infection. Proper technique, aftercare, and caregiver education are crucial for successful outcomes and preventing complications.

FURTHER READING

1. Armstrong BD. Lacerations of the mouth. Emerg Med Clin North Am. 2000;18(3): 471-80, v
2. Grunebaum LD, Smith JE, Hoosien GE. Lip and perioral trauma. Facial Plast Surg. 2010;26(6):433-44.
3. Attia MW, Loiselle J. Management of soft-tissue injuries of the mouth. In: Textbook of Pediatric Emergency Procedures, 2nd edition, King C, Henretig FM (Eds) (Eds), Lippincott, Williams & Wilkins, Philadelphia, PA 2008. p.680.
4. Gonsalves CL, Zhu JW, Kim GY, Leveille CF, Kam AJ. Surgical versus conservative management of tongue lacerations in the acute care setting: A systematic review of the literature. Paediatr Child Health. 2021;27(1):32-42.
5. Seiler M, Massaro SL, Staubli G, Schiestl C. Tongue lacerations in children: to suture or not? Swiss Med Wkly. 2018:148:w14683.

CHAPTER 26

Procedure for Management of Pencil Point Puncture in Children

INTRODUCTION

Pencil point punctures are common injuries in children, typically resulting from accidental stabs or pokes with a pencil. These injuries can introduce graphite and other contaminants into the skin, potentially leading to infection. Prompt and appropriate management is crucial to ensure proper healing and prevent complications.

INDICATIONS

- Puncture wound caused by a pencil
- Symptoms such as pain, bleeding, and visible graphite or pencil debris in the wound
- Swelling, redness, or tenderness around the site of the puncture.

CONTRAINDICATIONS

- Suspected deep tissue injury, requiring surgical intervention
- Signs of systemic infection (e.g., fever and chills), requiring antibiotic therapy
- Location near sensitive areas such as the eye or joints, requiring specialist care.

EQUIPMENT AND SUPPLIES

- Sterile gloves
- Antiseptic solution (e.g., povidone-iodine or chlorhexidine)
- Sterile gauze pads
- Cotton-tipped applicators
- Tweezers or fine-tipped forceps
- Needle (for stubborn debris removal)
- Magnifying glass or loupe (optional)
- Sterile saline solution
- Antibiotic ointment
- Adhesive bandage or sterile dressing
- Pain management (oral analgesics)
- Personal protective equipment (PPE).

PREPARATION

- *Explain the procedure:*
  - Inform the child (if age-appropriate) and caregivers about the injury, the removal procedure, its purpose, and what to expect.
  - Obtain informed consent from the caregivers.
- *Positioning:* Position the child comfortably, ideally seated or lying down with the affected area easily accessible.
- *Pain management:* Administer appropriate analgesics before the procedure if the child is in significant pain.

PROCEDURE STEPS

1. *Initial assessment:*
   a. Conduct a thorough history and physical examination to assess the location and extent of the injury.
   b. Inspect the affected area for signs of embedded graphite or other pencil debris.
2. *Cleansing:* Clean the area around the puncture wound with an antiseptic solution to reduce the risk of infection.

3. *Removal of debris:*
   a. *Visible and easily accessible debris*:
      i. *Procedure:*
         - Use tweezers or fine-tipped forceps to grasp and remove any visible graphite or pencil debris.
         - Gently lift and extract the debris without causing further injury to the surrounding tissue.
         - If the debris is difficult to grasp, use a magnifying glass or loupe to enhance visibility.
   b. *Partially embedded debris*:
      i. *Procedure:*
         - If part of the debris is embedded beneath the skin, use a sterile needle to gently lift the skin over the debris.
         - Once the debris is exposed, use tweezers or forceps to grasp and remove it.
         - Be careful to avoid breaking the debris, as this can make removal more difficult.
4. *Inspection and irrigation:*
   a. *Inspection:* Examine the wound to ensure no part of the debris remains.
   b. *Irrigation:* Irrigate the wound with sterile saline solution to flush out any remaining debris or contaminants.
5. *Postremoval care:*
   a. *Antibiotic ointment:* Apply a thin layer of antibiotic ointment to the wound.
   b. *Dressing:* Cover the wound with a nonadherent dressing or adhesive bandage to protect it and promote healing.

AFTERCARE

- *Monitoring:*
  - Observe the child for signs of infection, such as increased redness, swelling, warmth, or discharge.
  - Provide instructions to caregivers on monitoring the wound and ensuring proper wound care.
- *Pain management:*
  - Prescribe appropriate oral analgesics for pain relief.
  - Advise caregivers to keep the affected area clean and dry.
- *Wound care:*
  - Instruct caregivers on proper wound care, including changing the dressing daily and keeping the area clean.
  - Recommend avoiding activities that may cause further injury to the affected area until it has healed.
- *Follow-up:*
  - Schedule a follow-up appointment if there are concerns about infection or if the wound does not heal properly.
  - Further evaluation may be necessary if there are signs of persistent infection or delayed healing.

COMPLICATIONS

- *Infection:* Risk of secondary infection if the wound is not properly cared for
- *Retained debris:* Incomplete removal of graphite or pencil fragments may cause ongoing pain or infection.
- *Tissue damage:* Improper removal techniques can cause additional tissue damage.
- *Pain:* Persistent pain may require further evaluation and management.

PREVENTION

- *Safety measures:* Encourage the use of protective gear, such as pencil grips or covers, to reduce the risk of injury.
- *Education:* Teach children about the risks of playing with or handling pencils inappropriately.

- *Supervision:* Supervise young children during activities that may expose them to pencil injuries.

CONCLUSION

The management of pencil point punctures in children involves prompt and careful removal of debris to prevent further tissue damage and minimize pain. Proper technique, aftercare, and caregiver education are crucial for successful outcomes and preventing complications.

FURTHER READING

1. Bittencourt MJS, Santos JEBD, Barros JNDS Junior, Xerfan EMS. Pencil-core granuloma. An Bras Dermatol. 2017;92(4):578-9.
2. Chisholm CD, Schlesser JF. Plantar puncture wounds: controversies and treatment recommendations. Ann Emerg Med. 1989;18(12):1352-7.
3. Chudnofsky CR, Sebastian S. Special wounds. Nail bed, plantar puncture, and cartilage. Emerg Med Clin North Am. 1992;10(4):801-22.
4. Eidelman M, Bialik V, Miller Y, Kassis I. Plantar puncture wounds in children: analysis of 80 hospitalized patients and late sequelae. Isr Med Assoc J. 2003;5(4):268-7.
5. Orton E, Whitehead J, Mhizha-Murira J, Clarkson M, Watson MC, Mulvaney CA, Staniforth JU, Bhuchar M, Kendrick D. School-based education programmes for the prevention of unintentional injuries in children and young people. Cochrane Database Syst Rev. 2016;12(12):CD010246.

CHAPTER 27

First Aid Splint for Children with Fracture

INTRODUCTION

Fractures are common injuries in children and can result from falls, sports activities, or accidents. Proper first aid and immobilization using a splint are essential to prevent further injury, reduce pain, and prepare the child for transport to a healthcare facility for definitive care.

INDICATIONS

- Suspected fracture indicated by pain, swelling, deformity, or inability to use the affected limb
- Open fractures with visible bone protrusion
- Suspected fracture with neurovascular compromise (e.g., loss of pulse, numbness, or cyanosis distal to the injury)

CONTRAINDICATIONS

- Severe injuries requiring immediate medical attention without delay for splinting
- Lack of appropriate materials or training to apply a splint safely

EQUIPMENT AND SUPPLIES

- Sterile gloves
- Antiseptic solution (for open wounds)
- Sterile gauze pads and dressings
- Bandages or elastic wraps
- Rigid splinting materials (e.g., wooden boards, padded aluminum splints, and commercial splints)
- Soft padding materials (e.g., cloth and foam)
- Adhesive tape
- Scissors
- Personal protective equipment (PPE)

PREPARATION

- *Explain the procedure:*
  - Inform the child (if age-appropriate) and caregivers about the need for splinting, its purpose, and what to expect.
  - Obtain verbal consent from the caregivers.
- *Positioning:* Position the child comfortably, ensuring that the affected limb is supported and remains as still as possible.

PROCEDURE STEPS

1. *Initial assessment:*
   a. Conduct a brief history and physical examination to assess the injury.
   b. Check for signs of fracture, such as deformity, swelling, bruising, and inability to move the affected limb.
   c. Assess neurovascular status by checking for pulse, warmth, color, and sensation distal to the injury.
2. *Managing open wounds:*
   a. If there are open wounds, clean them with an antiseptic solution and cover them with sterile gauze pads.
   b. Do not attempt to push protruding bones back into place.

3. *Padding the splint:*
   a. Apply soft padding around the affected limb to protect the skin and provide additional comfort.
   b. Ensure that the padding extends beyond the ends of the splint to prevent pressure points.
4. *Applying the splint:*
   a. *Selection:* Choose a rigid splint that is long enough to immobilize the joints above and below the suspected fracture site.
   b. *Placement:* Gently place the splint along one side of the limb, ensuring it is in alignment with the limb.
   c. *Securing:*
      i. Use bandages or elastic wraps to secure the splint in place.
      ii. Start wrapping from the distal end (farthest from the heart) and move proximally (closer to the heart).
      iii. Ensure the wraps are snug but not so tight that they compromise circulation.
5. *Immobilizing the limb:*
   a. For upper limb fractures, use a sling to support the arm and hold it close to the body.
   b. For lower limb fractures, keep the child lying down with the leg elevated and supported.

USING A TRIANGULAR BANDAGE AS A SLING

- *Initial assessment:*
  - Conduct a brief history and physical examination to assess the injury.
  - Check for signs of fracture, dislocation, or other injuries.
- *Creating the sling:*
  - *Preparation:* Open the triangular bandage and fold it to create a broad fold (base at the top, point at the bottom).
  - *Placement:* Place the bandage under the injured arm, with the point of the triangle extending past the elbow.
  - *Securing:*
    - Bring the two ends of the bandage up and tie them around the neck, ensuring the knot is at the side of the neck for comfort.
    - Tuck the point of the bandage behind the elbow or secure it with a safety pin to create a comfortable, supportive sling.
- *Adjusting the sling:*
  - Ensure the hand is slightly elevated above the level of the elbow.
  - Check for comfort and proper support, making adjustments as necessary.

USING A TRIANGULAR BANDAGE FOR AN ARM OR LEG SPLINT (FIGS. 1A AND B)

- *Padding and aligning:*
  - Pad the splint (rigid material like a board) to make it more comfortable.
  - Align the splint with the injured limb, ensuring that it extends beyond the joints above and below the injury.
- *Securing the splint:*
  - *Preparation:* Fold the triangular bandage into a broad fold or leave it open, depending on the size of the splint and the injury.
  - *Placement:* Place the center of the bandage over the splint and injured area.
  - *Tying:*
    - Bring the ends of the bandage around the limb and tie them securely. Use additional bandages if needed to secure the splint.

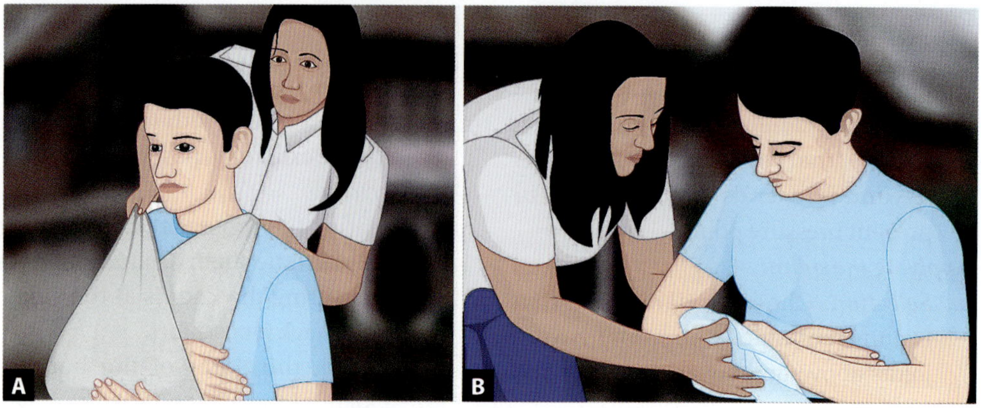

Figs. 1A and B: Triangular bandage first air arm sling.

- Ensure the ties are snug but not so tight that they compromise circulation.

- *Reassessing neurovascular status:*
  - Check for pulse, warmth, color, and sensation distal to the injury after applying the splint.
  - Adjust the bandage if there are signs of impaired circulation.

USING A TRIANGULAR BANDAGE TO CONTROL BLEEDING

- *Initial assessment and cleaning:*
  - Conduct a brief assessment of the wound.
  - Clean the wound with an antiseptic solution if available.
- *Applying a dressing:* Place a sterile gauze pad over the wound.
- *Securing the dressing with a bandage:*
  - *Preparation:* Open the triangular bandage and fold it as needed to create a broad or narrow fold, depending on the size of the wound.
  - *Placement:* Place the bandage over the gauze pad and wound.
  - *Tying:*
    - Bring the ends of the bandage around the limb or body and tie them securely to apply pressure and control bleeding.
    - Ensure the bandage is snug but not so tight that it compromises circulation.
- *Reassessing neurovascular status:*
  - After applying the splint, reassess the neurovascular status to ensure that circulation is not compromised.
  - Check for pulse, warmth, color, and sensation distal to the injury.
- *Transport:*
  - Keep the child calm and still while arranging for transport to a healthcare facility.
  - Provide ongoing support and reassurance to the child and caregivers.

AFTERCARE

- *Monitoring:*
  - Continuously monitor the child for signs of increased pain, swelling, or changes in neurovascular status.
  - Reassess the splint periodically to ensure it remains secure and does not cause discomfort.
- *Pain management:*
  - Provide appropriate pain relief with oral analgesics if needed.

- Advise caregivers on pain management strategies until medical help is obtained.
- *Follow-up:*
    - Ensure the child receives prompt medical evaluation and treatment at a healthcare facility.
    - Further imaging and definitive treatment, such as casting or surgical intervention, may be necessary.

COMPLICATIONS

- *Compartment syndrome:* Monitor for increased pain, swelling, or tightness, which may indicate compartment syndrome, a medical emergency requiring immediate attention.
- *Neurovascular compromise:* Ensure that the splint does not impair circulation or nerve function.
- *Infection:* Properly manage open fractures to prevent infection.

PREVENTION

- *Safety measures:* Encourage the use of protective gear during sports and physical activities to prevent fractures.
- *Education:* Teach children about safety practices to reduce the risk of falls and injuries.

CONCLUSION

The first aid management of fractures in children involves prompt and careful splinting to immobilize the injured limb, reduce pain, and prevent further injury. Proper technique, aftercare, and prompt transport to a healthcare facility are crucial for successful outcomes and preventing complications.

FURTHER READING

1. Chudnofsky C. Splinting techniques. In: Clinical Procedurs in Emergency Medicine, Roberts J, Hedges J (Eds), WB Saunders, Philadelphia 1998. p.852.
2. Geideman J. Orthopedic injuries: General principles. In: Rosen's Emergency Medicine: Concepts and Clinical Practice, 5th Ed, Marx J, Hockberger R, Walls R (Eds), Mosby, Philadelphia 2002. p.486.
3. Klig J. Splinting procedures. In: Textbook of Pediatric Emergency Procedures, Henretig F, King C, Joffe M (Eds), Lippincott, Williams & Wilkins, Baltimore 2008. p.919.
4. Kovan J, McKeag D. Ankle splinting, taping, and casting. In: Procedures for Primary Care Physicians, Pfenninger J, Fowler G (Eds), Mosby, St. Louis 1994. p.1004.
5. Steele P, Bush-Joseph C, Bach B Jr. Office management of trauma—management of acute fractures around the knee, ankle, and foot. Clin Fam Pract 2000;2:661.

CHAPTER 28

Procedure for Management of Pulled Elbow in Children

INTRODUCTION

A pulled elbow, also known as nursemaid's elbow or radial head subluxation, is a common injury in young children. It occurs when the radial head slips out of the annular ligament, usually due to a sudden pull on the child's outstretched arm. This condition is typically seen in children aged 1–4 years and can cause significant pain and reluctance to use the affected arm **(Fig. 1)**.

INDICATIONS

- Sudden onset of arm pain following a pulling mechanism (e.g., pulling on the child's hand or arm)
- Child holding the affected arm close to their body with the elbow slightly bent and forearm pronated
- Reluctance or refusal to use the affected arm

CONTRAINDICATIONS

- Suspected fracture or other serious injury requiring imaging and specialist intervention
- Significant swelling or deformity indicating a more severe injury

EQUIPMENT AND SUPPLIES

- Sterile gloves (if there are any open wounds)

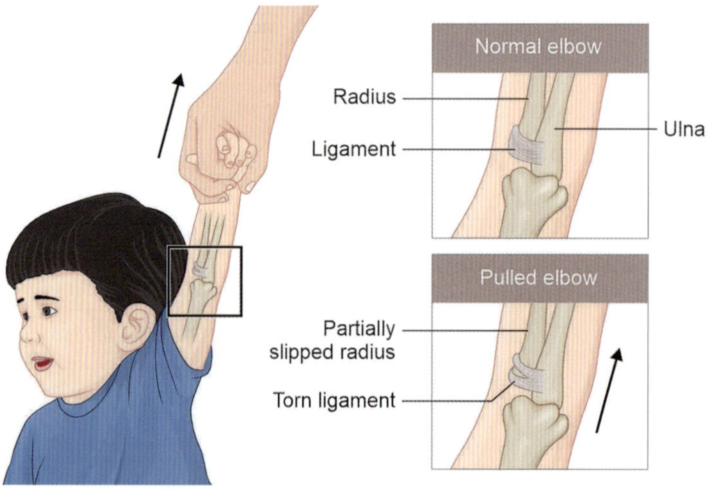

Fig. 1: Pulled elbow.

- Analgesics (if necessary)
- Personal protective equipment (PPE)

PREPARATION

- *Explain the procedure:*
  - Inform the child (if age-appropriate) and caregivers about the condition, the procedure, its purpose, and what to expect.
  - Obtain informed consent from the caregivers.
- *Positioning:* Position the child sitting comfortably on the caregiver's lap or on an examination table. Ensure the child is calm and supported.
- *Pain management:* Administer appropriate analgesics if the child is in significant pain.

PROCEDURE STEPS

1. *Initial assessment:*
   a. Conduct a thorough history and physical examination to confirm the diagnosis of a pulled elbow.
   b. Examine the affected arm for any signs of deformity, swelling, or tenderness suggesting a fracture or other injury.
2. *Reduction techniques:*
   a. *Supination-flexion method* ***(Figs. 2A and B)****:*
      i. *Preparation:* Hold the child's affected arm with one hand supporting the elbow and the other hand holding the wrist.
      ii. *Procedure:*
         - Supinate the forearm (turn the palm up) while simultaneously applying gentle traction.
         - Flex the elbow fully while maintaining supination.
         - You may feel a slight click or pop as the radial head repositions into place.
         - Observe the child for immediate relief and return of normal arm movement.
   b. *Hyperpronation method* ***(Figs. 3A and B)****:*
      i. *Preparation:* Hold the child's affected arm with one hand

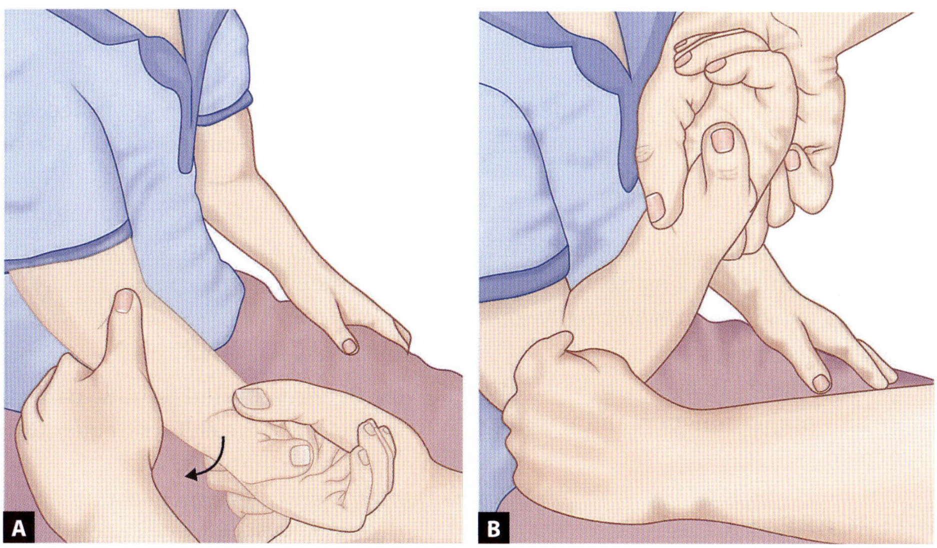

Figs. 2A and B: Supination technique for pulled elbow.

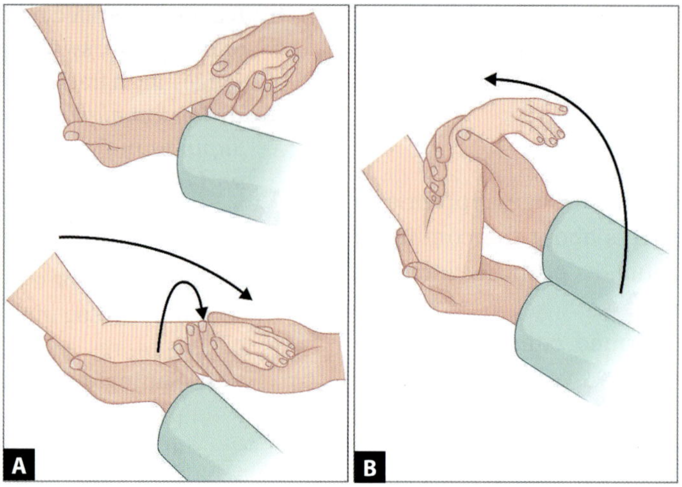

Figs. 3A and B: "Handshake" or hyperpronation maneuver. (A) Simultaneous pronation of the wrist and extension of the elbow; and (B) Followed by flexion of the elbow with the forearm maintained in pronation.

supporting the elbow and the other hand holding the wrist.

ii. *Procedure:*
   - Pronate the forearm (turn the palm down) while applying gentle traction.
   - Hyperpronate the forearm fully, which can help reposition the radial head.
   - Again, you may feel a slight click or pop indicating successful reduction.
   - Observe the child for immediate relief and return of normal arm movement.

3. *Postprocedure care:*
   a. *Observation:* Monitor the child for a few minutes to ensure the child begins using the arm normally and experiences pain relief.
   b. *Reassessment:* Reassess the arm to ensure proper function and absence of pain.

AFTERCARE

- *Monitoring:*
  - Observe the child for any signs of recurrence or complications.
  - Provide instructions to caregivers on monitoring for any issues and ensuring proper use of the arm.
- *Activity modification:*
  - Advise avoiding activities that involve pulling or lifting the child by the arms to prevent recurrence.
  - Educate caregivers on safe handling techniques.
- *Follow-up:*
  - Typically, no follow-up is necessary if the child resumes normal use of the arm without pain.
  - Schedule a follow-up appointment if there are concerns about recurrence or other injuries.

COMPLICATIONS

- *Recurrence:* Pulled elbow can recur, particularly if the child is frequently lifted or pulled by the arms.
- *Misdiagnosis:* Ensure accurate diagnosis to avoid missing fractures or other serious injuries.

- *Persistent pain:* Rarely, if pain persists or normal function does not return, further evaluation may be necessary to rule out other injuries.

PREVENTION

- *Safe handling:* Educate caregivers on proper techniques for lifting and handling young children, avoiding pulling or lifting with the arms.
- *Supervision:* Encourage close supervision during play and activities to prevent accidental pulls or falls.

CONCLUSION

The management of a pulled elbow in children involves prompt and gentle reduction to relieve pain and restore normal arm function. Proper technique, aftercare, and caregiver education are crucial for successful outcomes and preventing recurrence.

FURTHER READING

1. Genadry KC, Monuteaux MC, Neuman MI, Lipsett SC. Management and Outcomes of Children With Nursemaid's Elbow. Ann Emerg Me. 2021;77(2):154-62.
2. Macias CG, Bothner J, Wiebe R. A comparison of supination/flexion to hyperpronation in the reduction of radial head subluxations. Pediatrics. 1998l;102(1):e10.
3. Rudloe TF, Schutzman S, Lee LK, Kimia AA. No longer a "nursemaid's" elbow: mechanisms, caregivers, and prevention. Pediatr Emerg Care 2012;28:771.
4. Schunk JE. Radial head subluxation: epidemiology and treatment of 87 episodes. Pediatr Emerg Care. 2012;28(8):771-4.
5. Welch R, Chounthirath T, Smith GA. Radial Head Subluxation Among Young Children in the United States Associated With Consumer Products and Recreational Activities. Clin Pediatr (Phila). 2017;56(8):707-15. d

CHAPTER 29

Procedure for Management of Clavicle Fracture in Children

INTRODUCTION

Clavicle fractures are common pediatric injuries, often resulting from falls or direct trauma to the shoulder. Most clavicle fractures in children heal well with conservative management, but proper assessment and treatment are crucial to ensure optimal healing and function **(Fig. 1)**.

INDICATIONS

- Visible deformity or swelling over the clavicle
- Symptoms such as pain, tenderness, and limited range of motion in the shoulder
- History of trauma to the shoulder or clavicle area

CONTRAINDICATIONS

- Open fractures requiring surgical intervention
- Neurovascular compromise in the affected limb
- Severe displacement or comminuted fractures requiring orthopedic consultation

EQUIPMENT AND SUPPLIES

- Sterile gloves
- Antiseptic solution (if there are any open wounds)
- Sterile gauze pads
- Arm sling or figure-of-eight bandage
- Ice pack or cold compress
- Analgesics
- Personal protective equipment (PPE)

PREPARATION

- *Explain the procedure:*
    - Inform the child (if age-appropriate) and caregivers about the condition, the procedure, its purpose, and what to expect.

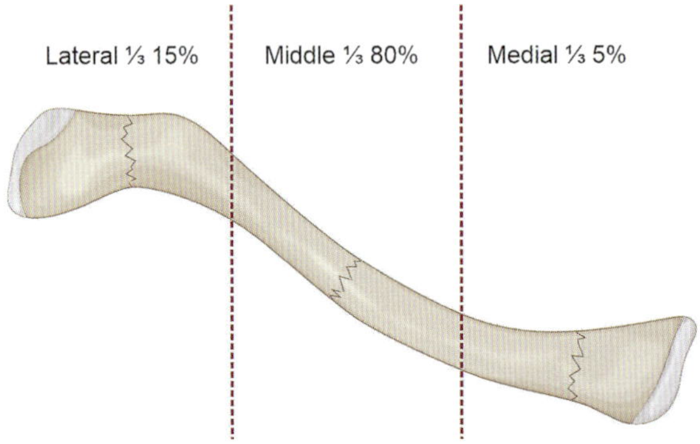

Fig. 1: Fractures of the clavicle can be classified by its anatomical location.

- Obtain informed consent from the caregivers.

- *Positioning:* Position the child in a comfortable sitting position to facilitate examination and treatment.
- *Pain management:* Administer appropriate analgesics if the child is in significant pain.

PROCEDURE STEPS

1. *Initial assessment:*
   a. Conduct a thorough history and physical examination to confirm the diagnosis of a clavicle fracture.
   b. Inspect the affected area for deformity, swelling, bruising, and tenderness.
   c. Assess the range of motion of the shoulder and look for any signs of neurovascular compromise (e.g., numbness, weakness, and diminished pulses).
2. *Imaging:* Obtain X-rays of the clavicle to confirm the fracture, assess the location and degree of displacement, and rule out associated injuries.
3. *Conservative management:*
   a. *Immobilization:*
      i. *Arm sling* ***(Fig. 2)***:
         - Place the child's arm in a sling to support the weight of the arm and reduce pain.
         - Ensure the sling is properly fitted to keep the arm close to the body and the elbow bent at a right angle.
      ii. *Figure-of-eight bandage (if needed)* ***(Fig. 3)***:
         - Apply a figure-of-eight bandage to immobilize the shoulder and clavicle if additional stabilization is required.

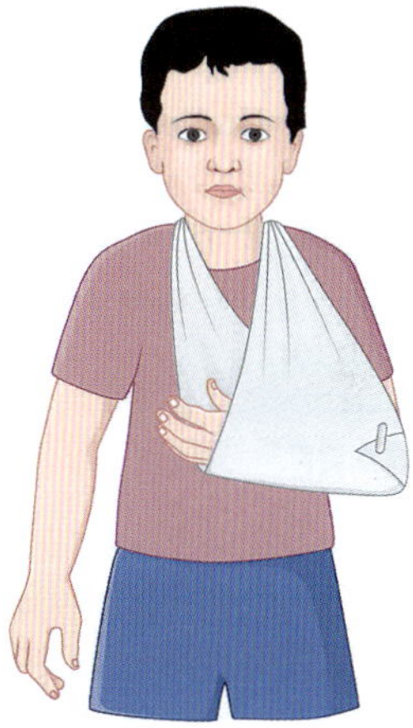

Fig. 2: Arm sling for clavicular fracture.

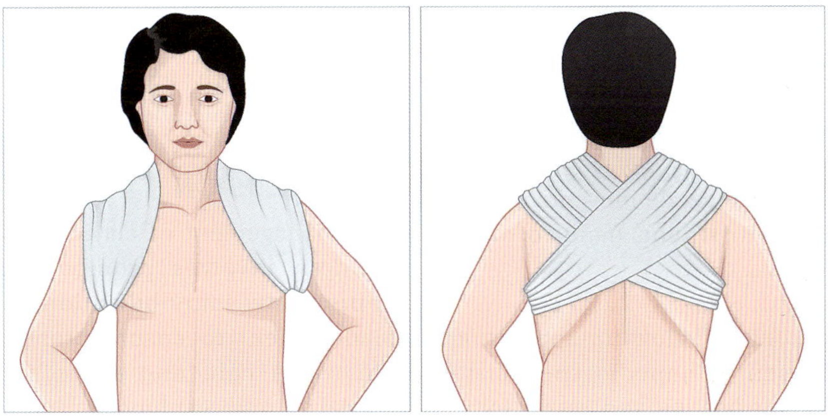

Fig. 3: Figure-of-eight bandage for clavicular fracture.

   - Ensure the bandage is snug but not too tight to avoid impairing circulation.
   b. *Pain management:* Administer oral analgesics (e.g., acetaminophen or ibuprofen) to manage pain and reduce inflammation.
   c. *Ice application:* Apply an ice pack or cold compress to the affected area for 15–20 minutes every 2–3 hours for the first 48 hours to reduce swelling and pain.
4. *Postprocedure care:*
   a. *Observation:* Monitor the child for signs of discomfort, pain, or complications.
   b. *Instructions:* Provide caregivers with detailed instructions on how to care for the child's injury, including the use of the sling or bandage, activity restrictions, and signs of complications to watch for.

AFTERCARE

- *Monitoring:*
  - Observe the child for signs of pain, swelling, or changes in neurovascular status.
  - Provide instructions to caregivers on monitoring for any delayed complications.
- *Activity modification*:
  - Advise the child to avoid strenuous activities, contact sports, and lifting heavy objects until the fracture has healed.
  - Encourage gentle movements of the elbow, wrist, and hand to prevent stiffness.
- *Follow-up:*
  - Schedule a follow-up appointment with an orthopedic specialist to monitor healing and assess for any complications.
  - Further imaging may be necessary to ensure proper healing and alignment of the clavicle.
- *Rehabilitation*:
  - Once the fracture has healed sufficiently, initiate a rehabilitation program to restore strength and range of motion in the shoulder.
  - Physical therapy may be recommended to facilitate recovery and prevent complications.

COMPLICATIONS

- *Nonunion or malunion:* Improper healing of the fracture may require further intervention.
- *Neurovascular injury:* Monitor for signs of nerve or blood vessel damage.
- *Infection:* Risk of infection if there are open wounds associated with the fracture.
- *Shoulder stiffness:* Prolonged immobilization can lead to decreased range of motion.

PREVENTION

- *Safety measures:* Encourage the use of protective gear during sports and physical activities.
- *Education:* Educate caregivers and children on the importance of safety and preventing falls and injuries.

CONCLUSION

The management of clavicle fractures in children involves prompt assessment, appropriate immobilization, and pain management to ensure proper healing. Follow-up care and rehabilitation are crucial for restoring function and preventing complications.

FURTHER READING

1. Eiff MP. Management of clavicle fractures. Am Fam Physician. 1997;55(1):121-8.
2. Hassankhani A, Amoukhteh M, Jannatdoust P, Valizadeh P, Gholamrezanezhad A. A systematic review and meta-analysis on the diagnostic utility of ultrasound for clavicle fractures. Skeletal Radiol. 2024;53(2):307-18.
3. Lenza M, Faloppa F. Conservative interventions for treating middle third clavicle fractures in adolescents and adults. Cochrane Database Syst Rev. 2016;12(12).
4. Pujalte GG, Housner JA. Management of clavicle fractures. Curr Sports Med Rep. 2008;7(5):275-80.
5. Serpico M, Tomberg S. The emergency medicine management of clavicle fractures. Am J Emerg Med. 2021;49:315-25.

CHAPTER 30

Procedure for Management of Ankle Sprain in Children

INTRODUCTION

Ankle sprains are common injuries in children, often resulting from sports activities, falls, or twisting motions. They involve the stretching or tearing of ligaments that support the ankle joint. Proper assessment and management are crucial to ensure optimal healing and prevent chronic instability.

INDICATIONS

- Acute pain in the ankle following an injury
- Swelling, bruising, and tenderness around the ankle
- Difficulty bearing weight on the affected foot
- History of twisting or rolling the ankle

CONTRAINDICATIONS

- Suspected fracture requiring imaging and orthopedic consultation
- Severe soft tissue injury or open wound requiring surgical intervention
- Signs of neurovascular compromise requiring immediate medical attention

IMAGING (FIG. 1)

Many ankle sprains do not require radiological investigations. Ottawa ankle rules perform well in children, provided they can communicate clearly and walk normally before the injury. Request an X-ray of the ankle/foot if the patient has one of the following:

- Tenderness of the lateral malleolus

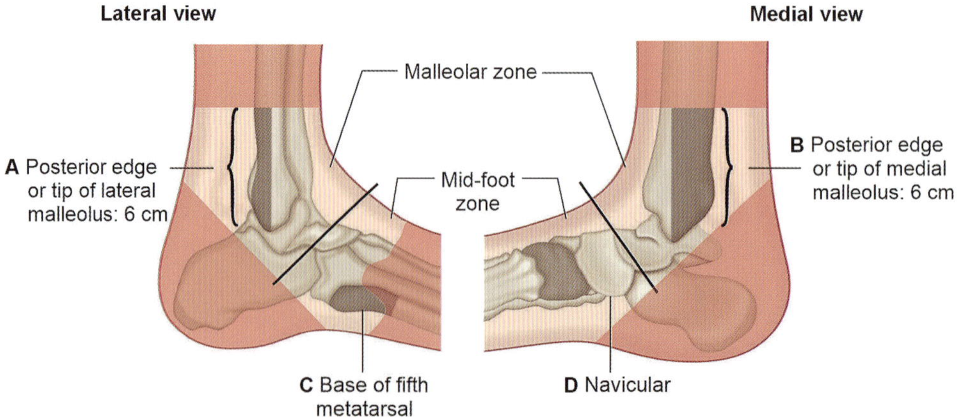

Fig. 1: Lateral and medial view of ankle sprain in children.
Source: Adapted from Stiell IG, McKnight RD, Greenberg GH, McDowell I, Nair RC, Wells GA, et al. Implementation of the Ottawa ankle rules. JAMA. 1994;271:827-32.

- Tenderness at the posterior aspect of the medial malleolus
- Inability to bear weight both at the time of the injury and for four steps at the time of evaluation.
- Tenderness at the base of the 5th metatarsal
- Tenderness at the navicular

All other children presenting with findings suggestive of an ankle sprain can be treated without the need for imaging.

EQUIPMENT AND SUPPLIES

- Sterile gloves
- Antiseptic solution (if there are any open wounds)
- Sterile gauze pads
- Ice pack or cold compress
- Elastic bandage or compression wrap
- Splint or brace (if necessary)
- Crutches (if necessary)
- Analgesics
- Personal protective equipment (PPE)

PREPARATION

- *Explain the procedure:*
    - Inform the child (if age-appropriate) and caregivers about the condition, the procedure, its purpose, and what to expect.
    - Obtain informed consent from the caregivers.
- *Positioning:* Position the child comfortably, ideally seated or lying down with the affected ankle elevated.
- *Pain management:* Administer appropriate analgesics if the child is in significant pain.

PROCEDURE STEPS

1. *Initial assessment:*
    a. Conduct a thorough history and physical examination to assess the extent of the injury.
    b. Inspect the affected area for swelling, bruising, and deformity.
    c. Palpate the ankle to identify areas of tenderness and assess the range of motion.
    d. Perform stability tests to assess ligament integrity (e.g., anterior drawer test and inversion stress test).
2. *Cleansing:* Clean any open wounds with an antiseptic solution to reduce the risk of infection.
3. *RICE protocol:*
    a. *Rest*:
        - Advise the child to avoid putting weight on the affected ankle to prevent further injury.
        - Use crutches if necessary to assist with ambulation.
    b. *Ice*:
        - Apply an ice pack or cold compress to the affected area for 15–20 minutes every 2–3 hours during the first 48 hours to reduce swelling and pain.
        - Ensure the ice pack is wrapped in a cloth to prevent direct contact with the skin.
    c. *Compression:*
        - Apply an elastic bandage or compression wrap to the ankle to minimize swelling and provide support.
        - Start wrapping from the toes and work up to the mid-calf, ensuring the wrap is snug but not too tight to avoid impairing circulation.
    d. *Elevation*: Elevate the affected ankle above heart level as much as possible to reduce swelling.
4. *Immobilization (if necessary):*
    a. *Splint or brace*:
        - If there is significant instability or a severe sprain, consider applying a splint or brace to immobilize the ankle.

- Ensure the splint or brace fits properly and provides adequate support.

5. *Pain management:* Administer oral analgesics (e.g., acetaminophen or ibuprofen) to manage pain and reduce inflammation.

POSTPROCEDURE CARE

- *Monitoring:*
  - Observe the child for signs of continued pain, swelling, or complications.
  - Provide instructions to caregivers on monitoring the injury and signs of complications to watch for.
- *Rehabilitation:*
  - After the initial acute phase (48–72 hours), encourage gradual weight bearing as tolerated.
  - Recommend gentle range-of-motion exercises to prevent stiffness and promote healing.
  - Advise starting with simple exercises such as ankle circles, toe flexion, and extension.
  - As pain and swelling subside, progress to strengthening exercises such as calf raises and resistance band exercises.
- *Follow-up:*
  - Schedule a follow-up appointment with a healthcare provider to monitor healing and assess for any complications.
  - Further imaging may be necessary if there are concerns about fracture or persistent instability.
- *Activity modification:*
  - Advise the child to avoid strenuous activities and sports until the ankle has fully healed.
  - Encourage the use of supportive footwear to prevent future injuries.

COMPLICATIONS

- *Chronic instability:* Improper healing may result in recurrent ankle sprains and chronic instability.
- *Persistent pain:* Ongoing pain may indicate improper healing or underlying issues requiring further evaluation.
- *Swelling:* Persistent swelling may indicate complications such as a fracture or soft tissue injury.
- *Joint stiffness:* Prolonged immobilization can lead to decreased range of motion and stiffness.

PREVENTION

- *Proper footwear:* Encourage the use of supportive footwear, especially during sports and physical activities.
- *Strengthening exercises:* Recommend regular exercises to strengthen the muscles around the ankle and improve balance.
- *Warm-up:* Emphasize the importance of proper warm-up and stretching before engaging in physical activities.

CONCLUSION

The management of ankle sprains in children involves prompt assessment, appropriate application of the RICE protocol, and pain management to ensure proper healing. Rehabilitation and follow-up care are crucial for restoring function and preventing complications.

FURTHER READING

1. Barelds I, Krijnen WP, van de Leur JP, van der Schans CP, Goddard RJ. Diagnostic Accuracy of Clinical Decision Rules to Exclude Fractures in Acute Ankle Injuries: Systematic Review and Meta-analysis. J Emerg Med. 2017;53(3):353-68.

2. Crocco A. Review: the Ottawa Ankle Rules are accurate for excluding fractures in acute blunt ankle/midfoot injury in children. Evid Based Med. 2009;14(6):184.
3. Dowling S, Spooner CH, Liang Y, Dryden DM, Friesen C, Klassen TP, et al. Accuracy of Ottawa Ankle Rules to exclude fractures of the ankle and midfoot in children: a meta-analysis. Acad Emerg Med. 2009;16(4):277-87.
4. Gomes YE, Chau M, Banwell HA, Causby RS. Diagnostic accuracy of the Ottawa ankle rule to exclude fractures in acute ankle injuries in adults: a systematic review and meta-analysis. BMC Musculoskelet Disord. 2022;23(1):885.
5. MacLellan J, Smith T, Baserman J, Dowling S. Accuracy of the Ottawa Ankle Rules applied by non-physician providers in a pediatric emergency department. CJEM. 2018;20(5):746-52.

CHAPTER 31

Procedure for Management of Avulsed Tooth in Children

INTRODUCTION

Tooth avulsion is a dental emergency where a tooth is completely displaced from its socket due to trauma. Immediate and appropriate management is crucial to increase the chances of successful reimplantation and long-term survival of the tooth. This chapter outlines the steps for managing an avulsed tooth in children.

INDICATIONS (FIGS. 1A AND B)

- Complete displacement of a tooth from its socket due to trauma
- Immediate intervention required for permanent teeth (primary teeth are not typically reimplanted).

CONTRAINDICATIONS

- Avulsion of primary (baby) teeth
- Severe trauma to the surrounding oral structures requiring surgical intervention
- Signs of infection or severe contamination of the avulsed tooth.

EQUIPMENT AND SUPPLIES

- Sterile gloves
- Saline solution or milk for tooth storage
- Sterile gauze pads
- Tooth preservation solution (Hank's Balanced Salt Solution, if available)
- Small container with lid (for tooth transport)
- Local anesthetic (if necessary)
- Dental mirror and probe
- Splinting materials (e.g., flexible wire and dental composite)
- Analgesics
- Antibiotics (if necessary)
- Tetanus prophylaxis (if indicated)
- Patient and caregiver education materials.

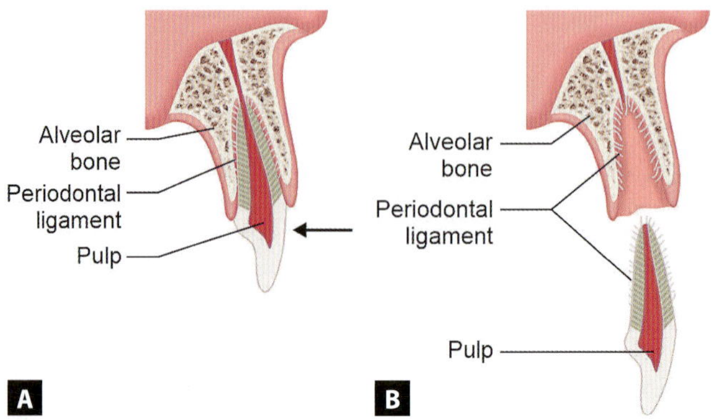

Figs. 1A and B: Tooth anatomy and a completely avulsed tooth.

PREPARATION

- *Explain the procedure:*
    - Inform the child (if age-appropriate) and caregivers about the avulsion, the importance of immediate action, and the procedure itself.
    - Obtain informed consent from the caregivers.
- *Immediate actions:*
    - *Find the tooth:* Locate the avulsed tooth. Handle the tooth by the crown (the white part), avoiding touching the root (the yellowish part).
    - *Clean the tooth:* If the tooth is dirty, rinse it gently with saline solution or milk. Do not scrub or use soap, as this can damage the periodontal ligament fibers necessary for reimplantation.
- *Temporary storage:* If immediate reimplantation is not possible, store the tooth in a suitable medium, such as Hank's Balanced Salt Solution, saline, or milk. If none of these are available, the tooth can be placed in the child's mouth between the cheek and gums, but this should only be done if the child is old enough not to swallow it.

PROCEDURE STEPS

1. *Reimplantation* **(Figs. 2A to D)**:
    a. *Clean the socket:* If there is debris in the socket, rinse it gently with saline solution.
    b. *Examine the tooth:* Check the avulsed tooth for fractures or damage.
    c. *Anesthesia:* If necessary, administer local anesthesia to the affected area for pain management.
    d. *Reimplant the tooth:* Gently insert the tooth into the socket. Use steady pressure to reposition the tooth into its natural alignment. Ensure the tooth

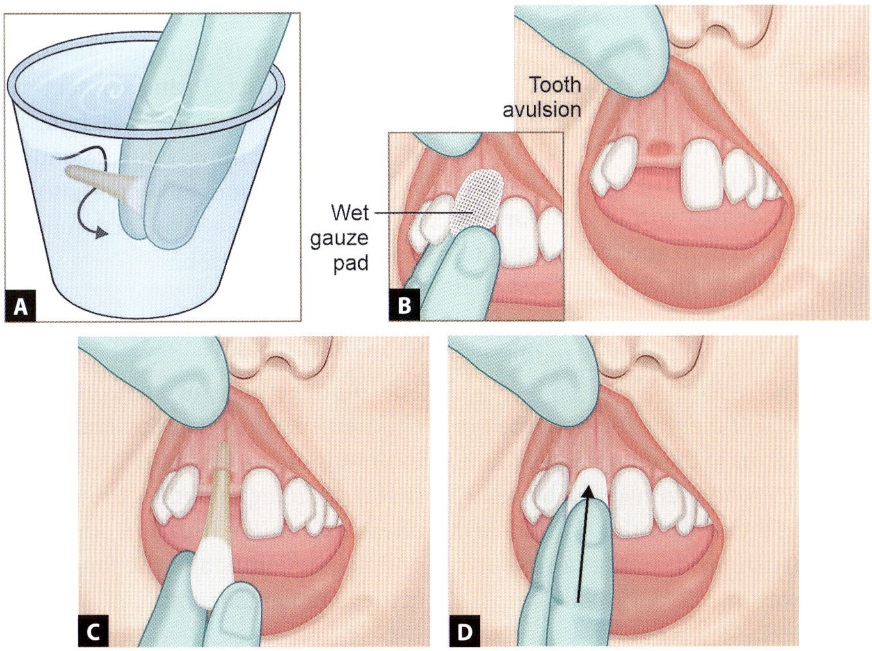

Figs. 2A to D: Reimplantation of avulsed tooth.

is correctly oriented and seated firmly in the socket.

2. *Stabilization:*
   a. *Splinting:* Apply a flexible splint to stabilize the tooth. This can be done using flexible wire and dental composite to attach the avulsed tooth to adjacent teeth.
   b. *Check occlusion:* Ensure that the splint does not interfere with the child's bite (occlusion).
3. *Postprocedure care:*
   a. *Wound care:* Clean any surrounding wounds or lacerations with saline and cover with sterile gauze if necessary.
   b. *Medication:* Prescribe appropriate analgesics for pain management. Antibiotics may be recommended to prevent infection.
   c. *Tetanus prophylaxis:* Assess the need for tetanus prophylaxis based on the child's immunization status and the nature of the injury.

AFTERCARE

- *Follow-up:*
  - Schedule an immediate follow-up appointment with a dentist or pediatric dentist within 24 hours for further evaluation and management.
  - Regular follow-up visits are essential to monitor the healing process and the stability of the reimplanted tooth.
- *Diet and oral hygiene:*
  - Advise a soft diet for the first week to avoid trauma to the reimplanted tooth.
  - Maintain good oral hygiene by gently cleaning the teeth with a soft-bristled toothbrush and using antiseptic mouthwash.
- *Activity modification:* Advise the child to avoid contact sports or activities that may risk further trauma to the mouth until the tooth is stable.
- *Signs of complications:* Educate caregivers on signs of complications, such as increased pain, swelling, pus, or changes in tooth color. Promptly report these signs to a dental professional.

COMPLICATIONS

- *Infection:* Risk of infection around the reimplanted tooth.
- *Ankylosis:* Fusion of the tooth to the bone, leading to the inability of the tooth to move.
- *Root resorption:* Gradual breakdown or loss of the root structure of the reimplanted tooth.
- *Tooth discoloration:* Possible darkening of the tooth indicating pulp necrosis.

PREVENTION

- *Mouthguards:* Encourage the use of mouthguards during contact sports or activities to prevent dental injuries.
- *Safety education:* Educate children and caregivers about the importance of dental safety and immediate action in the event of a tooth avulsion.

CONCLUSION

The management of an avulsed tooth in children requires prompt and appropriate intervention to increase the likelihood of successful reimplantation. Proper technique, aftercare, and education are crucial for optimal outcomes and the long-term health of the reimplanted tooth.

FURTHER READING

1. Emerich K, Wyszkowski J. Clinical practice: dental trauma. Eur J Pediatr. 2010;169:1045.
2. Fouad AF, Abbott PV, Tsilingaridis G, Cohenca N, Lauridsen E, Bourguignon C, et al. International Association of Dental Traumatology guidelines for the management of traumatic dental injuries: 2. Avulsion of permanent teeth. Dent Traumatol 2020; 36:331.
3. Layug ML, Barrett EJ, Kenny DJ. Interim storage of avulsed permanent teeth. J Can Dent Assoc. 1998;64:357.
4. Nelson LP, Shusterman S. Emergency management of oral trauma in children. Curr Opin Pediatr. 1997;9:242.
5. Wilson CF. Management of trauma to primary and developing teeth. Dent Clin North Am. 1995;39:133.

CHAPTER 32

Administration of Activated Charcoal in Children

INTRODUCTION

Activated charcoal is used in the management of certain types of poisoning. It works by adsorbing toxins in the gastrointestinal tract, preventing their absorption into the bloodstream. Prompt administration is crucial for its effectiveness **(Fig. 1)**.

INDICATIONS

- Known or suspected ingestion of toxic substances
- Ingestion of medications that are adsorbed by activated charcoal (e.g., acetaminophen, aspirin, and certain antidepressants)
- Recommended by a poison control center or healthcare professional

CONTRAINDICATIONS

- Altered mental status or decreased level of consciousness unless the airway is protected (risk of aspiration).

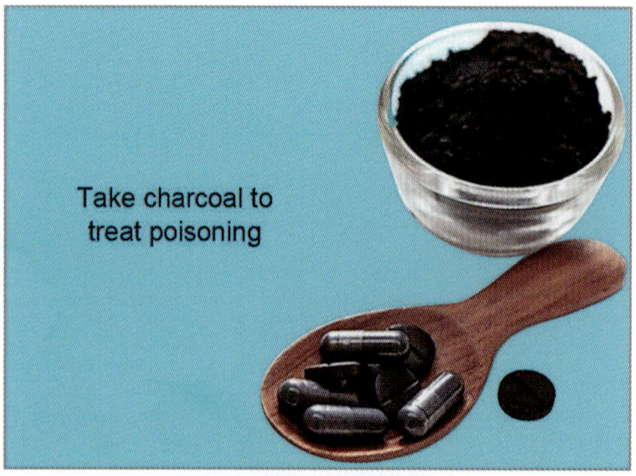

Fig. 1: Activated charcoal.

- Ingestion of corrosive substances (e.g., acids and alkalis) or hydrocarbons (e.g., gasoline) due to risk of aspiration and airway injury
- Known or suspected bowel obstruction or perforation

EQUIPMENT AND SUPPLIES

- Activated charcoal suspension (usually 15–50 g for children, based on weight and medical advice)
- Measuring device (e.g., syringe or cup) for accurate dosing
- Sterile gloves
- Oral or nasogastric administration set (if needed)
- Personal protective equipment (PPE)

PREPARATION

- *Explain the procedure:*
  - Inform the child (if age-appropriate) and caregivers about the purpose of activated charcoal, how it works, and what to expect during administration.
  - Obtain informed consent from the caregivers.
- *Positioning:*
  - Position the child comfortably, ideally sitting up or with the head elevated to reduce the risk of aspiration.
  - Ensure that the child is alert and able to swallow.

PROCEDURE STEPS

1. *Initial assessment:*
   a. Conduct a thorough history and physical examination to confirm the indication for activated charcoal.
   b. Determine the type and amount of substance ingested and the time since ingestion.
2. *Dose calculation:*
   a. Calculate the appropriate dose of activated charcoal, typically 1 g/kg of body weight.
   b. Standard doses are often 15–50 g depending on the child's age and weight.
3. *Preparation of charcoal suspension:*
   a. Shake the bottle of activated charcoal suspension well to ensure it is properly mixed.
   b. Measure the correct dose using a syringe or measuring cup.
4. *Administration:*
   a. *Oral administration*:
      i. *Procedure:*
         - Offer the activated charcoal suspension to the child to drink. Using a straw may help make it more palatable.
         - Encourage the child to drink the suspension slowly but steadily.
         - If the child is unable to drink the suspension voluntarily, use an oral syringe to administer it in small amounts.
   b. Nasogastric tube administration (if indicated and trained personnel available) **(Fig. 2)**
      i. *Preparation:* Confirm the correct placement of the nasogastric tube.
      ii. *Procedure:*
         - Attach the syringe containing the activated charcoal suspension to the nasogastric tube.

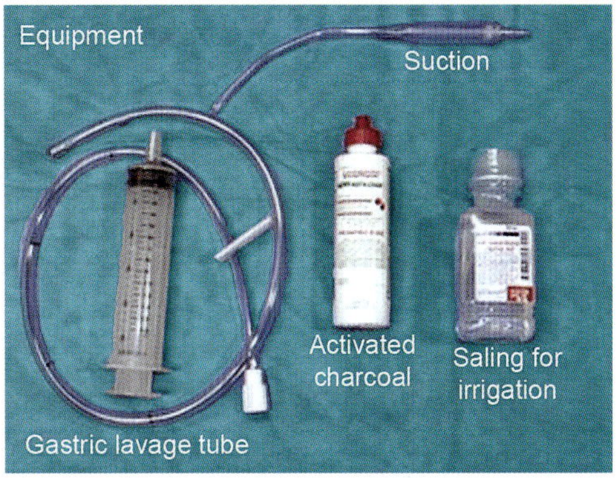

Fig. 2: Activated charcoal administration with nasogastric tube.

         - Administer the suspension slowly to avoid discomfort or aspiration.
         - Flush the tube with a small amount of water to ensure all the charcoal has been delivered.
5. *Monitoring:*
   a. Observe the child for any signs of adverse reactions, such as vomiting or aspiration.
   b. Ensure the child remains in an upright or slightly elevated position for at least 30 minutes after administration to reduce the risk of aspiration.

AFTERCARE

- *Monitoring:*
  - Continuously monitor the child for signs of complications, such as aspiration, respiratory distress, or worsening of the poisoning symptoms.
  - Check for bowel movements, as activated charcoal can cause constipation.
- *Supportive care:*
  - Provide supportive care as needed, including hydration and symptom management.
  - Follow up with a poison control center or healthcare provider for additional guidance and monitoring.

- *Documentation:*
  - Document the time, dose, and method of activated charcoal administration.
  - Record the child's response to the treatment and any adverse reactions.

COMPLICATIONS

- *Aspiration:* Risk of aspiration if the child vomits or has a decreased level of consciousness
- *Gastrointestinal issues:* Possible constipation or, rarely, bowel obstruction
- *Inadequate adsorption:* Ineffectiveness if administered too late after ingestion or for substances not adsorbed by activated charcoal.

PREVENTION

- *Poison prevention:* Educate caregivers and children about the safe storage of medications and toxic substances to prevent accidental ingestions.
- *Emergency preparedness:* Encourage caregivers to have emergency contact information for poison control centers readily available.

CONCLUSION

The administration of activated charcoal in children for the management of certain types of poisoning requires prompt and careful handling. Proper technique, aftercare, and monitoring are crucial to ensure effective treatment and prevent complications.

FURTHER READING

1. Canitrot E, Turgeon AF, Moore L, Diendéré E, St-Onge M. Effect of taste additives on the palatability of activated charcoal: a systematic review. J Med Toxicol. 2023; 19:268.
2. Chyka PA, Seger D, Krenzelok EP, Vale JA. Position paper: single-dose activated charcoal. Clin Toxicol (Phila). 2005;43:61.
3. Hoegberg LCG, Shepherd G, Wood DM, Johnson J, Hoffman RS, Caravati EM, et al. Systematic review on the use of activated charcoal for gastrointestinal decontamination following acute oral overdose. Clin Toxicol (Phila). 2021;59:1196.
4. Position statement and practice guidelines on the use of multi-dose activated charcoal in the treatment of acute poisoning. American Academy of Clinical Toxicology; European Association of Poisons Centres and Clinical Toxicologists. J Toxicol Clin Toxicol. 1999; 37:731.
5. Thanacoody R, Caravati EM, Troutman B, Höjer J, Benson B, Hoppu K, et al. Position paper update: whole bowel irrigation for gastrointestinal decontamination of overdose patients. Clin Toxicol (Phila). 2015; 53:5.

CHAPTER 33

Gastric Lavage for Poisoning in Children

INTRODUCTION

Gastric lavage, also known as stomach pumping or gastric irrigation, is a procedure used to remove toxic substances from the stomach. It is typically considered when a child has ingested a potentially life-threatening poison, and the procedure can be performed within an hour of ingestion.

INDICATIONS

- Ingestion of a potentially life-threatening substance
- Presentation within 1 hour of ingestion (optimal effectiveness)
- Directed by a poison control center or healthcare professional

CONTRAINDICATIONS

- Ingestion of corrosive substances (e.g., acids and alkalis) due to risk of further injury
- Ingestion of hydrocarbons (e.g., gasoline) due to risk of aspiration and chemical pneumonitis
- Compromised airway or risk of aspiration without protected airway (e.g., endotracheal intubation)
- Altered mental status without airway protection

EQUIPMENT AND SUPPLIES

- Sterile gloves
- Nasogastric or orogastric tube (appropriate size for the child)
- Lubricant (e.g., water-soluble gel)
- Suction apparatus
- Syringe (for water or saline)
- Normal saline or water (0.9% saline is preferred, especially in young children)
- Collection container
- Personal protective equipment (PPE)

PREPARATION (FIGS. 1A AND B)

- *Explain the procedure:*
  - Inform the child (if age-appropriate) and caregivers about the purpose of gastric lavage, how it works, and what to expect during the procedure.
  - Obtain informed consent from the caregivers.
- *Positioning:* Position the child lying on their side with the head slightly lower than the stomach (Trendelenburg position) to reduce the risk of aspiration.

PROCEDURE STEPS

1. *Initial assessment:*
   a. Conduct a thorough history and physical examination to confirm the indication for gastric lavage.
   b. Ensure that the child's airway is protected and they are hemodynamically stable.
2. *Prepare equipment:*
   a. Select an appropriate-sized nasogastric or orogastric tube for the child's age and size.
   b. Lubricate the tube with a water-soluble gel.

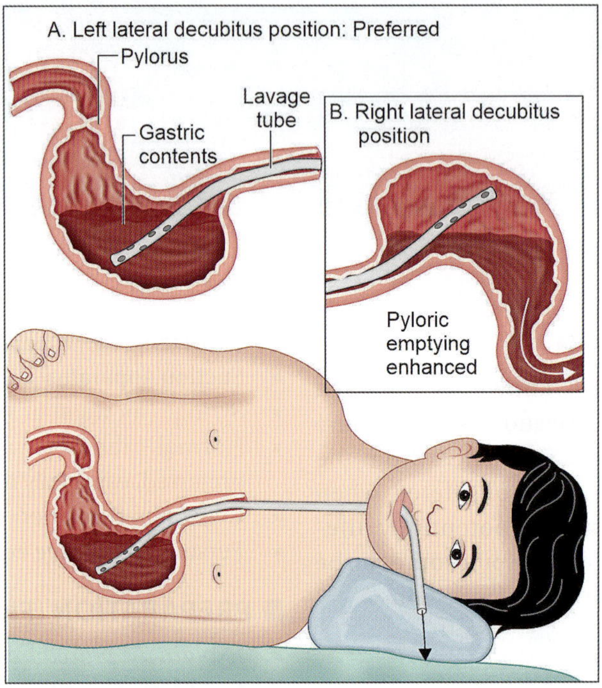

Figs. 1A and B: Gastric lavage position.

3. *Insertion of the tube:*
   a. *Nasogastric route*:
      i. Measure the tube from the child's nose to the earlobe and then to the xiphoid process to estimate the insertion length.
      ii. Insert the tube through the nostril, aiming toward the back of the throat.
      iii. Encourage the child to swallow as the tube passes down the esophagus.
      iv. Verify correct placement by aspirating stomach contents or injecting air and listening for a gurgling sound over the stomach.
   b. *Orogastric route*:
      i. Measure the tube from the child's mouth to the earlobe and then to the xiphoid process to estimate the insertion length.
      ii. Insert the tube through the mouth, aiming toward the back of the throat.
      iii. Encourage the child to swallow as the tube passes down the esophagus.
      iv. Verify correct placement by aspirating stomach contents or injecting air and listening for a gurgling sound over the stomach.
4. *Lavage procedure:*
   a. Connect the syringe to the tube.
   b. Instill small aliquots of normal saline or water (10–20 mL/kg for children) into the stomach.
   c. Allow the fluid to remain in the stomach for a short time before aspirating it back into the syringe.
   d. Repeat the process until the returning fluid is clear and free of particulate matter.

5. *Monitoring and safety:*
   a. Continuously monitor the child's vital signs, oxygen saturation, and overall condition during the procedure.
   b. Be prepared to manage complications such as vomiting, aspiration, or respiratory distress.
6. *Termination of procedure:*
   a. Once the lavage is complete, carefully remove the tube.
   b. Dispose of all used equipment and fluids according to biohazard protocols.

AFTERCARE

- *Monitoring:*
  - Observe the child for any signs of complications, such as respiratory distress, aspiration, or electrolyte imbalance.
  - Continuously monitor vital signs and oxygen saturation.
- *Supportive care:*
  - Provide supportive care, including hydration and symptom management.
  - Follow up with a poison control center or healthcare provider for additional guidance and monitoring.
- *Documentation:* Document the time, amount, and type of fluid used, as well as the child's response to the treatment and any complications encountered.

COMPLICATIONS

- *Aspiration:* Risk of aspiration if the procedure is not performed correctly or if the child vomits
- *Perforation:* Risk of esophageal or gastric perforation
- *Electrolyte imbalance:* Potential for electrolyte disturbances due to large volumes of lavage fluid.
- *Hypoxia:* Risk of hypoxia during the procedure, especially in children with compromised airways.

PREVENTION

- *Poison prevention:* Educate caregivers and children about the safe storage of medications and toxic substances to prevent accidental ingestions.
- *Emergency preparedness:* Encourage caregivers to have emergency contact information for poison control centers readily available.

CONCLUSION

Gastric lavage is a procedure used in the management of certain types of poisoning in children when performed within an hour of ingestion. Proper technique, aftercare, and monitoring are crucial to ensure effective treatment and prevent complications.

FURTHER READING

1. Benson BE, Hoppu K, Troutman WG, Bedry R, Erdman A, Höjer J, et al. Position paper update: gastric lavage for gastrointestinal decontamination. Clin Toxicol (Phila). 2013;51(3):140-6.
2. Christophersen AB, Levin D, Hoegberg LC, Angelo HR, Kampmann JP . Activated charcoal alone or after gastric lavage: a simulated large paracetamol intoxication. Br J Clin Pharmacol. 2002;53(3):312-7.
3. Hoffman RM, Maskell KF, Cumpston KL. A local survey of gastric lavage for gastrointestinal decontamination in a new century: The future marches on. Am J Emerg Med. 2018;36(6):1114-15.
4. Saetta JP, March S, Gaunt ME, Quinton DN. Gastric emptying procedures in the self-poisoned patient: are we forcing gastric content beyond the pylorus? J R Soc Med. 1991;84(5):274-6. d
5. Saetta JP, Quinton DN. Residual gastric content after gastric lavage and ipecacuanha-induced emesis in self-poisoned patients: an endoscopic study. J R Soc Med. 1991;84(1):35-8.

CHAPTER 34

Management of Hymenoptera and Bee Stings in Children

INTRODUCTION

Hymenoptera stings, including those from bees, wasps, hornets, and ants, are common in children. While most reactions are mild, some can be severe and potentially life-threatening, particularly in children with allergies. Proper management is essential to alleviate symptoms, prevent complications, and address any severe allergic reactions promptly.

INDICATIONS

- Visible sting with localized pain, redness, and swelling
- Symptoms such as itching, hives, or mild swelling around the sting site
- Systemic symptoms indicating a severe allergic reaction, such as difficulty breathing, swelling of the face or throat, rapid pulse, dizziness, or anaphylaxis.

CONTRAINDICATIONS

None specifically related to the initial management of stings, but severe allergic reactions require immediate emergency care.

EQUIPMENT AND SUPPLIES

- Sterile gloves
- Antiseptic solution (e.g., povidone-iodine or chlorhexidine)
- Sterile gauze pads
- Tweezers or a scraping tool (credit card or similar object)
- Ice pack or cold compress
- Antihistamine (oral or topical)
- Corticosteroid cream (if needed)
- Epinephrine autoinjector (for severe allergic reactions)
- Pain management (oral analgesics)
- Personal protective equipment (PPE)

PREPARATION

- *Explain the procedure:*
  - Inform the child (if age-appropriate) and caregivers about the sting, the management procedure, its purpose, and what to expect.
  - Obtain informed consent from the caregivers.
- *Positioning:* Position the child comfortably, ideally seated or lying down with the affected area easily accessible.
- *Pain management:* Administer appropriate analgesics before the procedure if the child is in significant pain.

PROCEDURE STEPS

1. Initial assessment:
   a. Conduct a thorough history and physical examination to assess the severity of the sting reaction.
   b. Look for signs of localized reactions (redness, swelling, and pain) or systemic reactions (difficulty breathing, swelling of the face or throat, hives, and dizziness).

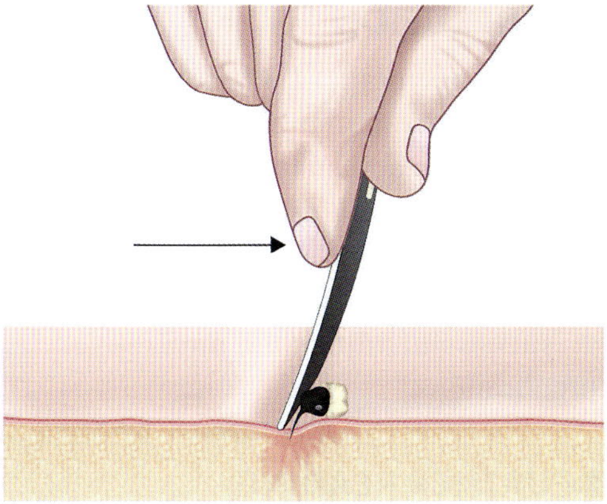

Fig. 1: Bee stinger removal using credit card.

2. *Stinger removal* ***(Fig. 1)****:*
   a. If the stinger is visible and still embedded in the skin (common with bee stings), remove it as quickly as possible to reduce the amount of venom injected.
   b. *Removal technique:* Scrape the stinger out using a flat object such as a credit card or the edge of a knife. Avoid using tweezers to squeeze the stinger, as this can inject more venom.
   c. *Cleaning:* Clean the area around the sting with an antiseptic solution to reduce the risk of infection.
3. *Apply ice pack:* Apply an ice pack or cold compress to the affected area for 15–20 minutes to reduce pain and swelling. Ensure the ice pack is wrapped in a cloth to prevent direct contact with the skin.
4. *Administer antihistamines:*
   a. *Oral antihistamines:* Administer an oral antihistamine such as diphenhydramine (Benadryl) to reduce itching and swelling.
   b. *Topical antihistamines:* Apply a topical antihistamine cream to the affected area for localized relief.
5. *Apply corticosteroid cream (if needed):* For more severe localized reactions, apply a corticosteroid cream to reduce inflammation and itching.
6. *Monitor for severe reactions:*
   a. *Signs of anaphylaxis:* Monitor for symptoms of a severe allergic reaction, including difficulty breathing, swelling of the face or throat, rapid pulse, dizziness, or loss of consciousness.
   b. *Epinephrine administration:* If anaphylaxis is suspected, administer an epinephrine autoinjector (e.g., EpiPen) immediately and call emergency services. Follow the instructions on the autoinjector for proper use.

POSTPROCEDURE CARE

- *Monitoring:*
  - Observe the child for signs of continued pain, swelling, or systemic reactions.
  - Provide instructions to caregivers on monitoring for any delayed allergic reactions or complications.
- *Pain management:*
  - Prescribe appropriate oral analgesics for pain relief.
  - Advise caregivers to keep the affected area elevated and apply cold compresses to reduce swelling and pain.
- *Wound care:*
  - Instruct caregivers on proper wound care, including cleaning the area and applying topical treatments as needed.
  - Recommend avoiding scratching or irritating the sting site to prevent infection.
- *Follow-up:*
  - Schedule a follow-up appointment if there are concerns about persistent reactions or if the child has a history of severe allergic reactions.

- Further evaluation by an allergist may be necessary for children with recurrent or severe reactions.

COMPLICATIONS

- *Infection:* Risk of secondary infection if the wound is not properly cared for
- *Severe allergic reaction:* Potential for anaphylaxis requiring emergency medical intervention
- *Persistent swelling or pain:* Ongoing symptoms may require further evaluation and management.
- *Serum sickness:* Rare delayed reaction to venom requiring medical attention

PREVENTION

- *Avoidance:* Educate children and caregivers on avoiding areas where stinging insects are common, such as near flowers, garbage, or uncovered food.
- *Protective clothing:* Encourage wearing protective clothing when outdoors in areas where stinging insects are present.
- *Allergy preparedness:* For children with known allergies, ensure they have access to an epinephrine autoinjector and that caregivers are trained in its use.
- *Safe environment:* Keep outdoor areas free from open food containers and sugary drinks that attract insects.

CONCLUSION

The management of Hymenoptera and bee stings in children involves prompt and appropriate treatment to alleviate symptoms, prevent complications, and address severe allergic reactions. Proper technique, aftercare, and caregiver education are crucial for successful outcomes and preventing complications.

FURTHER READING

1. Carlson J, Golden DB. Large local reactions to insect envenomation. Curr Opin Allergy Clin Immunol. 2016;16(4):366-9.
2. Goddard J. Physician's guide to arthropods of medical importance, 4th ed, CRC Press, Boca Raton 2003.
3. Golden DB, Demain J, Freeman T, Graft D, Tankersley M, Tracy J, et al. Stinging insect hypersensitivity: A practice parameter update 2016. Ann Allergy Asthma Immunol. 2017;118(1):28-54.
4. Gurlanick MW, Benton AW. Entomological aspects of insect sting allergy. In: Monograph on insect allergy, 4th ed, Levine MI, Lockey RF (Eds), Dave Lambert Associates, Pittsburgh 2003. p.11.
5. Severino M, Bonadonna P, Passalacqua G. Large local reactions from stinging insects: from epidemiology to management. Curr Opin Allergy Clin Immunol. 2009;9(4):334-7.

CHAPTER 35

Procedure for Rabies Immune Globulin Administration in Children

INTRODUCTION

Rabies immune globulin (RIG) is administered as part of postexposure prophylaxis for individuals exposed to rabies. This chapter outlines the procedure for the administration of RIG in children following potential rabies exposure, such as animal bites, to provide passive immunity and immediate protection against the virus.

INDICATIONS

- Bite or scratch from a suspected rabid animal (Class III bite—immunocompetent patients)
- Bite or scratch from a suspected rabid animal (Class II and Class III bite—immunocompromised patients)
- Exposure to a bat or other high-risk animals
- Postexposure RIG is given in conjunction with the rabies vaccine **(Fig. 1)**.

CONTRAINDICATIONS

- Known severe allergic reaction to human immunoglobulin products
- Previous completion of a rabies vaccination series with no new exposure

EQUIPMENT AND SUPPLIES

- Sterile gloves
- Antiseptic solution (e.g., povidone-iodine or chlorhexidine)
- Sterile gauze pads
- RIG
- Syringe and needle for intramuscular injection
- Syringe and needle for infiltration around the wound

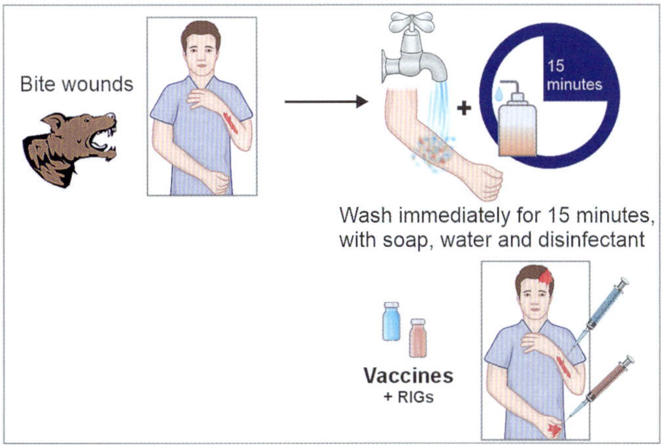

Fig. 1: Rabies postexposure prophylaxis.

- Adhesive bandage or sterile dressing
- Sharps container
- Personal protective equipment (PPE)

PREPARATION

- *Explain the procedure:*
  - Inform the child (if age-appropriate) and caregivers about the need for RIG, its purpose, and what to expect.
  - Obtain informed consent from the caregivers.
- *Positioning:* Position the child comfortably, either seated or lying down, with the wound site easily accessible for infiltration.
- *Pain management:* Administer appropriate analgesics before the procedure if necessary to alleviate pain.

PROCEDURE STEPS

1. *Initial assessment:*
   a. Conduct a thorough history and physical examination to assess the wound and determine the extent of rabies exposure.
   b. Clean the wound thoroughly with an antiseptic solution to reduce the risk of infection.
2. *Calculating the RIG dose:*
   a. The dose of RIG is calculated based on the child's weight: 20 IU/kg body weight.
   b. Use the entire dose of RIG for the child, even if it exceeds the volume that can be injected around the wound.
3. *Infiltration around the wound* ***(Figs. 2A to C)****:*
   a. *Preparation:* Draw the calculated dose of RIG into a syringe.
   b. *Procedure*:
      i. Infiltrate as much of the RIG as possible around and into the wound(s) where the virus is likely to be introduced.
      ii. Use multiple injection sites if necessary to ensure adequate infiltration around the wound.
      iii. Gently massage the area to aid the distribution of the RIG.
4. *Intramuscular injection:*
   a. *Preparation:* Any remaining RIG that cannot be infiltrated around the wound should be administered intramuscularly.
   b. *Procedure*:
      i. Administer the remaining RIG intramuscularly at a site distant from the site of rabies vaccine administration, typically in the anterolateral thigh or gluteal muscle.
      ii. Ensure proper technique to avoid intravascular injection.
5. *Postadministration care:*
   a. *Inspection:* Check the wound site and injection site for any immediate adverse reactions.
   b. *Cleaning:* Clean the wound area again and apply a sterile dressing or adhesive bandage if necessary.

AFTERCARE

- *Monitoring:*
  - Observe the child for signs of an allergic reaction or adverse effects, such as redness, swelling, or anaphylaxis.
  - Provide instructions to caregivers on monitoring the wound and the injection site for signs of infection or adverse reactions.
- *Pain management:*
  - Prescribe appropriate oral analgesics for pain relief if necessary.
  - Advise caregivers on the use of cold compresses to reduce swelling and pain at the injection site.

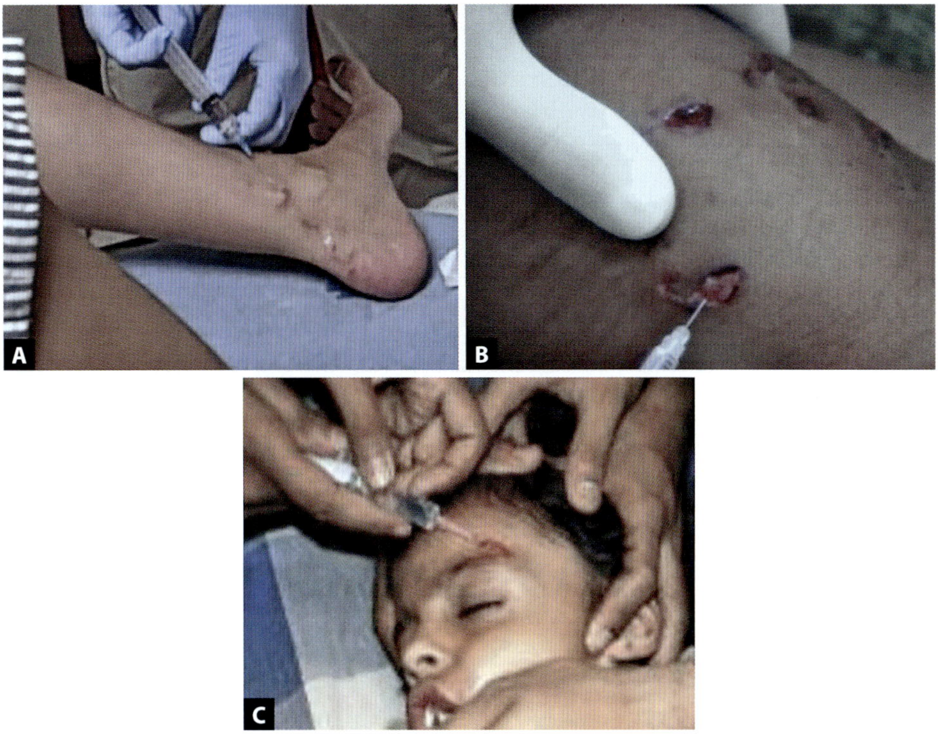

Figs. 2A to C: Rabies immunoglobulin administration.

- *Wound care:* Instruct caregivers on proper wound care, including keeping the wound clean and dry and watching for signs of infection.
- *Follow-up:*
    - Schedule follow-up appointments for the administration of the rabies vaccine series.
    - Further evaluation may be necessary if there are signs of infection or complications.

COMPLICATIONS

- *Allergic reaction:* There is a risk of an allergic reaction to the RIG. Emergency measures should be in place to manage anaphylaxis.
- *Infection:* Risk of infection at the wound or injection site if proper care is not taken
- *Pain and swelling:* Common at the injection site, typically managed with analgesics and cold compresses.

PREVENTION

- *Education:* Educate caregivers and children on avoiding contact with wild animals and unfamiliar domestic animals to prevent rabies exposure.
- *Vaccination:* Encourage rabies vaccination for high-risk individuals, including those who work with animals or in areas with high rabies prevalence.

CONCLUSION

The administration of RIG in children is a critical component of postexposure prophylaxis following potential rabies exposure. Proper technique, aftercare, and caregiver education are essential to ensure effective treatment and prevent complications.

FURTHER READING

1. Alberer M, Gnad-Vogt U, Hong HS, Mehr KT, Backert L, Finak G, et al. Safety and immunogenicity of a mRNA rabies vaccine in healthy adults: an open-label, non-randomised, prospective, first-in-human phase 1 clinical trial. Lancet 2017;390: 1511.
2. Aldrich C, Leroux-Roels I, Huang KB, Bica MA, Loeliger E, Schoenborn-Kellenberger O, et al. Proof-of-concept of a low-dose unmodified mRNA-based rabies vaccine formulated with lipid nanoparticles in human volunteers: A phase 1 trial. Vaccine 2021;39:1310.
3. General Best Practice Guidelines for Immunization. Centers for Disease Control and Prevention. Available at: https://www.cdc.gov/vaccines/hcp/acip-recs/general-recs/index.html.
4. Rabies vaccines: WHO position paper - April 2018. World Health Organization. Available at: https://iris.who.int/bitstream/handle/10665/272372/WER9316-201-219.pdf?sequence=1
5. World Health Organization. WHO Expert Consultation on Rabies, second report. Geneva, 2013. WHO Technical Report Series, No. 982. http://apps.who.int/iris/bitstream/10665/85346/1/9789240690943_eng.pdf.

CHAPTER 36

Intranasal Administration of Midazolam and Fentanyl in Children

INTRODUCTION

The nasal route is an effective alternative for administering medications such as midazolam and fentanyl in children, especially in emergency situations or when intravenous access is challenging. This route allows for rapid absorption and onset of action **(Flowchart 1)**.

INDICATIONS

- Acute seizure management (midazolam)
- Acute pain management (fentanyl)
- Situations where intravenous access is not feasible or delayed
- Preprocedural sedation

CONTRAINDICATIONS

- Known hypersensitivity to the medication
- Nasal trauma or severe nasal obstruction
- Recent nasal surgery
- Significant nasal bleeding

EQUIPMENT AND SUPPLIES

- Sterile gloves
- Midazolam nasal spray or solution (appropriate dose)
- Fentanyl nasal spray or solution (appropriate dose)
- Mucosal atomization device (MAD) if using a solution
- Syringe (if using solution)
- Gauze pads or tissues
- Personal protective equipment (PPE)

Flowchart 1: Drug delivery to central nervous system (CNS) via intranasal route.

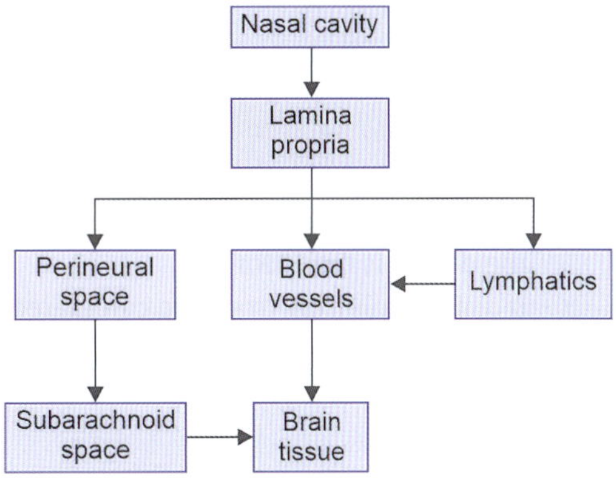

PREPARATION

- *Explain the procedure:*
  - Inform the child (if age-appropriate) and caregivers about the purpose of the medication, its effects, and what to expect during administration.
  - Obtain informed consent from the caregivers.
- *Positioning:* Position the child comfortably, ideally sitting up or lying with the head slightly elevated to prevent aspiration.

PROCEDURE STEPS

Midazolam Administration (Fig. 1)

- *Dose calculation:* Calculate the appropriate dose of midazolam based on the child's weight. The typical dose is 0.2 mg/kg.

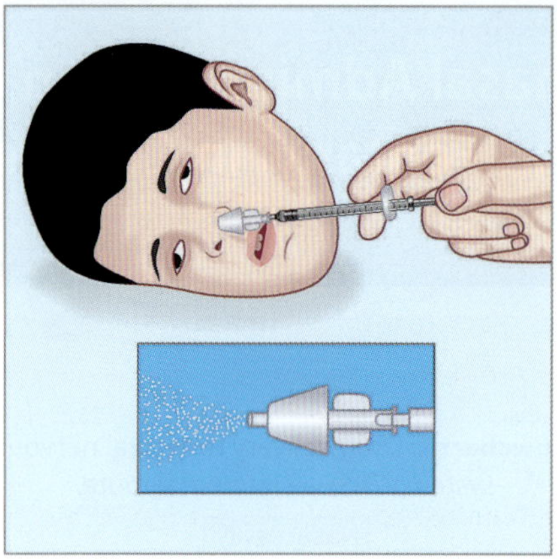

Fig. 1: Nasal drug administration.

- *Preparation of medication:*
  - If using a prefilled nasal spray, ensure the device is ready for use.
  - If using a solution, draw the calculated dose into a syringe and attach the MAD.
- *Administration:*
  - *Prefilled nasal spray:* Lay your child on their side (recovery position) or in the best position to allow easy administration of intranasal midazolam. Insert the MAD loosely into a nostril and press the plunger quickly to give half of the dose. Remove the device and insert it into the other nostril to give the remaining dose. Insert the tip of the nasal spray into one nostril and administer the full dose.
  - *Solution with MAD:*
    - Insert the MAD into one nostril and administer half of the dose.
    - Repeat in the other nostril with the remaining half of the dose to ensure optimal absorption.
- *Monitoring:*
  - Observe the child for signs of effectiveness and any adverse reactions.
  - Ensure the child remains in a safe position until the medication takes effect.

Fentanyl Administration

- *Dose calculation:* Calculate the appropriate dose of fentanyl based on the child's weight. The typical dose is 1.5–2 μg/kg.
- *Preparation of medication:*
  - If using a prefilled nasal spray, ensure the device is ready for use.
  - If using a solution, draw the calculated dose into a syringe and attach the MAD.
- *Administration:*
  - Prefilled nasal spray:
    - Tilt the child's head slightly back.
    - Insert the tip of the nasal spray into one nostril and administer the full dose.
  - *Solution with MAD:*
    - Tilt the child's head slightly back.
    - Insert the MAD into one nostril and administer half of the dose.
    - Repeat in the other nostril with the remaining half of the dose to ensure optimal absorption.
- *Monitoring:*
  - Observe the child for signs of pain relief and any adverse reactions.
  - Ensure the child remains in a safe position until the medication takes effect.

AFTERCARE

- *Monitoring:*
  - Continuously monitor the child's vital signs, including respiratory rate, oxygen saturation, heart rate, and level of consciousness.
  - Watch for signs of adverse reactions, such as respiratory depression, excessive sedation, or allergic reactions.

- *Supportive care:*
  - Provide supportive care as needed, including oxygen administration if required.
  - Ensure the child remains under close observation until the effects of the medication have worn off.
- *Documentation:*
  - Document the time, dose, and type of medication administered.
  - Record the child's response to the treatment and any adverse reactions.

COMPLICATIONS

- *Respiratory depression:* Risk of respiratory depression, particularly with fentanyl
- *Excessive sedation:* Potential for excessive sedation with midazolam
- *Nasal discomfort:* Possible nasal irritation or discomfort
- *Allergic reactions:* Risk of allergic reactions to the medication

PREVENTION

- *Proper technique:* Ensure correct administration technique to maximize absorption and minimize complications.
- *Dosing accuracy:* Calculate and administer the correct dose based on the child's weight.
- *Monitoring:* Continuously monitor the child's vital signs and response to the medication.

CONCLUSION

The nasal administration of midazolam and fentanyl in children is an effective alternative for managing acute seizures and pain, especially when intravenous access is challenging. Proper technique, monitoring, and aftercare are essential to ensure safe and effective treatment.

FURTHER READING

1. Ahmad S, Ellis JC, Kamwendo H, Molyneux E. Efficacy and safety of intranasal lorazepam versus intramuscular paraldehyde for protracted convulsions in children: an open randomised trial. Lancet . 2006;367:1591.
2. Arya R, Gulati S, Kabra M, Sahu JK, Kalra V. Intranasal versus intravenous lorazepam for control of acute seizures in children: a randomized open-label study. Epilepsia. 2011;52:788.
3. Chhabra R, Gupta R, Gupta LK. Intranasal midazolam versus intravenous/rectal benzodiazepines for acute seizure control in children: A systematic review and meta-analysis. Epilepsy Behav. 2021;125:108390.
4. Prescribing information Nayzilam (midazolam) nasal spray. https://www.accessdata.fda.gov/drugsatfda_docs/label/2019/211321s000lbl.pdf
5. Prescribing information Valtoco (diazepam nasal spray). https://www.accessdata.fda.gov/drugsatfda_docs/label/2020/211635s000lbl.pdf

CHAPTER 37

Buccal Drug Administration in Children

INTRODUCTION

Buccal drug administration involves placing a medication between the gums and the inner lining of the cheek, where it is absorbed through the mucous membranes. This route is particularly useful for rapid drug delivery and when oral or intravenous administration is not feasible **(Fig. 1)**.

INDICATIONS

- Rapid administration of medication in emergency situations (e.g., seizures)
- Inability to take medications orally due to vomiting, difficulty swallowing, or unconsciousness
- Situations where intravenous access is difficult or delayed

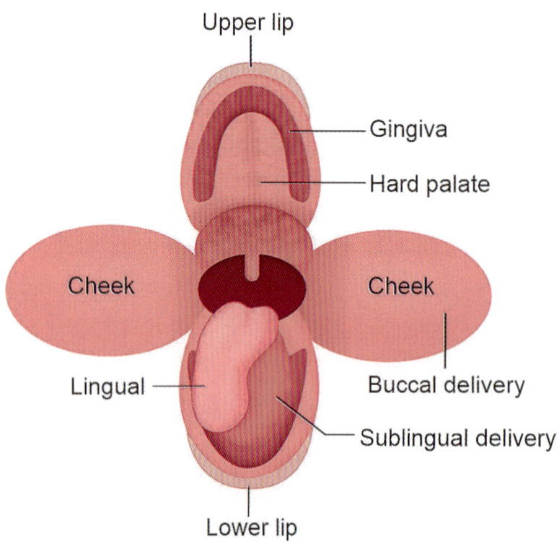

Fig. 1: Mouth and buccal cavity anatomy.

- Medications specifically designed for buccal absorption

CONTRAINDICATIONS

- Known hypersensitivity to the medication
- Severe oral lesions or infection
- Severe bleeding disorders or significant trauma to the buccal area

EQUIPMENT AND SUPPLIES

- Sterile gloves
- Medication in buccal form (e.g., midazolam buccal solution and lorazepam buccal tablet)
- Syringe (if using a liquid medication)
- Gauze pads or tissues
- Personal protective equipment (PPE)

PREPARATION

- *Explain the procedure:*
    - Inform the child (if age-appropriate) and caregivers about the purpose of the buccal medication, its effects, and what to expect during administration.
    - Obtain informed consent from the caregivers.
- *Positioning:*
    - Position the child comfortably, ideally sitting up or lying with the head slightly elevated to prevent aspiration.
    - Ensure the child's head is turned to one side to facilitate administration.

PROCEDURE STEPS

Midazolam Administration

- *Dose calculation:* Calculate the appropriate dose of midazolam based on the child's weight. The typical dose for buccal midazolam is 0.3–0.5 mg/kg.
- *Preparation of medication:*
  - If using a prefilled buccal solution, ensure the device is ready for use.
  - If using a liquid solution, draw the calculated dose into a syringe without a needle.
- *Administration:*
  - *Prefilled buccal solution* ***(Fig. 2)***:
    - Tilt the child's head slightly to the side.
    - Insert the tip of the prefilled device into the space between the gum and the cheek.
    - Slowly administer the medication, allowing it to be absorbed by the buccal mucosa.
  - *Solution with syringe*:
    - Tilt the child's head slightly to the side.
    - Insert the syringe into the space between the gum and the cheek.
    - Slowly depress the plunger to administer the medication, ensuring it is evenly distributed in the buccal area.
- *Monitoring:*
  - Observe the child for signs of effectiveness and any adverse reactions.
  - Ensure the child remains in a safe position until the medication takes effect.

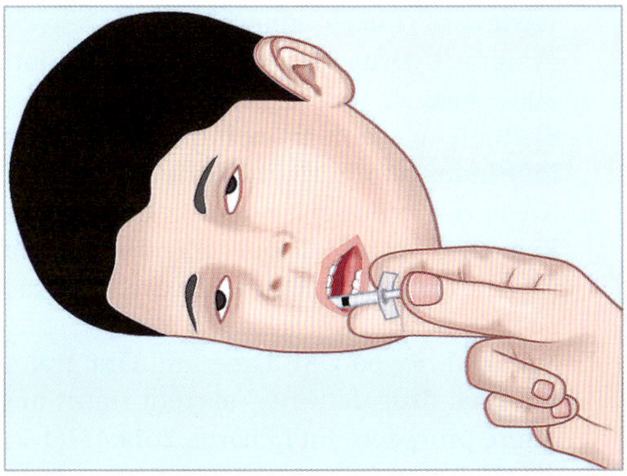

Fig. 2: Buccal drug administration. Lay your child on their side (recovery position). Open their lips and slowly trickle the midazolam from the syringe into the inside of the lower cheek (closest to the ground), between the lips and side teeth. There is no need to open your child's jaw. The solution does not need to be swallowed.

Lorazepam Administration

- *Dose calculation:* Calculate the appropriate dose of lorazepam based on the child's weight. The typical dose for buccal lorazepam is 0.1–0.2 mg/kg.
- *Preparation of medication:*
  - If using a buccal tablet, ensure it is at the correct dose.
  - If using a liquid solution, draw the calculated dose into a syringe without a needle.
- *Administration:*
  - *Buccal tablet:*
    - Tilt the child's head slightly to the side.
    - Place the tablet between the gum and the cheek.
    - Allow the tablet to dissolve and be absorbed by the buccal mucosa.
  - *Solution with syringe:*
    - Tilt the child's head slightly to the side.
    - Insert the syringe into the space between the gum and the cheek.
    - Slowly depress the plunger to administer the medication, ensuring it is evenly distributed in the buccal area.

- *Monitoring:*
  - Observe the child for signs of effectiveness and any adverse reactions.
  - Ensure the child remains in a safe position until the medication takes effect.

AFTERCARE

- *Monitoring:*
  - Continuously monitor the child's vital signs, including respiratory rate, oxygen saturation, heart rate, and level of consciousness.
  - Watch for signs of adverse reactions, such as respiratory depression, excessive sedation, or allergic reactions.
- *Supportive care:*
  - Provide supportive care as needed, including oxygen administration if required.
  - Ensure the child remains under close observation until the effects of the medication have worn off.
- *Documentation:*
  - Document the time, dose, and type of medication administered.
  - Record the child's response to the treatment and any adverse reactions.

COMPLICATIONS

- *Respiratory depression:* Risk of respiratory depression, particularly with midazolam and lorazepam
- *Excessive sedation:* Potential for excessive sedation with benzodiazepines
- *Oral discomfort:* Possible irritation or discomfort in the buccal area
- *Allergic reactions:* Risk of allergic reactions to the medication

PREVENTION

- *Proper technique:* Ensure correct administration technique to maximize absorption and minimize complications.
- *Dosing accuracy:* Calculate and administer the correct dose based on the child's weight.
- *Monitoring:* Continuously monitor the child's vital signs and response to the medication.

CONCLUSION

Buccal drug administration is a valuable alternative for delivering medications to children when oral or intravenous routes are not feasible. Proper technique, monitoring, and aftercare are essential to ensure safe and effective treatment.

FURTHER READING

1. Brigo F, Nardone R, Tezzon F, Trinka E. Nonintravenous midazolam versus intravenous or rectal diazepam for the treatment of early status epilepticus: A systematic review with meta-analysis. Epilepsy Behav. 2015;49:325-36.
2. Gupta S, Das S, Singh A, Ghosh S. A Brief Review on Bucco-adhesive Drug Delivery System. J. Drug Delivery Ther. [Internet]. 2021 Aug. 15 [cited 2024 Dec. 29];11(4-S):231-5. Available from: https://jddtonline.info/index.php/jddt/article/view/4934
3. Kraan H, Vrieling H, Czerkinsky C, Jiskoot W, Kersten G, Amorij JP. Buccal and sublingual vaccine delivery. J Control Release. 2014;190:580-92.
4. Sattar M, Sayed OM, Lane ME. Oral transmucosal drug delivery—current status and future prospects. Int J Pharm. 2014;471(1-2):498-506.
5. Targhotra M, Chauhan MK. An Overview on Various Approaches and Recent Patents on Buccal Drug Delivery Systems. Curr Pharm Des. 2020;26(39):5030-9.

CHAPTER 38

Making Intramuscular Injections Pain Free in Children

INTRODUCTION

Intramuscular (IM) injections are commonly used in pediatric care for administering vaccines, antibiotics, and other medications. However, the pain associated with IM injections can be distressing for children and their caregivers. Implementing strategies to minimize pain can improve the child's experience and cooperation with medical procedures.

INDICATIONS

- Administration of vaccines
- Delivery of antibiotics and other medications
- When oral or intravenous routes are not feasible or appropriate

CONTRAINDICATIONS

- Known hypersensitivity to the medication being administered
- Infection or inflammation at the injection site
- Muscle disorders or conditions affecting the injection site

EQUIPMENT AND SUPPLIES

- Sterile gloves
- Alcohol swabs
- Syringe and appropriate needle size for the child's age and weight
- Medication for injection
- Topical anesthetic (e.g., lidocaine cream) or vapocoolant spray
- Distraction tools (e.g., toys and videos)
- Comfort items (e.g., blanket and favorite toy)
- Buzzy Bee or NumBee device
- Personal protective equipment (PPE)

PREPARATION

- *Explain the procedure:*
  - Inform the child (if age-appropriate) and caregivers about the need for the injection, its purpose, and what to expect.
  - Obtain informed consent from the caregivers.
- *Preparation of the injection site:*
  - Choose an appropriate injection site based on the child's age and muscle mass:
    - *Infants:* Anterolateral thigh
    - *Older children:* Deltoid muscle or anterolateral thigh
- *Comfort measures:*
  - Allow the child to sit on a caregiver's lap or hold a comfort item.
  - Use distraction techniques such as playing videos, music, or engaging in conversation.

PROCEDURE STEPS

Step 1: Apply Topical Anesthetic

- *Topical anesthetic cream:*
  - Apply a topical anesthetic cream (e.g., lidocaine-prilocaine) to the injection

site at least 30–60 minutes before the procedure.
  - Cover the area with an occlusive dressing to enhance absorption.
- *Vapocoolant spray:*
  - If time does not allow for a topical cream, use a vapocoolant spray immediately before the injection.
  - Spray the vapocoolant on the injection site for a few seconds to numb the skin.

Step 2: Distraction and Comfort

- *Distraction:*
  - Use age-appropriate distraction techniques such as toys, videos, or conversation to divert the child's attention.
  - Engage the child in deep breathing exercises or have them blow bubbles to relax.
- *Comfort positioning:*
  - Have the child sit on a caregiver's lap or hold their favorite toy.
  - Use a comforting touch and reassuring words throughout the procedure.

Step 3: Using Buzzy Bee and NumBee

Buzzy Bee and NumBee devices are innovative tools designed to reduce pain and anxiety during medical procedures, including IM injections. These devices combine vibration and cold to block pain sensation.

- *Buzzy Bee **(Fig. 1)**:*
  - Place the Buzzy Bee device directly on the skin above the injection site.
  - Turn on the device to activate vibration and apply the cold wings to the skin.
  - Leave the device in place for about 30 seconds before administering the injection to ensure the area is numb.

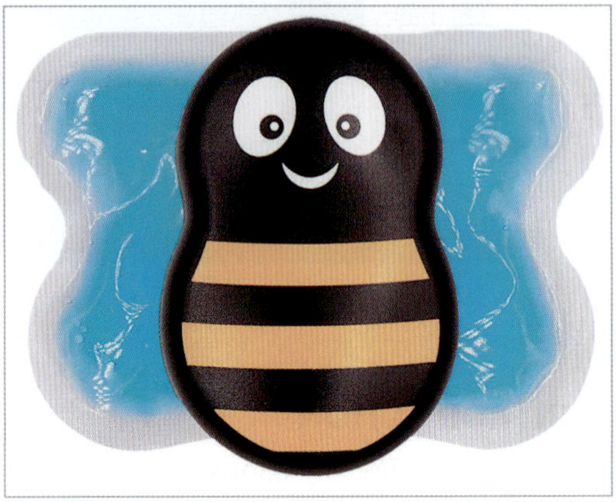

Fig. 1: Buzzy Bee for pain relief of injection.

- *NumBee:*
  - Apply the NumBee device similarly to the Buzzy Bee.
  - Activate the vibration and cooling functions.
  - Ensure the device is positioned correctly and left in place for the recommended time to achieve optimal numbing.

Step 4: Administer the Injection

- *Prepare the injection:*
  - Wash hands thoroughly and put on sterile gloves.
  - Draw the prescribed medication into the syringe, ensuring the correct dose.
  - Use an appropriate needle size for the child's age and weight (e.g., 22–25 gauge, 1 inch for older children, 5/8 inch for infants).
- *Clean the injection site:*
  - Clean the injection site with an alcohol swab, using a circular motion from the center outward.
  - Allow the site to air dry.
- *Injection technique:*
  - Hold the muscle firmly to stabilize it.
  - Insert the needle quickly and smoothly at a 90° angle to the skin.

- Aspirate (if indicated) to ensure the needle is not in a blood vessel, then slowly inject the medication.
- Withdraw the needle quickly and apply gentle pressure to the site with a gauze pad.

- *Postinjection care:*
  - Apply a bandage if needed.
  - Offer praise and reassurance to the child for their cooperation.
  - Encourage the child to move the limb gently to reduce soreness.

AFTERCARE

- *Monitoring:*
  - Observe the child for any immediate adverse reactions to the injection.
  - Monitor for pain, swelling, or redness at the injection site.
- *Comfort measures:*
  - Apply a cold pack to the injection site to reduce pain and inflammation.
  - Administer age-appropriate analgesics if needed.
- *Follow-up:*
  - Provide instructions to caregivers on monitoring the injection site and managing any discomfort.
  - Schedule follow-up appointments as necessary.

COMPLICATIONS

- *Injection site pain:* Common and usually mild, managed with analgesics and cold packs.
- *Infection:* Rare if proper aseptic technique is used; monitor for signs of infection.
- *Allergic reaction:* Potential for an allergic reaction to the medication; monitor closely after administration.

PREVENTION

- *Proper technique:* Ensure correct injection technique to minimize pain and discomfort.
- *Comfort measures:* Use topical anesthetics, distraction techniques, and comfort positioning.
- *Education:* Educate caregivers on the importance of staying calm and supportive during the procedure.

CONCLUSION

Making IM injections as pain free as possible for children involves a combination of proper technique, comfort measures, and distraction. Devices such as Buzzy Bee and NumBee offer additional tools to reduce pain and anxiety, enhancing the overall experience for the child and caregivers.

FURTHER READING

1. Ayinde O, Hayward RS, Ross JDC. The effect of intramuscular injection technique on injection associated pain; a systematic review and meta-analysis. PLoS One. 2021;16(5):e0250883.
2. Bartell JC, Roberts KA, Schutte NJ, Sherman KC, Muller D, Hayney MS. Needle temperature effect on pain ratings after injection. Clin J Pain. 2008;24(3):260-4.
3. Brazeau GA, Cooper B, Svetic KA, Smith CL, Gupta P. Current perspectives on pain upon injection of drugs. J Pharm Sci. 1998;87(6):667-77.
4. Cmc S, Lord H, Vargese SS, Kurian N, Cherian SA, Mathew E, et al. Effectiveness of physical stimulation for reducing injection pain in adults receiving intramuscular injections: a systematic review and meta-analysis. JBI Evid Synth. 2023;21(2):373-400.
5. Moura JWDS, Bitencourt AS, Silva TL, Carmo ACFD, Santos LMD, Rocha PK. Utilization of local pressure devices in pain management during injections: scoping review. Rev Bras Enferm. 2024;77(3):e20230399.

CHAPTER 39

Rectal Drug Administration in Children

INTRODUCTION

Rectal drug administration is an alternative route for delivering medications to children, especially when oral administration is not feasible due to vomiting, difficulty swallowing, or the need for rapid drug absorption. This chapter outlines the steps and considerations for administering drugs rectally in children.

INDICATIONS

- Inability to take medications orally due to vomiting, difficulty swallowing, or refusal
- Need for rapid absorption, such as in the case of febrile seizures
- Local treatment of rectal conditions
- Unconscious or uncooperative child when other routes are not available

CONTRAINDICATIONS

- Severe rectal or anal injury or disease (e.g., severe hemorrhoids and rectal prolapse)
- Recent rectal surgery
- Known hypersensitivity to the medication being administered
- Presence of active rectal bleeding

EQUIPMENT AND SUPPLIES

- Sterile gloves
- Lubricant (e.g., water-soluble gel)
- Medication in suppository form or liquid preparation with an appropriate applicator
- Gauze pads or tissues
- Personal protective equipment (PPE)

PREPARATION

- *Explain the procedure:*
  - Inform the child (if age-appropriate) and caregivers about the need for rectal drug administration, its purpose, and what to expect.
  - Obtain informed consent from the caregivers.
- *Positioning:* Position the child comfortably, either lying on their side with knees drawn up to the chest (Sims' position) or on their back with legs elevated and bent.

PROCEDURE STEPS

1. *Initial assessment:* Conduct a brief history and physical examination to ensure there are no contraindications to rectal drug administration.
2. *Preparation of medication:*
   a. If using a suppository, ensure it is at room temperature. Warm it slightly in your hands if it is too cold.
   b. If using a liquid medication, ensure it is in an appropriate applicator designed for rectal administration.
3. *Gloving and lubrication:*
   a. Wash your hands thoroughly and put on sterile gloves.
   b. Apply a generous amount of water-soluble lubricant to the gloved index finger (for suppository) or to the tip of the applicator (for liquid medication).
4. *Administration:*
   a. *Suppository administration*:

   i. *Preparation:* Remove the wrapper from the suppository if present.
   ii. *Procedure:*
      - Gently separate the child's buttocks with one hand.
      - With the other hand, insert the lubricated suppository into the rectum, aiming toward the navel.
      - Push the suppository in about 1 inch (2.5 cm) for infants and up to 2 inches (5 cm) for older children.
      - Hold the buttocks together for a few seconds to prevent the suppository from being expelled.
   b. *Liquid medication administration **(Fig. 1)**:*
      i. *Preparation:* Ensure the applicator is filled with the prescribed dose of medication.
      ii. *Procedure:*
         - Gently separate the child's buttocks with one hand.
         - Insert the lubricated applicator tip into the rectum, aiming toward the navel.
         - Slowly depress the plunger or squeeze the applicator to administer the medication.
         - Remove the applicator and hold the buttocks together for a few seconds to prevent expulsion of the medication.
5. *Postadministration care:*
   a. *Cleaning:* Wipe any excess lubricant or medication from the area with gauze pads or tissues.
   b. *Comfort:* Reposition the child to a comfortable position and provide reassurance.

AFTERCARE

- *Monitoring:*
   - Observe the child for any immediate adverse reactions to the medication.
   - Monitor for effectiveness of the medication as per the clinical indication (e.g., reduction in fever and cessation of seizures).
- *Hygiene:* Instruct caregivers on proper hygiene and care of the rectal area following medication administration.
- *Documentation:*
   - Document the time, dose, and type of medication administered.
   - Record any observations of the child's response to the treatment and any adverse reactions.

COMPLICATIONS

- *Rectal irritation:* Potential irritation or discomfort at the site of administration
- *Expulsion:* Risk of the medication being expelled before it can be absorbed
- *Infection:* Low risk if proper hygiene and technique are used

PREVENTION

- *Proper technique:* Ensure correct administration technique to minimize discomfort and maximize effectiveness.
- *Hygiene:* Maintain good hygiene to prevent infection or irritation.
- *Education:* Educate caregivers on the correct method of rectal drug administration if they need to perform it at home.

CONCLUSION

Rectal drug administration is a valuable alternative for delivering medications to children when oral administration is not feasible. Proper technique, aftercare, and caregiver education are essential to ensure effective treatment and minimize complications.

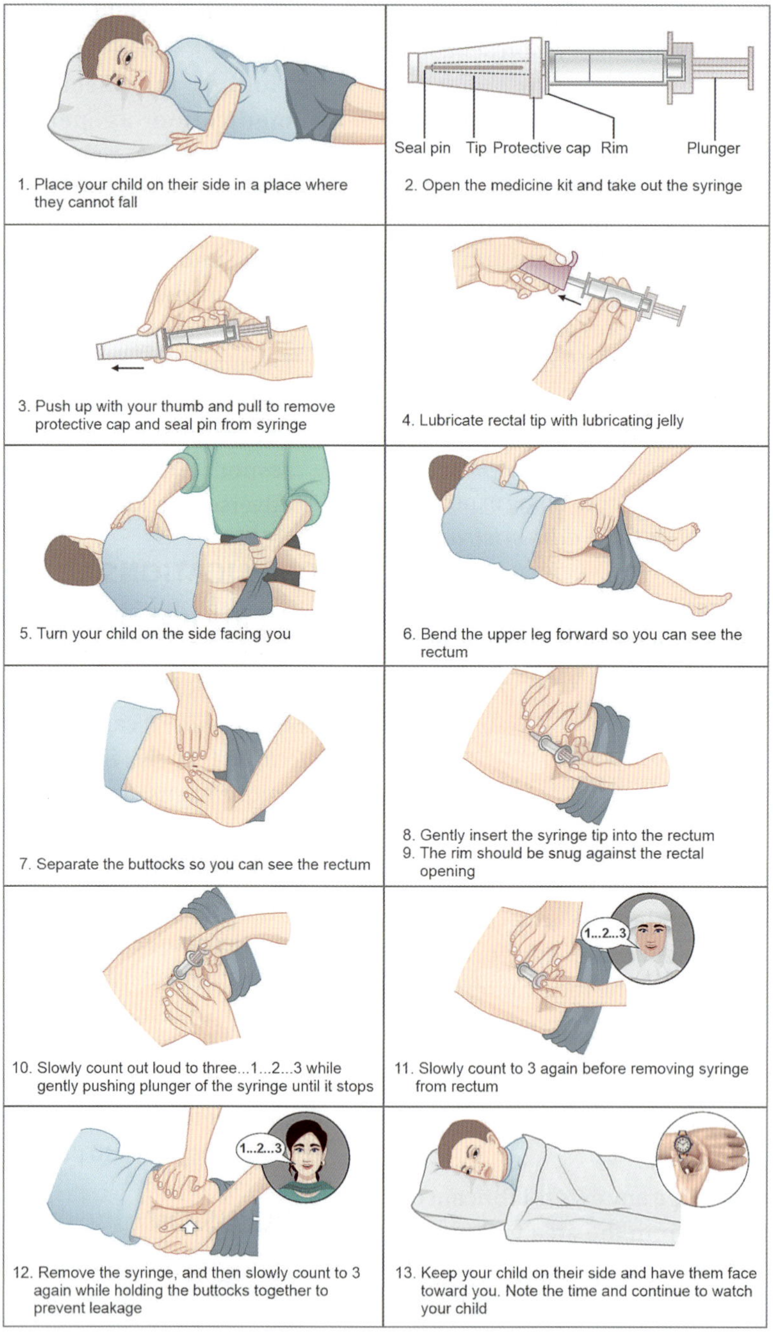

Fig. 1: Rectal diazepam administration.

FURTHER READING

1. Amidon S, Brown JE, Dave VS. Colon-targeted oral drug delivery systems: design trends and approaches. AAPS PharmSciTech. 2015;16(4):731-41.
2. Arévalo-Pérez R, Maderuelo C, Lanao JM. Recent advances in colon drug delivery systems. J Control Release. 2020;327:703-24
3. Dreifuss FE, Rosman NP, Cloyd JC, Pellock JM, Kuzniecky RI, Lo WD, et al. A comparison of rectal diazepam gel and placebo for acute repetitive seizures. N Engl J Med. 1998;338(26):1869-75.
4. Rathi R, Sanshita, Kumar A, Vishvakarma V, Huanbutta K, Singh I, et al. Advancements in Rectal Drug Delivery Systems: Clinical Trials, and Patents Perspective. Pharmaceutics. 2022;14(10):2210.
5. Rømsing J, Møiniche S, Dahl JB. Rectal and parenteral paracetamol, and paracetamol in combination with NSAIDs, for postoperative analgesia. Br J Anaesth. 2002; 88(2):215-26.

INDEX

Page numbers followed by *b* refer to box, *f* refer to figure, *fc* refer to flowchart, and *t* refer to table.

A

Abdomen 127
Abnormal cardiac evaluation 33
Absorbable hemostatic gauze 91
Abusive head trauma 61
Accidental drug 81
Accidental ingestion 81
Accidental poisoning 81
    causes of 80
Acetaminophen 192, 198
Acids 198, 201
Activated charcoal 198, 198*f*
    administration of 198, 199*f*
Acute abdomen 71
Acute angioedema 16
Acute asthma 19, 21*fc*, 22
    exacerbations, management of 22
Acute chest pain 29
Acute epiglottitis 16
Acute lead poisoning 83
Acute obstructive hydrocephalus 55
Acute pain management 211
Acute rectal prolapse 124
Acute seizure management 211
Adenovirus 15, 24
Adhesive bandage 148, 158, 165
Adhesive strips 165, 166
Adhesive tape 178
    application 166*f*
Administer antihistamines 205
Advanced pediatric life support 12
Advantages over traditional rabies immunoglobulin 67
Afebrile 66
Agitation 12, 51
Airflow, obstruction of 24
Airway 7, 46, 72
    management 13, 41, 45
    obstruction 15
    protection 201
Albuterol 20
Alcohol consumption 95
Aligning 179
Alkalis 198, 201
All out 80
Allergen immunotherapy 43
Allergic reaction 110, 209, 213, 219
    severe 206
Allergy 108
    preparedness 206
    referral 43
Alligator forceps 87, 99*f*
Altered mental status 12, 198, 201
Alternative closure materials 165
Aluminum phosphide 80
Amanita phalloides 82
Anal fissures 60
Analgesia 93, 114
Analgesics 91, 104, 117, 183, 186, 194
Anaphylaxis 32, 40, 43
    management 42*fc*
    signs of 205
Ancillary studies 29, 33
Anesthesia 114, 152, 195
Animal bites 207
Ankle sprain 190
    lateral of 190*f*
    management of 190, 192
    medial view of 190*f*
Ankylosis 196
Antibiotic 26
    eye drops 104
    ointment 91, 93, 104, 148, 158, 165
Anticonvulsant drug therapies 47*t*
Antiepileptic drug 45
Antihistamine 41, 204
Antipyretics 17
Antiseptic 67, 75
    solution 111, 148, 151, 158, 165, 175, 178, 186, 191, 204, 207
Antitubercular drugs 82
Antiviral therapy 26
Anxiety 39
Aortic dissection 31
Apnea 24
Arm
    pain, sudden onset of 182
    sling 186
    splint 179
Arrhythmias 37, 81
    kinds of 80
Artery forceps 169*f*
Aspiration 89
Asthma
    action plan 19
    exacerbations 19
    management of 19, 20
Atropine sulfate 13
Automated external defibrillator 4, 5
Avulsed nail, removal of 149
Avulsed tooth
    procedure for management of 194
    reimplantation of 195*f*

B

Back-out method 152
Bacterial infections 63
Baking soda 80
Balloon catheter 87
Bandages 178
    securing dressing with 180
Barbed hooks 152
Barbless hooks 152
Basic life support 11
Battery ingestion, management of 73*t*
Bayonet forceps 87
Benzodiazepines 47
Beta-agonists 41
Bleeding 114
Blood
    glucose 33, 47
    lead measurements 83
    pressure 7
    sugar level 64
    tests 48
Blunt object ingestion 72*t*

Bowel
  necrosis, risk for 72
  perforation, signs of 127
Brace 191
Brain
  injury, traumatic 50
  tumors 55, 57
Breathing 7, 36, 46, 72
Bright light source 87, 91, 104
Bromadiolone 80
Bronchiolitis 24, 25*fc*, 27
  management of 25
Bronchodilators 26, 41
Brue presentation
  assessment of 37
  risk stratification of 37
Brugada syndrome indicators 33
Bruising 114, 136
Buccal cavity anatomy 214*f*
Buccal drug administration 214, 215*f*
Bulb syringe 101
Buzzy bee and numbee 218

C

Calluses 162-164
  management of 164
Camphor 79
Cantharidin 163
Carbamazepine 81
Carbamide peroxide 101
Carbon monoxide 83
Cardiac arrhythmia 32
Cardiopulmonary resuscitation 4-7, 37
Cardiovascular disease 34
Cardiovascular systems 40
Cefotaxime 63
Ceftriaxone 63
Central nervous system 45, 78, 81, 211*fc*
  infections 48
Cerumen
  impaction 101
    procedure for management of 101
  loop 87
  removal 102*f*
Charcoal suspension, preparation of 199
Chemical
  burns 133
  cautery 92
Chemokines 24
Chest
  pain 32
    management of 30*fc*
  physiotherapy 27
  wall 29
    pain 29
  X-ray 30, 64
Chlorates 78
Chlorhexidine 111, 148, 151, 165, 175, 204, 207
Chronic constipation 127
Chronic instability 192
Circulation 7, 46
Clavicle fracture 186*f*, 187*f*, 218
  management of 186, 188
Clean injection site 218
Cluster headache 54, 55
Coin, management of 72*t*
Cold compress 92, 111, 112, 191, 204
Common household products 76*t*
Common primary headaches 54
Common respiratory emergency 15
Common warts 162
Compartment syndrome 181
Complete avulsion 149
Compression 112
Computed tomography 51, 56, 73
  pulmonary angiography 30
  scans 96
Conjunctival foreign body removal 106*f*
Consciousness
  loss of 32, 51
  prolonged loss of 33
  transient loss of 33
Constipated stool impaction, management of 127
Constipation 60
Constriction, signs of 155
Continuous positive airway pressure 3
Control bleeding 180
Convulsive status epilepticus 45, 47
  causes of 45
  incidence of 45
  management of 48
  pleocytosis 64
Corneal abrasion 60, 106
  assessment 104
Corns 163*f*
Coronavirus disease 2019 65
Corrosive 79
  substances, ingestion of 198, 201
Corticosteroids 13, 26, 41, 204, 205
Cotton-tipped applicator method 87, 101, 104, 105, 106*f*, 148, 158
Cough 24
C-reactive protein 64
Cream hair torniquet removal 156*f*
Croup
  management of 15, 18*f*, 18
  severe 16
  simple 16
  symptoms of 15
Crying, normal patterns of 58
Cryotherapy 162
Cyanosis 12, 24, 36, 178

D

Deep lacerations 172
Deep tissue injury, suspected 175
Deeper wounds 166
Deformity 178
Dehydration 130
  risk of 130
Dental mirror 194
Detergents 79
Detorsion, unsuccessful 119
Dexamethasone 17
Dextrose solution 111
Diazepam 47
Diet 196
Dietary modifications 62
Digital nerve block 142*f*
Digital rectal examination 128
Diphenhydramine 13
Discomfort 113
Disinfectants 75
Displaced fractures 96
Displacement, severe 186
Distal phalanx 137, 148
Dizziness 28
Doppler ultrasound 118
Dressings 178
  wound 149
Drooling 73
Drugs 47, 81
Duct tape occlusion therapy 162
Dysphagia 73
Ear
  canal
    damage 100
    injury 103
  curette 101

E

Echocardiogram 29
Edema 124
Elastic band method 135
Elastic wraps 178
Electrocardiogram 3, 7, 8, 29, 30, 33, 42
Electrocautery method 139
Electroencephalogram 48
Electrolyte imbalance 130, 203
Emergency
  department 16, 19, 54
    management 20
  management protocols 45
  medical services 12
  office equipment 13*b*
  preparedness 11, 200, 203
  situations 214
  use drugs 13*t*
Emotional stress 32
Emphasize 192
Empiric antimicrobials 65
Encephalitis 45
End-organ dysfunction 40
Endoscopy 72
Endotracheal tube 3
Enema administration 129
Epinephrine 13, 91
  administration 41, 205
  autoinjector 43, 204
Episodes 16, 36
Epistaxis 89, 91
  first aid pinch nose 92*f*
  management 91, 92*f*, 94
Epithelial cell necrosis 24
Equine rabies immunoglobulin 69
Esophageal perforation, risk of 203
Esophagus 73
Exacerbations, severe 20
Excessive crying 58, 59*fc*
Excessive sedation 213
Exercise-induced anaphylaxis 40
Exertional syncope 28
Expulsion 221
Eye 87
  conditions 60
  drop 108
    administration 108, 109, 109*f*
    medication 108
  irrigation 105*f*
  patch 104
  wash 104

F

Fatal asthma, risk factors for 20
Febrile infants, management of 63, 66
Fecal impaction 127*f*
  digital release of 128*f*
  manual of 128*f*
Feeding techniques 62
Fentanyl 211
  administration 212
  intranasal administration of 211
  nasal spray 211
Fever 63, 71
Figure-of-eight bandage 186, 187, 187*f*
Filiform warts 162
Filing 163
Fine-tipped forceps 158
Finger 112*f*, 155
  injury, severe 134
  paronychia 142*f*
Fingernail management of 148, 150
Fishhook injuries 151
Fishhook removal 152*f*, 153*f*
  procedure for 151
Fistula formation 72
Flat warts 162
Fluid 17, 41
  intake 34
  management 13
  resuscitation 41
Fluorescein strips 104
Food impaction 73
Foot hygiene 146
Forceps 105
Foreign body
  aspiration 16
  in ear, procedure for management of 98
  ingestion 71
    incidence of 71
    management of 71
  removal 99*f*
    spud 104
Formaldehyde exposure 78
Fosphenytoin 47
Fractures 60, 178, 186*f*
  management of 181
Full blood
  count 30
  examination 64

G

Gaping wounds 166
Gas embolism, risk of 79
Gasoline 201
Gastric
  lavage 201
    position 202*f*
  perforation, risk of 203
Gastroenteritis 60
Gastroesophageal reflux 60
Gastrointestinal issues 29, 200
Gastrointestinal obstructions 60
Gastrointestinal systems 40
Gastrointestinal tract 71
Gauze pads 91
Genitourinary conditions 60
Genitourinary tract 111
Gentle pressure 122
Gestational age 37
Glasgow coma scale 51
Glaucoma 60
Good night 80

H

Hair
  apposition technique 169*f*
  tourniquet 60, 155
    procedure for management of 155
Hand hygiene 27
Hank's balanced salt solution 194
Head injury
  symptoms of mild 50
  understanding mild 50
  vomiting after 12
Headache 50, 54
  characteristics 55
  management of 54
  primary 54, 55
  tension-type 54, 55
Headlamp 87, 91, 104
Heart 29
  failure 60
  rate 3, 5, 7
Heat illness 32
Heated paper clip method 138
Hematocrit 33
Hematoma 137
Hemostatic agents 91, 111
Herbal remedies 82
Herpes simplex virus 65
High-tension lacerations 167
Hospital emergency department 12

Household bleaches 79
Household poisoning 84
Human rabies immunoglobulin 69
Human rhinovirus 24
Humidification 93
Humidified air 18, 27
Hydration 26, 129
Hydrocarbons 75
  ingestion of 201
Hydrocephalus 57
Hydrogen peroxide 79, 101
  concentration of 79
Hygiene 110, 221
Hymenoptera
  management of 204, 206
  stings 204
Hyperpronation
  maneuver 184
  method 183
Hypersensitivity 108
Hypertonic saline 26
  nebulization 26
    role of 26
Hypertrophic cardiomyopathy 33
Hypoglycemia 45, 48
  management 47
Hyponatremia 45
Hypothyroidism 81
Hypovolemia 59
Hypoxemia 18, 22, 25
Hypoxia 203

I

Ibuprofen 192
Ice application 188
Ice pack 111, 191, 204, 205
Imiquimod 163
Immobilization 191
Immobilizing limb 179
Immunocompromised individuals 68
Immunotherapy 43
Important telephone numbers 13*t*
Infantile colic, diagnosis of 61
Infection 55, 73, 89, 93, 100, 103, 106, 110, 113, 149, 176, 181, 188, 196, 206, 219, 221
  presence of 163
  risk of secondary 160
  severe 111, 144
  signs of 131, 148, 172
Infertility 119
Infiltration around wound, syringe and needle for 207
Inflammatory cytokines 24
Influenza 65
Ingrowing toenail 144
  management of 144, 146
  spicule 145*f*
  trimming 145*f*
Inguinal hernia 60, 121
  anatomy of 121
  manual reduction of 122*f*
Inhalation, salbutamol for 13
Injection
  pain relief of 218*f*
  site pain 219
  technique 218
Injury, severe 178
Insecticides 80, 81
Intoxication 48
Intra-abdominal pressure 122
Intracranial hemorrhage 55, 57
Intracranial pressure 59
Intramuscular injection
  pain free 217
  syringe and needle for 207
Intramuscular regimen 68, 70
Intranasal route 211*fc*
Intravenous access 41
Intravenous pain medication 117
Invasive bacterial infection 63
  risk factors for 65
Ipratropium bromide 20
Iron 82
Irrigation
  kit 101
  method 89, 99, 102, 105
  syringe 87, 104
Ischemia 113, 124

J

Jeweler's forceps 104
Joint stiffness 192

L

Lacerations 172
  superficial 166
Large coins 72
Laryngotracheobronchitis 15
Lateral malleolus, tenderness of 190
Lavage procedure 202
Left coronary artery, anomalous origin of 60
Leg splint 179
L-epinephrine 17
Levetiracetam 47
Licks 68
Lidocaine 91, 98, 151, 165
  gel 111
  spray 87
Lignocaine 115*f*
Lip laceration 171
Liquid medication administration 221
Local anesthesia 115
  syringe and needle for 111, 148, 165
Lorazepam 47
  administration 215
Loud noise 32
Low-grade fever 24
Lubricant 111, 201
  method 115
Lubrication method 112, 125, 134
Lumbar puncture 48, 55, 64
Lungs 29
Magnetic resonance
  angiography 56
  imaging 56, 73

M

Magnifying glass 87, 104, 158
Malunion 188
Manual cerumen removal 102*f*
Manual detorsion technique 118
Manual hair torniquet removal 156*f*
Manual rectal prolapse reduction 125
Manual reduction
  complications of 123
  technique of 121
Martial nail avulsion 146*f*
Meatal ulcers 60
Mechanical ventilation 22
Medical emergency pathways 9
Medication
  ingestion of 198
  preparation of 108, 215, 220
Meningitis 46, 61
Mental disorders, diagnostic and statistical manual of 59
Mental status, signs of altered 51
Metabolic diseases 61
Metal zippers 115

Metapneumovirus 24
Methane 83
Microscopy 64
Midazolam 47, 211, 215*f*
 administration 211, 215
 intranasal administration of 211
 nasal spray 211
Migraine 54, 55
Mild croup 16
 outpatient treatment for 16
Mild head injuries 50, 53
 management of 53
Mild-to-moderate exacerbations 20
Moderate-to-severe croup, management of 16
Monoclonal antibody 67
Mortein
 mosquito repellents 80
 rodenticide 80
Mosquito 80
 repellents 80
Mucosal atomization device 211, 212
Mucosal damage 89
Mucus production 24

N

Nail
 avulsion 148
 deformity 149
 nippers 148
 wedge removal 145*f*
Naphthalene 79
Naphthalene 79
Nasal balloon catheter 91
Nasal care 93
Nasal decongestant spray 87
Nasal deformity 96
Nasal discomfort 213
Nasal drug administration 212*f*
Nasal flaring 24
Nasal foreign body
 insertion 87
 management of 87
 removal 88*f*
Nasal fractures 95-97
 effective management of 97
 management of 96
Nasal injuries 95
 procedure for management of 95
Nasal packing 92
Nasal speculum 87, 91
Nasal structure 95*f*
Nasal tampon 92*f*
Nasal tampons 91
Nasal-packing materials 91
Nasogastric route 202
Nasogastric tube 199*f*, 201
 administration 199
Nasopharyngeal swab 24
N-diethyl-benzamide 81
Nebulized epinephrine 17
Nebulizer 17
Necrosis 113
Needle 158
Needle-cover method 152
Neonatal abstinence syndrome 60
Neuroimaging 55
Neurologic conditions 61
Neurologic examination 33
Neurologic findings 34
Neuromuscular diseases 61
Neurovascular compromise 178, 181, 186
Neurovascular injury 188
Neutralization 132
Nocturnal enuresis 82
Noisy breathing 12
Nonadherent dressing 148
Nonconvulsive status epilepticus 48
Nondisplaced fractures 96
Nonpharmacologic interventions 27
Nonradiopaque objects 71
Nontoxic
 accidental ingestions 83
 ingestion 75
 substances 83*b*
Nontraumatic chest pain 28
Nontraumatic headaches 54
Nonunion 188
Normal cardiac examination 33
Nosebleed 91
Numbness 178
Nutritional support 26

O

Obstructed inguinal hernia, manual reduction of 121, 123
Ocular foreign body, procedure for management of 104
Odomos cream 81
Office preparedness components 11
Office-based assessment 11
Ointment 104
Onychocryptosis 144
Open fractures 178, 186
Open wounds 178, 186
Oral analgesics 158, 165
Oral antihistamines 205
Oral hygiene 196
Oral laxatives 129
Oral pain medication 117
Orogastric route 202
Orogastric tube 201
Orthostatic hypotension 34
Orthostatic symptoms 33
Osmotic agents 111, 112
Osteomyelitis 60
Otitis media 60
Otoscope 98, 101
Outpatient
 management 20
 visits 18
Ovarian torsion 60
Oxygen 13, 41
 saturation 3, 42
 therapy 22, 25, 41
Oxymetazoline 87
 spray 91

P

Padded aluminum splints 178
Padding 179
 splint 179
Pain 32, 103, 113, 114, 146, 150, 160, 176, 204, 206
 description 28
 management 112, 116, 118, 119, 148, 149, 151, 158, 165, 180, 183, 187, 188, 192, 204, 205, 208
  analgesics for 196
 persistent 192
 relief 114
Palivizumab prophylaxis 27
Pallor 36
Palpable mass 127
Palpitations 32
Paracetamol 81
 tolerant of 81
Paradichlorobenzene 79
Parainfluenza virus 24
Paraphimosis 111, 111*f*
 manual reduction of 112
 procedure for management of 111
Parent's kiss method 88, 88*f*

Paronychia 141
  procedure for management of 141
Partial avulsion 149
Partial nail avulsion 145
Peak expiratory flow 21
Pecarn guidelines 50
Pediatric advanced life support 12, 29
Pediatric considerations 43
Pediatric emergency 11
  care 51
Pediatric headache approach 56*fc*
Pediatric intensive care unit 12, 46
Pediatric medical care 11
Pediatric office
  emergency procedures 85
  practice 11
Pediatric resuscitation pathways 1
Pediatric subspecialty consultation, indications for 31
Pediatric syncope, management of 34
Pencil point puncture 175
  management of 177
  procedure for management of 175
Penile zipper injury management 115, 115*f*
Penis 111, 155
Perforation 72
Peripheral vascular disease 163
Peritonsillar abscess 16
Periungual tissues, infection of 141
Persistent swelling 206
Persistent symptoms 18
Personal protective equipment 87, 91, 98, 101, 104, 108, 112, 141, 148, 158, 165, 178, 183, 186, 191, 198, 201, 204, 208, 211
Pesticides 75, 80
Pharmacologic interventions 26
Phenol 78
Phenytoin 47, 81
Phimosis 111*f*
Physical activity 130
Physical examination 19, 28, 33
Plantar warts 162
Plants and fungi 75, 82
Plumbism 83
Pneumothorax 31
Pointed object ingestion, management of 74*t*
Poison prevention 200
Poisoning 12, 75, 201
  severe 82
  types of 198
Polypharmacy 43
Portal vein thrombosis 6
Positive pressure technique 88
Postadministration care 109
Postprocedure care 89, 93, 105, 113, 119, 122, 125, 142, 149, 192, 205
Postremoval care 73, 115, 136
Postural changes 32
Potential sequelae 61
Povidone-iodine 111, 148, 151, 165, 175, 204, 207
Preexcitation syndromes 33
Pre-exposure prophylaxis 68
Prefilled buccal solution 215
Prefilled nasal spray 212
Pregnancy 43, 68
  test 33
Premature infants 27
Prepare injection 218
Preprocedural sedation 211
Pressurized metered-dose inhaler 21
Prilocaine 115
Primary care provider 38
  visits 38
Probiotics 62
Prolapse 124
Prolapsed tissue
  ischemia of 124
  strangulation of 124
Proparacaine 104
Proper footwear 192
Proper foreskin care 113
Proper nail care 146
Proper technique 213, 221
Prophylactic orchiopexy 119
Protective clothing 206
Protective eyewear 107
Proton pump inhibitors 30, 62
Protruding intestine 121
Psychogenic pain 29
Public health measures 68
Pulled elbow 182*f*
  management of 185
Pulmonary embolism 31
Pulse
  loss of 178
  oximetry 20
  pressure variation 3
Pulseless electrical activity 6
Puncture wound 175
Purulence 155
Pus 172
Pyrethrins 80
Pyrethroids 80

Q

QT interval
  prolonged 33
  short 33
Rabies 67
  immunoglobulin 67, 207
  immunoglobulin administration 209*f*
    procedure for 207
  postexposure prophylaxis 207*f*
    guidelines 69*fc*
    protocol 67
  vaccine 68

R

Rabishield 67
Racemic epinephrine 17
Radial head subluxation 182
Radiologic evaluation 71
Raised intracranial pressure 48
Reassessing neurovascular status 180
Receive pre-exposure prophylaxis 68
Recent nasal surgery 211
Rectal bleeding 127
Rectal diazepam administration 222
Rectal drug administration 220
Rectal irritation 221
Rectal prolapse
  manual reduction of 126
  reduction 124
    procedure for 124
Rectum 127
Recurrent bleeding 93
Recurrent granuloma 133
Recurrent symptoms 18
Reduction techniques 183
Re-exposure prophylaxis 70
Refractory status epilepticus 48
Regular bowel habits 130
Regular ear hygiene 103

Regular monitoring 113
Rehabilitation 192
Reimplant tooth 195
Removal technique 88, 152, 205
Requiring surgical intervention 111
Residual hearing loss 100
Respiratory 40
  conditions 29
  depression 213
  distress, signs of 19
  failure 22
  illness 15
  syncytial virus 15, 24, 65
Retained debris 176
Retractions 24
Retropharyngeal abscess 16
Rhinorrhea 24
Rhinovirus 15
Ribbon method 134
Rifampicin 81
Right-angle hook 87
Rigid splinting materials 178
Ring cutter method 135
Ring removal
  procedure for 134
  string method 135, 135*f*
Ring stuck 134
Ringer's solution 13
Rodenticide 80
Root resorption 196

S

Safe ear care 103
Safe environment 206
Safety education 196
Safety measures 181, 188
Salicylic acid 162
Saline 101
  solution 194
Saliva 68
Salt application 133
Scarring 106
Scissors 148, 165, 178
Screwdriver method 115
Scrotal pain, acute onset of 117
Securing 179
  splint 179
Sedation 118
Seizure 12, 214
  termination 47
Septal hematoma 96
Septal perforation 93
Septic arthritis 60
Septic shock 65
Serum sickness 206
Severity assessment 16
Short-acting beta agonist 20, 21
Shoulder stiffness 188
Shushing sounds 61
Sickle cell disease 31
Silver nitrate sticks 91
Simethicone drops 62
Simple lacerations 165
  management of 165, 169
Simple lip laceration, procedure for 172
Simple tongue
  and lip lacerations, management of 171, 174
  laceration, procedure for 171
Skeletal conditions 60
Skin 40
  abrasions 136
  and mucosa 40
  conditions 60
Small forceps 104, 148
Small hemostat 112
Small lacerations 166
Soaking 163
Sodium bicarbonate 80
Soft padding materials 178
Solution with syringe 215
Somnolence 51
Soothing techniques 61
Splinting 148, 149, 191, 196
  materials 194
Spud method 105
Squeeze bottle 105*f*
Stabilization 196
Stable patients 31
Staple removal technique 168*f*
Stapler and staple remover 165
Steeple sign 15
Sterilants 75
Sterile dressing 158, 165
Sterile gauze pads 101, 104, 111, 148, 151, 158, 178, 186, 191, 194, 204, 207
Sterile gloves 87, 91, 98, 101, 104, 111, 117, 148, 151, 158, 165, 178, 182, 186, 191, 194, 201, 204, 207, 211, 220
  optional 108
  personal protection 108
Sterile saline 104
  solution 104, 141, 158, 165
Stinger removal 205
Stomach 72, 73
  position 61
Stool
  impaction 127
    management of 130
  softeners 129
Strangulation 126
  signs of 124
Strengthening exercises 192
Stridor 12
String wrapping 135
String-Yank
  method 152
  technique 152*f*
Structural cardiac disease 32
Stubborn splinters 158
Stuck ring, management of 136
Subsequent therapy 22
Subungual hematoma 137, 137*f*
  drainage 138*f*
  management of 139
Sucking 61
Suction apparatus 201
Suction device 87, 91, 98
Sudden infant death syndrome 36
Superficial splinter 158
  management of 161
  removal 159*f*
Supervision 107
Superwarfarin 80
Supination technique 185*f*
Supination-flexion method 183
Supplemental oxygen 22
Supporting anxious caregivers 39
Supportive care 17, 25, 199, 203, 216
Suppository administration 220
Suprapubic aspirate 64
Supraventricular tachycardia 60
Surgical intervention 155
Surgical treatment 145
Suture kit 165
Suturing 166
Swaddling 61
Swelling 114, 136, 155, 175, 178, 186, 192, 204
  acute onset of 117
Swinging 61
Sympathomimetics 81
Symptom evaluation 19
Symptomatic coins 72
Syncope 32
  causes of 32
  management of 34*fc*

Systemic glucocorticoids 20, 22
Systemic infection, signs of 175

T

Tachypnea 24
Taxis maneuver 122
Tenderness 191
Testes
  manual detorsion of 118
  procedure for detorsion of 117
  torsion of 117*f*
Testicular atrophy 119
Testicular torsion 60, 117
Tetanus prophylaxis 194, 196
Thrush 60
Thumbs 112*f*
Thyroxin 81
Tissue
  adhesive 165, 166
  damage 160, 176
    severe 148, 155
  glue application 267*f*
Toe 155
Toenail avulsion
  management of 150
  procedure for management of 148
Toenail grows 144
Tongue laceration 171
Tooth
  anatomy 194*f*
  avulsion 194
  complete displacement of 194
  discoloration 196
  preservation solution 194
  storage, milk for 194
  transport 194
Topical anesthesia 92
Topical anesthetic 87, 91, 92
  cream 217
  eye drops 104
Topical antihistamines 205
Topical vasoconstriction 92
Toxicity 76-78
Toxicology screen 33, 48
Tranexamic acid 91
Trauma 60
Traumatic brain injury 51
Traumatic injury 45
  suspected 111
Trephination techniques 138
Triangular bandage 179, 180
  first air arm sling 180*f*
Tricyclic antidepressants 82
Triggers 32
Trim toenail straight 145
Tweezers 158
Tying 179
Tympanic membrane perforation 100

U

Ulceration 111, 124, 163
  and infection 126
Umbilical granuloma 131
  ligation 132*f*
  management of 133
  procedure for 131
Umbilical polyp, presence of 131
Umbilical venous catheter 3
Uncontrolled bleeding 12
Understanding anaphylaxis 40
Unstable patients 29, 31
Upper airway 16
  injury 16
  obstruction, causes of 18
Urgent consultation 34
Urgent medical attention 19
Urinary tract
  infection 59, 60
    suspected 65
  obstruction 60
Urological emergency 111

V

Vaccination schedule 68, 70
Vaccines, administration of 217
Valproate 47
Vascular access 13
Vasoconstrictive agent 91, 92
Venous pooling, prevent 35
Ventricular fibrillation 6
Ventricular tachycardia 6
Verbal communication 51
Verruca vulgaris 162
Vertigo 103
Viral bronchiolitis
  diagnosis of 26*b*
  history of 26*b*
  signs of 26*b*
  symptoms of 26*b*
Viral infections 65
Visible deformity 186
Visible nasal deformity 96
Visible sting 204
Vision changes 106
Visual inspection 92
Vital signs 28, 33, 47

W

Warm compress 125
Warm water 101
Warts 162, 163*f*, 164
  management of 164
Waterproof drape 101
Water-soluble gel 201
Wearable identification 43
Wheezing 12, 24, 26*b*
Wooden boards 178
Wound
  care 67, 70, 89, 100, 113, 116, 133, 136, 149, 196, 205, 209
  closure 166, 167*f*
  remaining open sections of 166*f*

Z

Zagreb regimen 68
Zinc phosphide 80
Zipper injuries 114
  management of 116
  procedure for 114
Zipper, interlocking teeth of 115*f*